Advisors
Anita DeAngelis
Daniel Goldman, J.D.
James Hale Sr.
Jacqueline Heying
Vicki Moore

Mayo Medical Ventures
Gregory Anderson, M.D.
Michael Casey
Marne Gade
Laura Long
S. Rebecca Roberts
Gayle Rock
Richard Van Ert
John Schmidt

Literary Agent
Arthur Klebanoff

Media Support Services
Nancy Moltaji

preface

This book is for people who will soon be having a baby. If that is you, please accept our warmest congratulations! There are few events in anyone's life that rival the importance — and the joy — of childbirth. This new person will be so important to you as a parent that you will do anything to nurture, protect and give love to this special baby. Undoubtedly, your desire to start that care is reflected in your interest in this book, a guide to starting out a new life in good health for both mother and baby.

Although pregnancy is a normal event, it is marvelously complex, involving changes in mother's anatomy and physiology and in the entire family's relationships. These changes are tiny compared to the miracle of development of a single cell formed from the sperm and egg to a brand-new, one-of-a-kind, important human being. I know of nothing in medicine that is more exciting, fascinating or satisfying to observe.

There has never been a time when there was a better opportunity to start a life in good health, and wisdom dictates that you should seek information from people you can trust. This book is a compilation of expertise from many viewpoints and approaches to care. Mayo Clinic has at the core of its greatness an approach to every medical issue by a team of caregivers, each with special insight and gifts. This book reflects that philosophy. Not only does it come to you from a team of obstetricians with specialized medical knowledge related to problems of pregnancy, but Mary Murry, C.N.M., is the principal co-editor, lending the wisdom and experience of a scientifically grounded midwife to its pages. This team has brought its multiple skills to bear to help you have a healthier, happier pregnancy.

It is our sincere wish that you find this book informative, helpful and meaningful as you anticipate your new baby. It is our hope that your need for solid information is met in its pages. It is also our hope that your pregnancy will be a wonderful experience, and your new baby will have the blessing of good health.

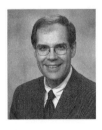

Roger W. Harms, M.D.
Editor in Chief

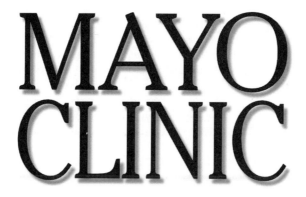

MAYO CLINIC

GUIDE TO A
HEALTHY
PREGNANCY

Roger W. Harms, M.D.
Editor in Chief

Associate Medical Editors

Robert V. Johnson, M.D.
Mary M. Murry, C.N.M.

HarperResource
An Imprint of HarperCollins*Publishers*

Copyright © 2004 Mayo Foundation for Medical Education and Research

Layout and production by Mayo Clinic Health Information, Rochester, Minn.

Stock photography for lifestyle and cover photos from PhotoDisc, Stockbyte, and © Thinkstock. The individuals pictured in these photos are models, and the photos are used for illustrative purposes only. There is no correlation between the individuals portrayed and the condition or subject being discussed.

First Edition

Library of Congress Cataloging-in-Publication Data has been applied for.

ISBN: 0-06-074637-8

Printed in the United States of America

08 09 RRD 30 29 28 27 26 25 24 23

About this book

To use *Mayo Clinic Guide to a Healthy Pregnancy*, you may find it helpful to understand how the information is arranged. The book is divided into four parts:

Part 1: Pregnancy, Childbirth and Your Newborn
This section offers month-by-month insights into your baby's development as well as your own physical and emotional changes. It also gives detailed information on labor, childbirth, and newborn and postpartum care.

Part 2: Decision Guides for Pregnancy, Childbirth and Parenthood
Each guide is designed to help you reach a decision that's best for you and your situation.

Part 3: Pregnancy Reference Guide
Here, you'll find helpful self-care tips for heartburn, nausea, back pain, fatigue and many more of the common concerns of pregnancy.

Part 4: Complications of Pregnancy and Childbirth
This section provides details on complications that can occur with pregnancy, along with information on being pregnant when you have a health condition.

Throughout this book, the term *health care provider* covers the many kinds of medical professionals who provide pregnancy care. When the term *doctor* is used, it indicates that a doctor of medicine (M.D.) is likely the best type of health care professional to provide this type of care.

About Mayo Clinic

Mayo Clinic evolved from the frontier practice of Dr. William Worrall Mayo and the partnership of his two sons, William J. and Charles H. Mayo, in the early 1900s. Pressed by the demands of their busy practice in Rochester, Minn., the Mayo brothers invited other physicians to join them, pioneering the private group practice of medicine. Today, with more than 2,000 physicians and scientists at its three major locations in Rochester, Minn., Jacksonville, Fla., and Scottsdale, Ariz., Mayo Clinic is dedicated to providing comprehensive diagnoses, accurate answers and effective treatments.

With this depth of medical knowledge, experience and expertise, Mayo Clinic occupies an unparalleled position as a health information resource. Since 1983 Mayo Clinic has published reliable health information for millions of consumers through award-winning newsletters, books and online services. Revenue from the publishing activities supports Mayo Clinic programs, including medical education and research.

Editorial Staff

contents

Part 1

pregnancy, childbirth and your newborn

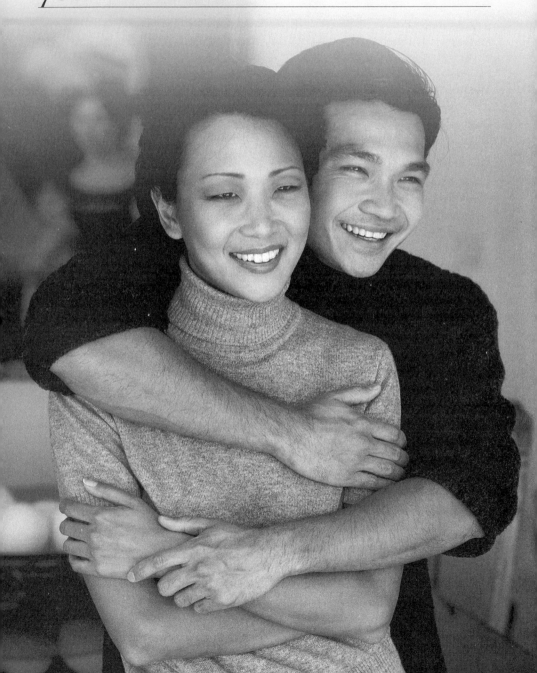

Pregnancy brings change. From the moment of conception, your body begins to transform in ways that accommodate the new life starting within you. As your baby grows and develops, you adjust, too, both physically and emotionally. Late in your pregnancy, you prepare for labor and childbirth. And after your baby arrives, you begin the transition to life as a parent of this unique new person.

"Pregnancy, Childbirth and Your Newborn" offers guidance on the many changes of pregnancy, from planning for pregnancy to the first weeks at home with your newborn.

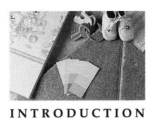

preparing to have a baby

Are you ready to have a baby?

Maybe you're thinking about starting a family. Maybe you're trying to conceive. Or perhaps you already know that you're pregnant. If so, congratulations!

When you decide to have a child, your life changes. The choices you make now — even if you haven't yet conceived — can have a lasting effect on your future child.

The changes pregnancy brings can be exhilarating and unsettling, blissful and exhausting. As you prepare for this sometimes unpredictable journey, let this book serve as your guide. Part 1, "Pregnancy, Childbirth and Your Newborn," helps you plan and prepare for pregnancy. In four-week segments, it walks you through your baby's development and the changes you may experience physically and emotionally during pregnancy. It offers guidance on labor and childbirth. Finally, it provides information and advice on your newborn and your transition to parenthood.

Part 2, "Decision Guides for Pregnancy, Childbirth and Parenthood," includes information to help you make informed decisions on issues such as selecting a health care provider for your pregnancy, understanding prenatal testing options and choosing pain relief for labor. Part 3, "Pregnancy Reference Guide," offers explanations and self-care advice for many of the common concerns of pregnancy. Part 4, "Complications of Pregnancy and Childbirth," provides insight into some of the problems that can develop with pregnancy.

Think of pregnancy as a wonderful opportunity to nurture your child in every way, and use this book to prepare for the exciting changes ahead.

Before pregnancy: Giving baby the best

When it comes to pregnancy, thinking ahead can give you and your baby the best possible beginning. Whatever point you're at in planning a family, the decisions you make today can make a difference in your baby's health as well as your own.

If you're thinking about having a baby, you might want to ask yourself some key questions, such as:

- Why do I want to have a baby?
- Does my partner feel the same way I do about having a child?
- How will having a baby affect my current and future lifestyles? Am I ready and willing to make those changes?
- Do I have the emotional and financial support I need to raise a child?
- Will I be able to provide my baby with proper child care?

At the same time, think about your physical health. Indeed, the better your health before you conceive, the better your chances of avoiding problems that can affect you and your baby.

If you haven't thought about any of these issues so far, it doesn't mean you'll have an unhealthy pregnancy. But the sooner you set the stage for a successful outcome, the better your odds. That's true whether you are still in the planning stages, are trying to conceive or already have a baby on the way.

The following sections offer more information on how to do the best for you and your baby before, during and, in some cases, after your pregnancy.

Nutrition: Make every bite count

Good nutrition isn't only important during pregnancy. Even if you're just planning to become pregnant, eating a healthy, well-balanced diet is one of the best things you can do for yourself and your future child.

Once you're pregnant, you'll be eating for two, but if you think this means eating twice as much, you may be disappointed. Eating for two (you and your baby) means that you need to focus on eating twice as well as in the past.

If you already follow good eating habits, you have a head start in providing your baby with the nutrition he or she will need. Over the course of your pregnancy, you'll want to increase your intake of iron, calcium, folic acid and other essential vitamins and nutrients, since these nutrients are important to your baby's development. You'll also need to avoid certain foods that pose a safety risk so that neither you nor your baby gets sick. Yet, for the most part, you simply may have to do more of what you're already doing.

If your nutrition is poor or you often diet, skip meals or eat a limited variety of foods, start making changes now. In fact, it's critical to make good eating habits a part of your pregnancy planning from the start. The reason: Most of your baby's major organs form during the first few weeks of pregnancy — before you may even know you're pregnant. With too few calories or nutrients, cell development can be less than ideal and your baby may be underweight at birth, which may increase his or her risk of short- and long-term health problems.

Preconception visit: What to share

✔ It's a good idea to make a preconception appointment with your doctor, nurse-midwife or other medical health care provider. Be ready to talk about the following subjects.

❑ **Birth control.** If you've been taking birth control pills, your health care provider may want you to switch to another birth control method for the first month or two after you stop taking them. That's because it often takes several months for your menstrual periods to return to a regular pattern. Until this happens, it's more difficult to pinpoint when ovulation occurs or to estimate your due date.

❑ **Immunities.** The earlier you determine if you're immune to infections that can cause serious birth defects in babies, the better. If you aren't immune to infectious diseases such as chickenpox (varicella) and German measles (rubella), your health care provider may recommend that you be vaccinated at least one month before you try to become pregnant.

❑ **Current and past health issues.** If you have an ongoing medical condition such as diabetes, asthma or high blood pressure (hypertension), you'll want to make sure it's under control. Even if you've had no problem maintaining your health for some time, chronic conditions may require special care during pregnancy. That's because a growing baby can put new demands on your body.

❑ **Family history.** Tell your health care provider if your or your partner's family medical history puts you at greater risk of having a child with a birth defect.

❑ **Medications.** Your health care provider may recommend stopping certain prescription medications or changing doses before you become pregnant. Make sure he or she is aware of any nonprescription medications you take regularly. That includes herbal products such as St. John's wort, kava, valerian and ginkgo. If you're not taking a multivitamin, you'll want to begin taking one. Make sure it includes folic acid, which is a B vitamin that can help prevent serious birth defects in early pregnancy.

❑ **Age.** If you're over 35, you're at increased risk of fertility problems, miscarriage and pregnancy-related problems such as high blood pressure and gestational diabetes. You may want to discuss these increased risks with your health care provider and develop a plan for avoiding complications. (For more information, see "Pregnancy timing: Does age matter?" on page 35.)

❑ **Pregnancy difficulties.** If you've had previous miscarriages or trouble becoming pregnant, talk to your health care provider about it. He or she may be able to determine possible causes that might be corrected. At the very least, the two of you can discuss your concerns and fears about conception.

❑ **Lifestyle.** If you smoke, drink, eat a poor diet or don't have a regular exercise program, now is the perfect time to drop bad habits and adopt a healthier lifestyle. If you smoke and want to quit, your health care provider can connect you with the help you may need to stop smoking. He or she can also give you advice on improving your eating habits, starting an exercise program and reducing stress.

❑ **Your partner.** If possible, have your partner attend the preconception visit with you. He can answer questions about his family medical conditions and risk factors for infections or birth defects. Your partner's health and lifestyle are important because they can affect yours.

Eating right doesn't mean that you have to follow a rigid diet. To get proper nourishment and gain the weight you need to have a healthy pregnancy, you'll want to eat many different types of food. Just remember: What you eat and drink will have a direct effect on your developing baby.

Putting on pounds

It's important for you to gain weight throughout your pregnancy. Depending on your pre-pregnancy height and weight, your health care provider may recommend a range for weight gain during your pregnancy. You're expected to gain weight during pregnancy, but this doesn't mean you can gain an unlimited number of pounds. On the other hand, adequate weight gain is necessary for a healthy pregnancy.

Over the years, the recommendations for weight gain have changed dramatically. Not too long ago, medical experts thought a minimal weight gain was best for mother and child. Your mother probably was told to gain no more than 15 pounds! Now, if you're at a normal weight for your size when you conceive, research suggests that gaining 25 to 35 pounds is healthiest for you and your baby.

The weight you put on in pregnancy doesn't all come from fat. The weight from the baby you're carrying and an increase in blood and body fluids all contribute to your weight gain.

Although this range may be considered ideal, it's best to work with your health care provider to determine what's right for you. That decision will be based on your pre-pregnancy weight, your body mass index (BMI), your medical history, your health, the health of your developing baby and whether you're carrying twins or other multiples. During your prenatal visits, your health care provider can track how much weight you're gaining over time.

If possible, strive to put on your weight gradually with most of your gain in the second and third trimesters. During your first trimester, an

PREGNANCY AND WEIGHT GAIN

Here's a quick breakdown of where the weight goes if you were to gain 24 to 32½ pounds during your pregnancy:
- Your baby: 6½ to 9 pounds
- Placenta: 1½ pounds
- Amniotic fluid: 2 pounds
- Breast enlargement: 1 to 3 pounds
- Uterus enlargement: 2 pounds
- Fat stores and muscle development: 6 to 8 pounds
- Increased blood volume: 3 to 4 pounds
- Increased fluid volume: 2 to 3 pounds

extra 150 to 200 calories a day will help keep your weight gain between 1 to 1½ pounds a month. The more active you are, the more calories you'll need to consume.

In your second and third trimesters, you'll need a total of 400 to 500 extra calories a day beyond your normal diet. Guidelines suggest gaining ½ to 1 pound a week in the second and third trimester. Lack of weight gain during the second trimester is associated with low birth weight in the baby if you start out at a normal weight or are underweight to begin with. If you're overweight, but otherwise healthy, below average weight gain isn't likely to affect fetal growth.

How you obtain your added calories is as important as how many pounds you see on the scale. Even though you can easily obtain 200 or more calories by eating a candy bar, this choice doesn't offer the nutrition you need. You'll get the same calorie boost — as well as valuable carbohydrates, calcium, protein and iron — by adding to your daily diet a slice of whole-grain bread, a glass of skim milk and 1 ounce of lean meat.

WHAT'S MY BMI?

Body mass index (BMI) is one measurement health care providers use to assess your weight and health. Use this chart to determine your BMI.

	HEALTHY		OVERWEIGHT		OBESE			
BMI	19	24	25	29	30	35	40	45
HEIGHT	**WEIGHT IN POUNDS**							
4'10"	91	115	119	138	143	167	191	215
4'11"	94	119	124	143	148	173	198	222
5'0"	97	123	128	148	153	179	204	230
5'1"	100	127	132	153	158	185	211	238
5'2"	104	131	136	158	164	191	218	246
5'3"	107	135	141	163	169	197	225	254
5'4"	110	140	145	169	174	204	232	262
5'5"	114	144	150	174	180	210	240	270
5'6"	118	148	155	179	186	216	247	278
5'7"	121	153	159	185	191	223	255	287
5'8"	125	158	164	190	197	230	262	295
5'9"	128	162	169	196	203	236	270	304
5'10"	132	167	174	202	209	243	278	313
5'11"	136	172	179	208	215	250	286	322
6'0"	140	177	184	213	221	258	294	331
6'1"	144	182	189	219	227	265	302	340
6'2"	148	186	194	225	233	272	311	350
6'3"	152	192	200	232	240	279	319	359
6'4"	156	197	205	238	246	287	328	369

(Source: National Institutes of Health)

A BMI over 30 before pregnancy can increase the risks to you and your baby. Your chances of having gestational diabetes and delivery by Caesarean birth are greater. For your baby, it can increase the risk of birth defects such as spina bifida and heart problems. It can also increase your chances of having a baby with a high birth weight (macrosomia), which can make it more difficult to deliver the baby through the birth canal.

If you enter pregnancy with a BMI of more than 30, work closely with your health care provider to monitor your weight gain and your health. You may be asked to limit your weight gain to 15 to 25 pounds or even less during pregnancy. Guidelines call for about a 2-pound weight gain in the first trimester and a 2/3 pound gain each week in the second and third trimesters.

A low BMI — less than 18.5 — also can put you and your baby at risk of some problems. You may be more likely to have a preterm (before 37th week) delivery, which means the baby is born before he or she is fully developed. Low maternal BMI may also increase your likelihood of having a low-birth-weight baby (under 5 1/2 pounds).

Again, it's best to talk with your health care provider about weight gain. If you have a low BMI, you may be asked to gain 28 to 40 pounds, which is slightly more than the normal range. Guidelines suggest a 5-pound gain in the first trimester and at least a 1-pound gain each week in the second and third trimesters.

Abuse during pregnancy

For some women, pregnancy isn't a time of happy anticipation. It's a time of fear. Studies show that 4 percent to 8 percent of pregnant women report being physically abused during their pregnancy.

Physical abuse may include having your partner beat, slap, kick or punch you. Sexual abuse may include rape or being forced to perform other sexual acts against your will.

Abuse can also be verbal or emotional. Emotional and verbal abuse may include shouting at you, scaring you or saying things that make you feel ashamed or unimportant.

If you're pregnant and in an abusive situation, it's more important than ever for you to seek help. Remember, you have to consider not only your health but the health of your unborn baby. Talk to your health care provider or a member of his or her professional staff.

You can also contact the National Domestic Violence Hotline at (800) 799-SAFE or (800) 799-7233 or (800) 787-3224 (TTY) or on the Web at *www.ndvh.org*. In addition, many states and communities have domestic violence hot lines.

Embracing nutrition basics

During pregnancy, it's important to eat a variety of healthy foods. Eating at least three meals a day and healthy snacks is probably the best way to consume a greater variety of foods. If morning sickness makes this impossible, try eating a series of snacks or small meals throughout the day. Remember that you can get servings from several food groups at once if you eat them in combination. A slice of cheese pizza, for example, would count toward servings in the grain (crust), vegetable (tomato sauce) and dairy (cheese) groups.

When you're pregnant, aim to eat more than the minimum number of servings typically recommended in each category of the food pyramid. The increased minimum serving suggestions listed on the next page will provide you with 1,800 to 2,800 calories daily.

To become more aware of your food selections and keep track of your servings, you may want to make copies of the "Minimum daily serving suggestions" sheet and write down what you eat throughout the day. If you find you're low in one category and high in others, try to balance your selections. You can also use this list to point out concerns to your health care provider. If you're unable to meet the recommendations because of allergies, personal aversions or confusion over serving sizes, your health care provider can help you.

Pay close attention to ingredient lists and nutrition facts on food labels. This information can help you keep track of sugars and fats, which add calories but little nutrition to your diet. Labels also reveal the amount of artificial sweeteners and sodium in packaged foods. Although most commercially used sweeteners are thought to be safe, try to limit your intake of artificially sweetened foods and drinks. These may include candy, yogurt, sodas and drink mixes.

Salt needs increase during pregnancy. However, it's still not wise to eat too many salty foods and snacks. That may be especially true if you have high blood pressure or if you develop complications in your pregnancy. In general, don't make any drastic changes in your sodium intake unless directed to do so by your health care provider.

Taking vitamin and mineral supplements

The best place to get the vitamins and minerals you need is from food sources. Yet during pregnancy, you may find it difficult to eat enough foods to supply you with enough folic acid, iron and calcium. That's why many health care providers prescribe prenatal vitamins.

Even if you take a prenatal vitamin or other supplements, the need for a well-balanced diet remains. In fact, taking supplements in no way makes up for bad eating habits. Here's more information about the nutrients that are the most critical to the health of you and your baby:

- **Folic acid.** Folic acid is a B vitamin that's essential in early pregnancy. The Centers for Disease Control and Prevention (CDC) and U.S. Public Health Service recommend that all women of childbearing age consume

MINIMUM DAILY SERVING SUGGESTIONS

Here's a guide to the types and amounts of foods you can eat for good nutrition during pregnancy.

Food category	Number of daily servings during pregnancy	Good choices
Breads and cereals	At least 9 servings 1 serving = 1/2 cup pasta, cooked cereal or rice; 1 slice bread; 6 crackers; 1/2 hamburger bun, 1/2 English muffin or 1/2 small bagel	Cereals, bagels, brown rice, whole-grain breads, rolls and crackers, whole-wheat pasta At least 3 servings of whole grains a day
Vegetables	4 or more servings 1 serving = 1/2 cup cooked or 1 cup raw vegetables	Leaf lettuce (romaine, endive), spinach, red and green peppers, sweet potatoes, winter squash, peas, green beans, broccoli, carrots, corn, tomatoes
Fruits	3 or more servings 1 serving = 1/2 cup cooked fruit or 1 medium-sized piece of fruit	Apples, apricots, bananas, grapes, mango, pineapple, strawberries, raspberries, orange, grapefruit, melon, peach, raisins
Milk, yogurt, cheese	3 or more servings 1 serving = 1 cup milk or yogurt; 1 ounce cheese	Skim milk, low-fat cheese, low-fat yogurt, low-fat cottage cheese
Meat, fish, eggs, dry beans	At least 3 servings 1 serving = 2 to 3 ounces	Chicken, dried peas and beans, fish, lean beef, lean pork, peanut butter, turkey
Fats and sugars	Use sparingly	Butter, margarine, sour cream, nuts, avocado, olive oil, salad dressing, sugar, syrup, honey, candy, desserts

600 micrograms (0.6 milligrams) of folic acid each day, whether or not they intend to become pregnant. Why? Studies have shown that this amount significantly decreases the risk of neural tube defects. Such defects include incomplete closure of the spine (spina bifida) and a partially or completely missing brain (anencephaly). Yet this protection

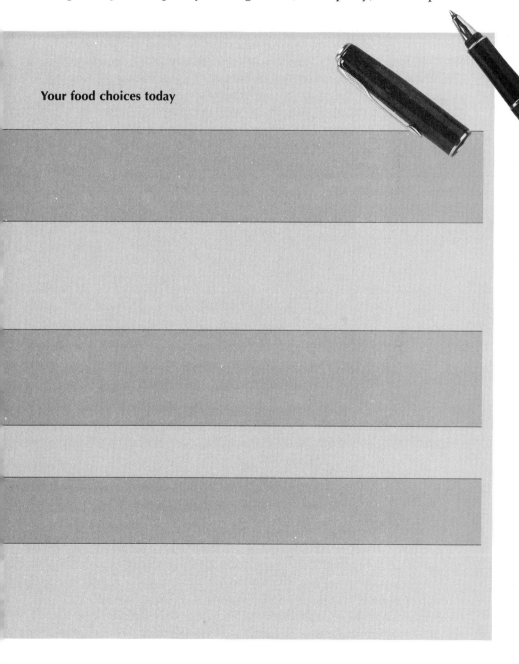

Your food choices today

may not come soon enough if you don't take folic acid until after you find out you're pregnant. That's because neural tube defects occur in the first four weeks of pregnancy, before you may realize you're having a baby.

Fortunately, many ways exist to get the folic acid you need — including taking a supplement or multivitamin and eating foods high in folate.

If you have had a fetus with a neural tube defect in a previous pregnancy, your health care provider may prescribe a daily supplement of 4,000 micrograms (4 mg) of folic acid. You'll likely take it one month before you plan to become pregnant through the first three months of pregnancy. Do not, however, consume more than 1,000 micrograms (1 mg) of folic acid a day without an OK from your health care provider. Too much folic acid in your diet can make it difficult to spot symptoms of vitamin B-12 deficiency.

GOOD DIETARY SOURCES OF FOLIC ACID (FOLATE) INCLUDE:

- Fortified breakfast cereals
- Fortified whole-grain breads
- Leafy green vegetables
- Dried peas and beans
- Citrus fruits and juices, such as oranges and grapefruits
- Bananas
- Cantaloupe
- Tomatoes

- **Iron.** This mineral, which is found in red blood cells, is always an important part of your diet. But it becomes even more important during pregnancy — when your blood volume expands to accommodate changes in your body. If you don't get enough iron, you may develop iron deficiency anemia, a condition that can cause fatigue and lowered resistance to infection. Iron is also required to form tissue for your baby and the placenta. In fact, at birth your newborn needs enough stored iron to last for the first six months of life.

  It's nearly impossible to eat enough foods to get the 30 mg of iron you need daily during pregnancy. This is double the amount of iron needed by adult women who aren't pregnant. Therefore, an iron supplement — along with a diet that includes iron-rich foods — is necessary.

  To help your body absorb the iron in your prenatal or iron supplement, take it with beverages high in vitamin C. Orange, tomato and vegetable juices are your best bets. You can also enhance iron absorption by eating foods high in vitamin C at the same time you eat iron-containing foods. For example, put some strawberries on top of iron-fortified breakfast cereal.

GOOD DIETARY SOURCES OF IRON INCLUDE:

- Lean red meat
- Poultry
- Fish
- Spinach
- Tofu
- Dried fruits, such as raisins and prunes
- Nuts, such as almonds, cashews and peanuts
- Whole-grain and fortified breads and cereals

- **Calcium.** This mineral helps form strong bones and teeth. When you're pregnant and breast-feeding, you need 1,000 to 1,500 mg a day. That's about 40 percent more than most adult women require. If you enjoy and regularly eat dairy products, it's easy to get the added calcium. If you don't, try eating other foods containing calcium.

  Most prenatal supplements also contain calcium, but they usually don't contain enough of the mineral to meet your daily requirements. Several forms of calcium supplements are available. If your health care provider recommends that you take one, be sure it's made from calcium carbonate or calcium citrate, which are highly absorbable. Never take oyster shell or bone meal calcium — also known as dolomite and calcium appetite — because it may be contaminated with lead and other harmful chemicals.

  During pregnancy, you also need protein, carbohydrates and fat in your diet to maintain your energy level and provide the material for cell building, tissue growth and brain development. Vitamins A and C also are important. Vitamin A promotes healthy skin, eyesight and bone growth. Vitamin C forms healthy gums, teeth and bones for your baby. It also keeps your tissues healthy and improves iron absorption. Whole-grain breads, cereals, rice and pasta are good sources of vitamin A, and fruits such as mango, kiwi and oranges provide vitamin C.

  If you can't get enough of these nutrients from your diet, supplements may help. Work with your health care provider to make sure that you don't take excessive amounts of any vitamins or minerals. Big doses of vitamins may harm your baby. For example, large amounts of vitamin A — more than 10,000 international units (IU) — taken daily can cause defects in your baby's bones, heart, nervous system, head and face. Avoid supplementing more than the 5,000 IU.

GOOD DIETARY SOURCES OF CALCIUM INCLUDE:

- Milk
- Cheese
- Yogurt
- Salmon
- Canned sardines with bones
- Spinach
- Broccoli
- Dried beans
- Papaya
- Oranges
- Calcium-fortified foods such as some fruit juices and breakfast cereals

Following a vegetarian diet

If you're a vegetarian, you can continue to follow your diet during pregnancy and have a healthy baby. But you'll need to plan and review your food intake. To get the nutrition you need, eat a wide variety of foods and balance your intake each day.

If you normally include fish, milk and eggs in your diet, you'll have an easier time getting the iron, calcium and protein you need. If you don't eat any animal products at all, that is, you're a vegan, you'll need to carefully plan your daily food intake. Vegans often have difficulty getting enough zinc, vitamin B-12, iron, calcium and folic acid. To avoid this problem, try the following:

- **Eat at least four servings of calcium-rich foods each day.** Nondairy sources include broccoli, kale, dried beans, and calcium-fortified juices, cereals and soy products.
- **Add more energy-rich foods to your diet.** This is particularly important if you're having trouble gaining enough weight. Good sources include nuts, nut butters, seeds and dried fruit.
- **Seek advice on supplements.** Many vegans need a vitamin B-12 supplement. A prenatal vitamin that supplements other nutritional needs also may be necessary. To be sure what's right for you, consult with your health care provider and, if recommended, a registered dietitian.

Eating and cooking safely

There's an old adage that says, "Keep hot foods hot, cold foods cold and keep everything clean." During pregnancy, this saying could help keep you and your baby from becoming quite sick. The changes in your metabolism and circulation while pregnant may increase your risk of bacterial food poisoning.

If you do become sick from bacteria in your food, your reaction will probably be more severe than if you weren't pregnant. Whether or not you have signs and symptoms of food poisoning, your baby can become sick. That's because bacterial toxins pass from mother to baby through the placenta.

Salmonella and listeria are two common food-borne bacteria. Salmonella bacteria are often found in raw poultry, fish, eggs, milk and products containing these ingredients. With salmonella poisoning, you'll experience signs and symptoms within 24 hours after eating contaminated food. They include vomiting, diarrhea, fever, headache and abdominal pain. Most people recover in two to four days. During pregnancy, it may take longer.

Listeria bacteria are common. A particular species called *Listeria monocytogenes* can cause the food-borne illness known as listeriosis. The main sources of the bacteria are raw (unpasteurized) milk, soft cheeses such as brie and feta, undercooked poultry, and hot dogs and deli meats. Avoid these foods during pregnancy.

The signs and symptoms of listeriosis are similar to those of the flu (influenza). They include fever, fatigue, nausea, vomiting and diarrhea. About one-third of all cases of the illness occur during pregnancy. Severe cases may lead to miscarriage or newborn infections in the bloodstream or in the fluid surrounding the brain (meningitis).

To protect yourself and your developing baby, take these precautions:

Shop smart

When you go grocery shopping, pick up the highly perishable items last to reduce the amount of time they aren't refrigerated. These items include meat, poultry, fish and eggs. Once you get home, unpack and store these foods immediately.

Check your refrigerator

To keep bacterial growth at bay, set the temperature in your refrigerator between 34 and 40 F. Keep your freezer at or below 0 F. Monitor these temperatures with an inexpensive refrigerator thermometer. In addition, keep your refrigerator and freezer free of food that's past its expiration date. If you haven't cleaned out the contents in a while, now is a good time to do so.

Keep hands and surfaces clean

Always wash your hands and under your fingernails before you begin any food preparation. It's perhaps the best way to prevent food-borne disease. Keep raw and cooked foods separate when preparing a meal. Use different cutting boards for meats and produce. Wash cutting boards, cutting utensils and other work surfaces with hot, soapy water after each use. To help prevent contamination during food preparation, wash your hands after handling raw foods.

During your pregnancy, when you're selecting the foods you eat and deciding how to prepare them, changes may have to be made, especially with the following items:

Raw fruits and vegetables
Always wash them thoroughly with water before eating. In some cases, you even may want to scrub or peel away the skin. Don't eat alfalfa sprouts.

Ground meat
Hamburger, ground chicken and sausage require special handling. That's because *Escherichia coli (E. coli)* bacteria are commonly found on the surface of meat and distributed throughout the whole product during the grinding process. Unless you cook ground meat until it's well-done, you may not raise its internal temperature high enough to kill all the *E. coli*. Therefore, skip medium or rare burgers or sausages. Cooked ground meat is well-done when the meat is light gray and the juices run clear. All other meats and poultry also should be fully cooked before eating. Use a meat thermometer to ensure doneness.

Fish and shellfish
Seafood is highly nutritious and can continue to be part of your diet during pregnancy. Fish is a great source of omega-3 fatty acids, which are good for brain development in the growing baby.

Both fresh and frozen fish must be properly prepared to eliminate viral or bacterial contamination. When cooking, use the 10-minute rule. This involves measuring fish at its thickest part and cooking for 10 minutes per inch at 450 F. Shellfish such as clams, oysters and shrimp should be boiled for four to six minutes.

While you're pregnant, avoid all raw and undercooked seafood. It's also a good idea to buy fresh fish and seafood the same day you plan to eat it. Be aware that environmental toxins can be a problem with some freshwater fish and ocean seafood.

Despite being banned in 1979, polychlorinated biphenyls (PCBs) remain in our waterways. PCBs can accumulate to potentially dangerous levels in fish. Equally hazardous is methyl mercury, a byproduct of industrial waste and fuel burning that's released into the air and eventually pollutes waterways.

Pregnant or nursing women who consume mercury can harm their baby's developing brain and nervous system. Young children are also more sensitive to the harmful effects of methyl mercury than are older children or adults, who have more fully developed nervous systems.

If you are pregnant, could become pregnant or are nursing, the Environmental Protection Agency (EPA) recommends taking the following steps to limit your exposure to environmental contaminants that may be present in some seafood:

- Choose fish with low mercury levels, such as Pacific salmon, haddock, flounder, shrimp, and farmed trout and catfish. Avoid shark, swordfish, king mackerel or tilefish, since these species tend to have the most chemical contaminants.
- Limit freshwater fish caught by family or friends to no more than 6 ounces a week.
- Limit consumption of fish purchased in a store or restaurant to no more than 12 ounces a week.
- Pay close attention to local advisories concerning the safety of eating fish from certain recreational lakes, rivers and streams. Warnings may be posted at the water's edge or included with information in local fishing licenses. Also watch for advisories issued by the Food and Drug Administration (FDA) regarding any hazards posed by fish sold in stores and restaurants.

To keep up with the latest freshwater fish consumption advisories across the country and in your area, check the EPA Web site at *www.epa.gov/ waterscience/fishadvice/advice.html.* For current advice on any hazards posed by coastal and ocean fish caught by family or friends, visit the FDA's Web site at *www.cfsan.fda.gov/~lrd/tphgfish.html.*

Exercise: Pace it for pregnancy

Pregnancy seems like a perfect time to sit back and relax. Once your body begins changing, you'll notice that you feel more tired than usual. You may also have to deal with such pregnancy-related problems as back pain, muscle cramps, swelling and constipation.

But guess what? Sitting around won't help matters. In fact, pregnancy offers a great reason to get active. Exercise can help lessen common pregnancy complaints. It can boost your energy level and improve your overall health. Perhaps best of all, it can help you prepare for labor and childbirth by increasing your stamina and muscle strength. If you're in good physical condition before giving birth, you may even shorten your labor and recovery times.

Still, it's natural to wonder if exercise is safe during pregnancy. The answer is yes, with a few cautions. Before starting or continuing any exercise program, talk with your health care provider. That's especially important if you have a known medical condition, such as thyroid disease.

It's also important to know that pregnancy itself is physically demanding. You can expect to gain 25 to 35 pounds. Pregnancy is not a time to try losing weight or maintaining your current weight. In addition, your heart will pump about 50 percent more blood. Your body will consume up to 20 percent more oxygen while you rest and even more when you exercise.

As your abdomen increases in size, your posture will shift, putting new strain on your back muscles and changing your balance. Toward the end of your pregnancy, the joints and ligaments in your pelvis will loosen in preparation for labor. All of these changes will affect the way your body responds to exercise. Muscle and joint injuries are more likely to occur if you're not careful.

Good ways to start

For the average person, the Centers for Disease Control and Prevention and the American College of Sports Medicine recommend getting 30 minutes or more of moderate exercise on most, if not all, days of the week. If you are pregnant and have no complications, you may want to meet this goal. However, exercising even three or four days a week for 20 minutes or more can offer health benefits.

Walking is an excellent exercise for beginners. It provides moderate aerobic conditioning and puts minimal stress on your joints. Other good choices are nonweight-bearing activities, such as swimming or cycling on a stationary bike. Before you begin any activity, check with your health care provider.

You're more likely to stick with an exercise plan if it involves activities that you enjoy. Choose activities that can be included easily in your daily schedule. Programs held at inconvenient times and places may discourage you from exercising at all. If you need help with motivation, contact your local hospital or birthing center. Many offer prenatal fitness classes. There, you can learn safe ways to exercise while working out with other pregnant women.

Sports and activities to approach with care

Usually, it's safe to do some form of exercise throughout pregnancy. After the first trimester, though, avoid floor exercises that require you to be on your back for a long period of time. The weight of the baby can cause problems with blood circulation. Standing motionless for a long period of time also can be hard on the circulatory system.

As soon as you learn you're pregnant, be especially careful with activities that carry a high risk of falling or abdominal injury. Gymnastics, horseback riding, downhill or water skiing, and vigorous racket sports have greater risk of injury. It also may be wise to take care if you play high contact sports such as soccer and basketball. These sports involve the risk of falling or colliding with another person. Plus, they often require you to jump or change

MEDICAL CONDITIONS REQUIRING CAUTION WITH EXERCISE

Exercising is good for your health during pregnancy. But if you have a medical condition, you may need to take a more cautious approach to physical activity. Conditions that may require caution include:

- Anemia
- Thyroid disease
- Diabetes
- A seizure disorder, such as epilepsy
- An irregular heartbeat
- A history of preterm labor

Other conditions require special monitoring during exercise or prohibit all forms of exercise. Examples of these conditions include:

- Heart disease
- An infectious disease such as hepatitis
- Severe high blood pressure
- Lung disease
- A history of multiple miscarriages
- Uterine bleeding
- Placenta previa

Other circumstances can affect your exercise program. If you are expecting twins or other multiples, have a condition that places you at high risk of premature labor or are carrying a baby that shows poor weight gain, you will need to carefully review with your health care provider what is and isn't permissible. However, that doesn't mean all exercise will be out of the question. If you're not restricted to bed rest, walking may be OK.

directions quickly. You may run a greater risk of straining the cartilage and ligaments that support your joints because these soften during pregnancy.

Underwater and high-altitude activities also can be a problem. Snorkeling is generally OK. However, avoid scuba diving during pregnancy because the air decompression poses a potential risk to the fetus. Physical activities such as hiking at altitudes higher than 6,000 feet above sea level can put you at risk of altitude sickness if you haven't had a chance to acclimate, which could endanger your health and that of your baby.

Listen to your body

If you're in good condition, you can probably work out safely at about the same level you did before you became pregnant, as long as you're feeling comfortable and your health care provider has given approval.

While exercising, listen to the messages your body sends you. If your body is telling you to slow down, follow its advice, no matter how fit you are. Watch for dizziness, nausea, blurred vision, fatigue and shortness of breath. These can be signs of heat stroke, which can threaten the life of you and your baby.

Chest pain, abdominal pain and vaginal bleeding are other danger signs telling you to slow down, stop and get help if you need it. Never exercise through pain. Pain is your body's way of telling you to slow down or stop. Discuss pain and other danger signs with your health care provider.

Along with listening to your body, it pays to take some preventive measures. Injury and muscle cramps often can be avoided if you stretch muscles before and after exercise. To avoid dehydration, drink fluids during exercise whether you're thirsty or not. Take measures to prevent overheating your body. During warm weather, exercise outside in the early morning or late evening. With indoor exercises, work out in rooms with good ventilation or use a fan.

No matter how dedicated you are to being in shape, don't exercise to the point of exhaustion.

Lifestyle: Living for two

Once you become pregnant, everyone has advice about what you should and shouldn't do. Every day seems to bring a new health warning. To make matters worse, the information sometimes conflicts with what you might have heard last year or last week. It can make you question what changes, if any, you should make in your life.

You might wonder: Is an occasional glass of wine at dinner all right? Should I avoid people who smoke? Do I have to give up caffeine? Can I take a soak in the hot tub without harming my baby? Will sexual intercourse cause me to miscarry?

Your body will undergo major changes during your pregnancy. How much you need to change your lifestyle depends on your current habits. High-risk activities such as smoking, drinking alcohol and using recreational drugs should be off limits during pregnancy. Other habits and activities may simply need to be approached with caution or avoided for a time.

If you have any questions about how lifestyle issues can affect your health or the health of your baby, talk to your health care provider. In the meantime, think of pregnancy as the perfect time to kick bad habits and adopt new ones.

Drinking alcohol

The question: One little drink won't hurt my baby, will it? The answer: Maybe not. But experts agree that no level of alcohol has been proved safe during pregnancy. Although you have a greater chance of harming your baby if you drink excessively, even moderate or minimal alcohol use can be damaging.

The reason: If you drink alcohol, so does your baby. It doesn't matter if you drink beer, wine or other forms of liquor. Once in your bloodstream, alcohol passes through the placenta to your baby. Sustained drinking during pregnancy increases your risk of miscarriage and fetal death. It also can cause permanent damage to your baby.

Fetal alcohol syndrome (FAS) is the most serious problem caused by excessive alcohol consumption during pregnancy. Each year, between 1,300 and 8,000 babies are born in the United States with the condition. FAS can cause such birth defects as facial deformities, heart problems, low birth weight and mental retardation. Babies born with FAS may also have permanent growth problems, short attention spans, learning disabilities and behavioral problems.

Children whose mothers drink even moderately can be born with fetal alcohol effect (FAE). This condition can cause some, but not all, of the defects of FAS. Depending on the damage done, these children may be referred to as having alcohol-related birth defects (ARBDs) or alcohol-related neurodevelopmental disorders (ARNDs).

The damage caused by alcohol is permanent. It's also completely preventable. As soon as you know you're pregnant, don't drink alcohol. If you're planning to get pregnant, it's a good idea to stop drinking. Alcohol exposure can cause birth defects in the early weeks of your pregnancy, before you may know you're carrying a child.

Small amounts of alcohol can wind up in breast milk and be passed on to your baby. You may want to abstain from alcohol use until you're finished breast-feeding.

If you think you might need help to stop drinking alcohol, talk with your health care provider.

Smoking

There's no question about it: Smoking is dangerous for you and your baby. Smoking during pregnancy increases your risk of:

- Preterm birth, which means delivering your baby before the 37th week of pregnancy. Preterm birth puts your baby at risk of low birth weight and other health problems.
- Problems with the placenta, which nourishes your baby during pregnancy.
- Stillbirth, in which the baby dies in the uterus before it's born.
- Having a low-birth-weight baby. Babies born at weights lower than $5\frac{1}{2}$ pounds are more likely to have health problems and chronic disabilities.
- Having a child with certain birth defects.

- Having your baby die of sudden infant death syndrome (SIDS) after birth. SIDS occurs when an apparently healthy baby dies unexpectedly during sleep.
- Having a baby with behavioral difficulties and chronic respiratory problems, such as asthma.

How does smoking cause so much damage? Cigarette smoke contains thousands of chemicals. Two of them — carbon monoxide and nicotine — are toxins that can move through your bloodstream and harm your developing baby. Both can reduce the flow of oxygen to the fetus. And nicotine, which causes your heartbeat and blood pressure to increase and your blood vessels to constrict, can also decrease your baby's supply of nutrients.

It's best to stop smoking before you become pregnant and give up the habit completely, even after the baby is born. It's also wise to keep you and your baby away from the smoke of other smokers. Regular exposure to secondhand smoke appears to be capable of causing health problems for your child before and after birth.

If you're still smoking after becoming pregnant, remember that it's never too late to quit. Even if you stop late in pregnancy, you can reduce your baby's exposure to dangerous chemicals. Quitting for good also reduces your risk of developing cancer, heart disease and other serious illnesses.

Smoking is an addiction and a habit. Stopping can be very difficult. If you're ready to break the habit, ask your health care provider for help. It's especially important to consult with your health care provider before using products such as nicotine patches and gum. Although these products can help you stop smoking, risks are associated with using them during pregnancy. Your health care provider can help you weigh the benefits and risks of smoking cessation products and help you find support or classes in your area.

Using illicit drugs

If you're pregnant, the rule about using illicit drugs is simple: Don't do it. Any and all illicit drug use can harm your baby. This includes cocaine, marijuana, heroin, methadone, LSD, phencyclidine (PCP), methamphetamine and any other kind of recreational or street drug.

While you're pregnant, the drugs you take can pass from you to your baby. This can affect the development of the fetus and the future of your child as he or she grows up. It can also cause the death of your fetus or withdrawal symptoms in newborns that if untreated can lead to death.

For instance, if you use cocaine during pregnancy, you risk miscarriage, problems with the placenta, and preterm labor and childbirth. Cocaine also can cause growth restriction and birth defects. After delivery, cocaine can be passed from you to your baby in breast milk.

Dangers associated with drug use can harm you and your baby. Drugs that are used intravenously may cause infections, including human immuno-deficiency virus (HIV), the AIDS virus. Money spent on drugs can take away from what's needed to provide you and your family with health care, housing and nutrition.

If you find it difficult to stop using drugs, talk to your health care provider. He or she can help you find the help you need.

Drinking caffeinated beverages

It's best to avoid caffeine whenever possible during pregnancy. At the very least, limit how much caffeine you consume. Research has been mixed on the subject. But overall, studies show a moderate intake — 200 milligrams (mg) or less a day, about the amount found in one to two cups of coffee — has no negative effects on pregnant women and their babies.

However, the same doesn't hold true for high amounts of caffeine — 500 mg or more daily, or five or more cups of coffee. Regular intake of this much caffeine may cause a decrease in your baby's birth weight and head circum-ference. Low birth weight can make it difficult for the baby to maintain a healthy body temperature and appropriate blood sugar levels, which can lead to other problems.

Coffee is the most common source of caffeine. Tea, carbonated beverages, cocoa and chocolate also contain caffeine. To reduce the amount of caffeine you consume in a day, consider switching to decaffeinated beverages. Or with hot, brewed beverages, shorten the time you brew them. For instance, brewing a tea bag for just one minute instead of several minutes can reduce caffeine content by as much as half.

Although herbal teas may seem like a safe alternative during pregnancy, avoid them. Little is known about herbs and their effects on pregnancy. In some cases, they can do damage. The herb comfrey, for example, can cause serious liver disease. For more information on herbal products, see page 455.

Precautions around the house

There's plenty to do to get ready for the baby, along with the usual work that continues despite your pregnancy. But is it safe to repaint walls, use household cleaning products, clean up after pets, sit in front of a computer screen or take a warm bath to relieve sore muscles? Yes, as long as you take some simple precautions in the following areas:
- **Painting.** In general, avoid exposure to oil-based paints, lead and mercury — all of which may be found in old paints that you may be

stripping from surfaces. Also avoid other substances that have solvents, such as paint removers. Even if you're just painting a small room or piece of baby furniture, be careful. Work in a well-ventilated area to minimize breathing fumes and wear protective clothing and gloves. Don't eat or drink in the area where you're painting. In addition, be extra careful if you use a ladder. Your changing body shape may throw off your sense of balance.

- **Housecleaning.** The use of normal household cleaners hasn't been shown to harm a developing baby. Still, it's a good idea to stay away from oven cleaners that emit strong fumes in a contained space. Don't mix chemicals such as ammonia and bleach because the combination can produce toxic fumes. When cleaning, avoid inhaling any strong, caustic fumes. Wear protective gloves to avoid absorbing any chemicals through your skin. You might also consider switching to cleaners such as vinegar and baking soda or other products that contain no harsh, toxic chemicals.

- **Cleaning the litter box.** Cats who hunt rodents may harbor a parasite that causes an infection known as toxoplasmosis. Some women cat owners are immune to the illness before pregnancy. Usually, your own cat isn't much of a risk. But if you're not immune and you were to pass on a first-time, active infection to your baby, it could result in birth defects such as blindness, deafness and mental retardation. When disposing of used litter, wear rubber gloves or, better yet, get someone else to do it. Change the litter frequently to avoid a buildup of cat feces dust.

- **Soaking in hot water.** A bath can help you relax and relieve sore muscles without posing any health hazards. But be careful to avoid long exposures to hot tubs with temperatures greater than 101 F. Warm temperatures may also cause your blood pressure to drop, increasing your risk of fainting. In short, if you're in warm or hot water and you get dizzy, you've been in too long.

Sex

Usually, you can have sex well into your third trimester, as long as you're having no problems with your pregnancy. But you may not always want to. During the early stage of pregnancy, changing hormones, new weight gain and decreased energy levels may take their toll on sexual desire. Lack of interest may continue through the first trimester, when exhaustion and nausea are most likely to occur.

During the second trimester, increased blood flow to your sexual organs and breasts may rekindle your desire. It may even increase your normal interest in sex. As you enter your final trimester, however, interest may wane once again and your growing abdomen can make sex physically challenging. Plus, increased fatigue and back pain can dampen your mood.

Fear about harming your baby also can make many expectant mothers and fathers shy away from sex. Some may worry that intercourse will cause a miscarriage, especially in the first trimester. But intercourse isn't a concern. Miscarriages that occur during this time commonly result from genetic defects, not from anything you do or don't do.

Orgasms can cause uterine contractions. Most research indicates that if you have a normal pregnancy, orgasms — with or without intercourse — don't lead to premature labor. Nor are they connected with your water breaking or premature birth. Intercourse more than once a week late in pregnancy might increase the risk of intrauterine infection. In that case, your health care provider may recommend abstinence during the last weeks.

If you have certain problems during pregnancy, your health care provider may ask you to stop having intercourse. That may be the case if you have preterm labor, vaginal bleeding or problems with your cervix or placenta. Special conditions such as carrying two or more babies may rule out intercourse late in pregnancy.

Pregnancy doesn't have to mean an end to physical closeness with your partner. If intercourse is difficult or off-limits, try cuddling, touching and massage.

Medications: Take with care

Should you avoid all medicines when you're pregnant? No. Although some medicines should be avoided, others may be recommended because of your needs.

That doesn't mean all medicines are safe as long as you need them. Even over-the-counter (OTC) products such as aspirin and cough syrup may cause side effects for you and your baby. Check with your health care provider before taking any medication — including OTC medicines, prescription drugs and herbal products.

If you have a health condition that requires regular medication — such as asthma, hypothyroidism, high blood pressure or depression — don't stop these until you talk with your health care provider. He or she can help you evaluate what's safe to take before, during and after pregnancy. In many cases, continuing your medication may be the best choice. In others, you may be advised to discontinue taking a certain medication. Or you may be advised to switch to one that eliminates the risk or poses less risk to you or your baby.

In some cases, studies may help determine whether a particular drug is safe for pregnant women. Yet it's not always easy or even possible to determine the short- and long-term effects of medications. The FDA rates drugs in terms of their safety during pregnancy. But most medications haven't been studied on pregnant women. Therefore, it isn't known for certain if they cause damage to growing fetuses or can affect a child later in life.

Some medications have been shown to be extremely harmful to a developing fetus, even in the early weeks of pregnancy. Some of the most dangerous drugs include:

- The acne drug isotretinoin (Accutane)
- The multiuse drug thalidomide (Thalomid)
- The psoriasis drug acitretin (Soriatane)

If you're taking one of these medications, avoid becoming pregnant until you discontinue its use. Your health care provider will advise you on the best way to stop taking a medication and how long you may need to wait before it's safe to conceive. Don't restart a drug without talking to your health care provider.

For more specific information on medications, see "Medications," on page 463, in Part 3, "Pregnancy Reference Guide." Talk with your health care provider about any specific questions you have regarding medications.

Vaccines

During pregnancy, you may be at increased risk of complications from infectious diseases and illnesses, such as the flu. In fact, the flu can prove deadly. That's why the flu shot is recommended during pregnancy. The shot, which is made from inactivated viruses, is thought to be safe at any stage of conception. But some experts recommend that pregnant women wait until their second trimester, when the highest risk of miscarriage has passed. If you're still in your first three months of pregnancy when the flu season hits, ask your health care provider if he or she recommends waiting or going forward with the shot.

Other vaccines for chickenpox (varicella), German measles (rubella) and measles (rubeola) haven't been approved for women who are pregnant. Most of these illnesses occur early in life. They're now relatively rare because of childhood immunization programs. But you're at increased risk of serious complications if you contract them during pregnancy. If you're susceptible to chickenpox and are planning to conceive, your health care provider may recommend that you have the vaccination and put off pregnancy for a month or more.

If you're already pregnant and found not to be immune from serious infectious diseases, you'll need to avoid exposure to them. After pregnancy, your health care provider may recommend that you be vaccinated against such illnesses as German measles so that you'll be immune in future pregnancies. Once vaccinated, though, you shouldn't become pregnant again for at least one month.

Work: Plan ahead

If you're planning to work throughout your pregnancy, you're not alone. Many women stay on the job until they're ready to give birth.

Pregnancy does raise some serious questions that you typically need to answer before too much time passes. Some of these questions may include:

- When should I tell my boss and co-workers?
- How do I deal with fatigue or morning sickness on the job?
- Will continuing to work hurt my baby or endanger my pregnancy?
- How much maternity leave can I take?

You might have many more questions and concerns about working during pregnancy. Feel free to ask your health care provider. In addition, seek help if you're having trouble keeping up with daily demands.

Breaking the news at work

Everyone has a different idea about the perfect time to tell others that she is pregnant. Many women wait to tell anyone except their partner until after their first trimester, when the highest risk of miscarriage has passed. Others can't wait to share the news.

At work, there's no perfect time to tell others. It's wise not to wait too long, especially if you have health issues or other complications to sort through with your supervisor. No matter when you break the news, consider the following tips:

- **Tell your boss personally.** Your boss deserves to hear the news directly from you instead of overhearing it in the break room. Even if you tell only one or two people you trust, secrets can be hard to keep. If you begin having trouble keeping your eyes open at meetings or are constantly running to the bathroom, it's better to let your boss know that you're pregnant instead of letting him or her think that you are ill or have lost interest in work.
- **Watch out for potential conflicts.** These days, it's illegal to withhold a promotion, reduce the amount of a raise or take back a job offer just because a woman is pregnant. Nevertheless, if you have an upcoming salary review or are under consideration for a new position or important project, you may want to wait to share your news. After all, these decisions should be based on your performance up until now. If, however, you want to avoid taking on a special assignment that would be impossible to finish before your baby arrives, you may want to speak up sooner.
- **Keep your options open.** Your boss and co-workers may want to know exactly how long you plan to work and when you intend to come back.

Share some general plans at the start of your pregnancy, but leave enough room for negotiation in case the idea of working until your water breaks loses its appeal by your final trimester. For instance, you could say, "My goal is to work straight through pregnancy, but I probably can't make a final decision until I reach my third trimester." Even if you decide to state your plans in detail, be sure to acknowledge that unforeseen problems or circumstances could result in changes.

- **Know what your options are.** Once you make your big announcement at work, go to your company's personnel office. Collect information on health insurance, disability benefits, and family or maternity leave policies. You may also want to check into company policies regarding flextime or telecommuting, which may allow you to shorten your hours before your baby arrives or work from home after your maternity leave.
- **Offer solutions.** Before you share your baby news, think about how your work might be split up. Consider who could be trained to take your spot for a few months, if necessary. This is particularly important if you're in a management position or will need to change job responsibilities because your current position might pose health hazards to your baby. The bottom line: If you help come up with solutions, your boss and colleagues are less likely to focus on the challenges your pregnancy might create.
- **Know the law.** Although policies regarding work hours, sick leave and health care benefits vary from company to company, federal laws offer protections for pregnant women and those who can't work because of the need to care for a newborn. These laws are known as the Pregnancy Discrimination Act of 1978 and the Family Medical Leave Act of 1993.

  Be aware, however, that some small companies may be exempt from these laws. Also, you may not qualify for certain benefits if you're a relatively new employee. Consult your company handbook and your human resources office if you're in doubt about what's available to you.

Surviving sickness and sleepiness

The myth of superwoman is just that — a myth. Even though it's safe for almost all women to work while pregnant, at times it may not be easy to keep up the same pace as before you were pregnant.

One reason for that is morning sickness. Up to 70 percent of pregnant women experience nausea and vomiting in early pregnancy. Usually, it begins early on and subsides during the second trimester. But some women continue to be sick beyond the first trimester. An unlucky few have trouble throughout their pregnancy. To top it off, the condition — commonly known as morning sickness — can occur anytime of day.

You can take steps to help keep morning sickness under better control:

- **Avoid nausea triggers.** A lot of women find certain foods and smells can aggravate nausea during pregnancy. If this is the case for you, steer clear of whatever triggers queasiness. For instance, if the smells of the hot dishes in the company cafeteria turn your stomach, start brown bagging it or eating at your desk. Strong colognes or perfumes that set you off may be harder to eliminate. But if your co-worker in the next cubicle wears a particularly strong scent, see if you can enlist his or her help. For instance, you might say, "Normally, I love the after-shave you wear, but since I became pregnant, all colognes seem to make my morning sickness worse. Because we sit so close, would you consider not using any after-shave for a while?"

- **Eat snacks and light meals.** Crackers and other bland foods can be life-savers when you start to feel nauseated. Once you find what items work best for you, keep a stash in your desk drawer or in your purse for emergencies. Snacking on light bites can keep your stomach from being completely empty or full, two conditions that can make nausea worse. Nibbling a few crackers before getting out of bed might keep you from feeling sick first thing in the morning.

- **Drink enough fluids.** Your body uses more water in early pregnancy. If you don't drink enough fluids, it can worsen your nausea. A good goal is six to eight 8-ounce cups throughout the day. Caffeinated drinks don't count.

- **Get enough rest.** The more tired you are, the more nauseated you can become. Therefore, it's important to get a good night's sleep. Rushing around in the morning also can make you queasy. Try going to bed earlier and getting up a little sooner to maximize the amount of sleep you get and minimize the stress you feel when preparing for your workday.

Even with a little more sleep at night, you still may notice that you have less energy during the day. This is especially true in the first and third trimesters, when you may feel tired much of the time. Fatigue is your body's way of telling you to slow down, but this can be tough during the workday. To make it through the day, try the following:

- **Take short, frequent breaks.** Regular rest periods can improve your productivity, especially if fatigue is interfering with your ability to concentrate or make decisions. Even 10 minutes spent with the lights off, your eyes closed and your feet up can help you recharge. Getting up and moving around for a few minutes also can make you feel refreshed.

- **Rethink your schedule.** If you're exhausted by the afternoon, get your toughest or high-concentration tasks done earlier in the day. If it takes you longer to regain energy in the morning, try to put off energy-draining chores until the afternoon. You may want to see if you can arrange more flexible work hours that allow you to start work later in the day.

Consider cutting back on commitments and activities outside the office to get more rest in the evening. If you have a physically strenuous job, it's even more important to take it easier on evenings and weekends. If you sit at a desk all day long, though, a walk, a prenatal exercise class or a night out could be the best way to keep from feeling drained. The rule of thumb: Maintain a balance.

- **Accept and use help.** You may be used to cleaning your own house, mowing your own yard and running errands after work. But to get in some extra rest and relaxation, you might consider hiring services or the teenager down the street to help with cleaning or yardwork. You might even want to take advantage of online shopping sites and home deliveries to gain extra time.

  During work hours, don't be too proud to accept help and support from co-workers. If colleagues offer to answer your phone while you close your office door to take a 10-minute nap or reschedule late afternoon meetings so that you can attend birthing classes, let them. By letting them show their support for you, you'll strengthen the bond you share with your colleagues.

Staying comfortable

Carrying around a growing baby can make everyday activities like sitting, standing, bending and lifting uncomfortable. It can also cause constant pressure on your bladder, strain on your back and fluid retention in your legs and feet.

Emptying your bladder frequently can help relieve pressure. Moving around every few hours can ease muscle tension and help prevent fluid buildup. But you may need to try other strategies to make yourself comfortable throughout your workday and prevent potential health hazards. Here's how to handle common on-the-job activities:

- **Sitting.** If you have an office job, the chair you sit in is important, and not just during pregnancy. While the weight of your body is increasing and shifting, it helps to have a seat you can adjust for height and tilt. Adjustable armrests, a firm seat and back cushions, and good back support can make long hours of sitting much easier and facilitate exits from the chair.

  If a chair with these options isn't available, take steps to improve what you do have. For instance, if you need more cushioning or back support, use a small pillow or invest in a cushion designed to support the lower back. This type of cushion can also serve as a car seat support, which might make driving easier if you have a long commute.

While sitting, it's best to elevate your feet on a footrest or box to help take some of the strain off your back. This may also reduce your chance of developing varicose veins or clots in the veins of your legs. Using a footrest may also help reduce the swelling in the feet and legs. Round-bottomed footrests even can be rocked gently with your feet. This motion is good for your circulation and may be soothing if you feel restless. Skip crossing your legs as well.

- **Standing.** Standing for long periods may not seem like a risky proposition. But during pregnancy, you have increased dilation of blood vessels. This can cause blood to pool in the legs with too much standing, which could lead to pain, dizziness and even fainting.

    Standing can also put pressure on your back. If standing is part of your job, put one foot on a box or low stool to take pressure off your back and decrease blood pooling. Switch feet every so often. It may help to wear support hose and take frequent breaks throughout the day. Most health care providers recommend wearing shoes with low, wide heels rather than high heels or flats.

    If your job requires you to stand for four or more hours a day, ask your health care provider if he or she has any specific recommendations or concerns that might require you to stop working earlier in your pregnancy or modify your job duties.

- **Bending and lifting.** To prevent or ease back pain, follow proper form when bending and lifting. To pick up something off the floor, stand with your feet shoulder-width apart and lower your body by bending at the knees, not the waist. Keep your back as straight as possible when you grasp the load. Then keep the load close to your body while you use your leg muscles to lift you and the item. Don't twist the body as you rise to a standing position.

Keeping stress under control

Stress on the job can be exhilarating in some cases. It can inspire you to push harder and achieve more than you ever thought possible. However, it can also exhaust you and take away the time and energy you need to care for yourself and your unborn baby. Eating right and exercising, for instance, can go out the window when you spend a great deal of time dealing with stressful workplace issues.

Although it may be impossible to eliminate job-related stress, you can try to minimize it. Talk out problems with a supportive co-worker, friend or spouse. Your health care provider might be another source of support. Or he or she may be able to refer you to other professionals or support groups that can help you deal with stress before it affects your well-being.

A good sense of humor and the company of positive, optimistic people also can help. So can keeping your eye on the big picture. When you feel yourself getting angry or upset as a result of stress, stop and ask yourself if you can do anything to change the situation. If not, you may just need to let it go.

Relaxation exercises also can help you release pressure that may build up during the course of a day. Most of these exercises can be done anywhere at any time. They include:

- **Breathing.** Inhale slowly through your nose and then hold your breath while you count to five. Exhale slowly and deeply when you're finished counting. Repeat this exercise three or four times.
- **Refocusing your thoughts.** Think about a positive experience or a place you enjoy. If you need help or inspiration, look at a picture or object that has a pleasant meaning for you. Listening to music also can help you relax and take your mind off what's troubling you for a few moments. If this isn't possible while you're working, try this exercise on your break, during your commute or when you get home.
- **Keeping a journal.** Write in a notebook for 10 minutes whenever you get frustrated or need to get rid of the stress of the day. Forget about grammar and spelling. Just write whatever thoughts or feelings you want to express. Once you're done, read what you wrote. You may be surprised to find insights or solutions to your problems. At the very least, you'll blow off some steam.

Taking proper job precautions

If heavy physical labor isn't part of your job, you may think that you can continue working with no worries while pregnant. This may be true. But several studies indicate that certain activities and working conditions can increase your risk of preterm labor and giving birth to a low-birth-weight baby. These activities and conditions include:

- Heavy, repetitive lifting
- Prolonged standing
- Heavy vibrations, such as from large machines
- Long, stressful commutes to and from work

Other job conditions also may be cause for concern. Frequent shift changes, for instance, may make it hard for you to get the proper rest. A hot working environment may decrease your stamina and ability to perform strenuous physical tasks. Activities that require agility and good balance may become more difficult later in pregnancy.

If any of these issues apply to you, you may need to review them with your health care provider and, possibly, your employer. Your health care provider will be able to tell you if you need to take any special precautions or modify your responsibilities. He or she can also make specific recommendations throughout the stages of pregnancy and, if needed, provide documents for your employer explaining any work restrictions you might need.

Other workplace issues that you may have concerns and questions about include the following.

Exposure to harmful substances

The good news: As long as you and the company you work for follow standard Occupational Safety & Health Administration (OSHA) practices regarding harmful substances, it's unlikely that your fetus will be harmed.

To be safe, be aware of any substances you're exposed to at work — especially if you're in health care or manufacturing. Industries in the United States are required by federal law to have material safety data sheets on file that report hazardous substances in the workplace and to make this information available to employees.

Substances known to be harmful to a developing fetus include lead, mercury, ionizing radiation (X-rays) and drugs used to treat cancer. Chemicals such as anesthetic gases and organic solvents such as benzene are suspected to be harmful, although results of studies are inconclusive.

Tell your health care provider about any part of your job that exposes you to chemicals, drugs or radiation. Also tell your health care provider about any equipment you use to minimize your exposure. This may include gowns, gloves, masks and ventilation systems.

Your health care provider can use this information to determine whether a risk exists and, if so, what can be done to eliminate or reduce it. To help assess the risk, you might be asked to keep a diary of your workplace activities for a week or two.

Fortunately, it appears that environmental agents cause few birth defects. Of the small percentage of birth defects that can be traced to an environmental cause, most involve alcohol, tobacco or drugs used during pregnancy — not substances in the workplace. Nevertheless, avoid exposure to known or suspected harmful substances.

A high risk of infections

If you're a health care professional, child-care worker, school teacher, veterinary worker or meat handler, you may be exposed to infections during the course of your job. When you're pregnant, several infections are of great concern. They include German measles (rubella), chickenpox (varicella), fifth disease (parvovirus), cytomegalovirus (CMV), toxoplasmosis, herpes simplex, hepatitis B and AIDS.

You already may be immune to some of these diseases, either because you have had them or have been vaccinated against them. If you don't have immunity, avoid situations in which you're exposed to these diseases, and practice infection-control measures whenever possible.

If you work in a health care setting, wear gloves, wash your hands regularly and avoid eating on the job. If you work in child care, wash your hands after changing diapers, after helping children use the bathroom and before eating. Don't kiss or share food with the children you supervise.

If you're concerned about or at high risk of getting an infection at work, talk with your health care provider. After reviewing your health, immune status and job duties, he or she may advise you to take special precautions to avoid exposure.

Computers in the workplace

As computers have become more common in the workplace, concerns have arisen about the risks associated with sitting for hours in front of a computer screen — also known as a video display terminal (VDT). Computer screens do emit a small amount of nonionizing radiation, but so far studies indicate that this low level of radiation isn't dangerous to a developing fetus.

If you're still worried or you just want to be cautious, take a few simple precautions: Sit 22 to 28 inches — about an arm's length — from your terminal and 3 to 4 feet from the back and sides of your co-workers' terminals. At these distances, the amount of nonionizing radiation that reaches you drops off dramatically.

Another form of energy — called electromagnetic fields (EMFs) — also are produced by VDTs. This same energy comes from such sources as power lines and electric appliances. Some studies have suggested that being exposed to high levels of EMFs can pose health concerns. Yet research has shown that working with VDTs doesn't expose workers to EMFs that are any higher than those they tend to experience from other sources. Better yet, recent studies haven't shown that VDTs pose health risks for pregnant women — even if they work at a computer all day long.

Some computer workers complain of straining everything from their neck and back to their wrists and hands. However, many of these problems can be avoided or helped by taking regularly scheduled work breaks. In addition, use proper hand positioning and adjust office equipment for your height and comfort.

Preparing for maternity and paternity leave

Plan ahead to determine how long you can take off work. In most cases, the time you're away will be unpaid, unless you can use paid sick leave, vacation days or personal days to substitute as part of your maternity leave.

Before you have your baby, be sure to check on which benefits will continue during your leave and which ones, if any, will cease. If the father of your baby plans to take paternity leave, he needs to ask the same questions at his workplace.

Child care is another issue that requires some planning. Some child-care providers have long waiting lists or may not take infants. Don't wait until your maternity leave is almost over to investigate your options. To avoid this problem, talk to family, friends and co-workers who have faced the same issue. Through their experiences, you can start thinking about your child-care options and what steps you need to take.

Pregnancy timing: Does age matter?

About 4 million American women give birth each year. Although some are teenagers, most are in their 20s and 30s. With today's advances in assisted reproductive technologies, some new moms are even in their late 40s or 50s. In 2000, for example, 255 American women in their 50s gave birth.

Over the past three decades, the average age of first-time moms in the United States has increased. In 1970, the average first-time mom was 21.4 years old. In 2002, the average first-time mom was just past her 25th birthday, 25.1 years old. Though the numbers vary quite widely from state to state and for different ethnic groups, this upward trend is widespread, occurring in all ethnic groups and all 50 states.

Why the increase in the average age of new moms? The reasons are likely twofold. Over the past three decades, the percentage of babies born to teenage mothers has decreased. In 1970, these births made up 17.6 percent of the total. By 2000, this percentage had fallen to 11.8 percent. One possible reason for this is the use of contraceptives. Between the 1970s and 1990s, the number of couples using contraception, especially condoms, during their first sexual experience rose dramatically.

The other reason has to do with women on the other end of the age spectrum — those age 35 and older. Over the past three decades, the percentage of babies born to these women has increased from 6.3 percent in 1970 to 13.4 percent in 2000. Educational and career opportunities are often cited as reasons that American women are waiting longer to become moms. In fact, from 1970 to 2000, the percentage of women having completed four or more years of college nearly tripled. During the same period, women's participation in the American workforce increased by nearly 40 percent.

The years from ages 20 to 34 are still the most "popular" for childbearing, accounting for about three-fourths of all births. That hasn't changed much in 30 years, although the percentage of women becoming new moms in their early 20s has decreased, and the percentage of women becoming new moms in their early 30s has increased. When you tally up all the births in the United States each year, women in their 20s still account for more than half.

Fertility and age

If you're in your 30s or 40s, you may be wondering whether you'll have trouble getting pregnant. Fertility does decline with age. A woman is at her peak fertility between ages 20 and 24. If you're in your early to mid-30s, you're probably about 15 percent to 20 percent less fertile than you were in your early 20s. If you're in your mid- to late 30s, you may be 25 percent to 50 percent less fertile than you were at your peak. If you're in your early to mid-40s, your decline in fertility may be as much as 95 percent.

Here's another way of thinking about it: In the United States, about 10 percent of women in their 20s report some difficulty getting pregnant. This percentage increases to 25 percent among women in their 30s and to more than 50 percent among women age 40 and older.

Studies suggest that your fertility declines slowly through your mid- to late 20s and early 30s. It then drops off more steeply once you reach age 35. Statistics bear this out: About one-third of couples in which the woman is over 35 have trouble conceiving a child. However, some research suggests that while this age-related drop in fertility decreases your chances of becoming pregnant in a given month, it doesn't reduce your overall chances of conceiving. In other words, if you're in your mid- to late 30s, getting pregnant may just take a bit longer than it would have earlier in your life.

Why does fertility decline as you get older? Researchers think it mainly has to do with the quality and quantity of your eggs. The receptiveness of your uterus and age-related hormonal changes also may play a role.

Egg quality

When you're born, your ovaries contain all the eggs you're ever going to have — about 2 million — although they're in an undeveloped form. As you mature, most of the undeveloped eggs disappear, leaving only about 40,000 by puberty. During your reproductive life — about 30 years for most women — only about 400 of these eggs will develop fully, typically about one a month. When you've used up all your eggs and your ovaries no longer produce enough estrogen to properly stimulate the lining of your uterus and vagina, you've reached menopause.

Studies suggest that as you reach your mid-30s and your eggs get older, they decline in quality. They don't look any different from younger eggs, and their advanced age doesn't seem to make them less likely to be successfully

DOES A MAN'S FERTILITY DECLINE OVER TIME?

You hear stories about men fathering children well into their 60s and 70s — sometimes even into their 80s. This may be true in isolated cases. But scientists are finding that men experience an age-related decline in fertility, too. It occurs later than it does in women, typically starting in the late 30s. One study found a 40 percent decline in the probability of a man impregnating his partner from ages 35 to 40.

What causes reduced fertility in men? In order for your partner's sperm to fertilize your egg, it must mature properly, survive intercourse and the passage through your reproductive tract, and remain viable until your egg is ready. It then must penetrate the firm capsule (zona pellucida) of the egg, fertilize the egg and provide normal genetic material for the early development of your baby. That's a tall order anytime. Under the best circumstances, a sperm cell is capable of fertilizing an egg for only two to three days after ejaculation.

As a man gets older, his sperm have a harder time completing all these tasks. Starting even as early as his 30s, his sperm are more likely to have chromosome problems, which can adversely affect sperm function and the early development of the embryo. In addition, his sperm may not swim as well as they used to, although unless he also has a low sperm count, this isn't likely to affect his fertility. Doctors and scientists are investigating whether changes in the testes and prostate may adversely affect sperm production and the biochemical properties of semen. Although a man's age doesn't seem to have much effect on the biochemistry of his semen, researchers are identifying new substances that may affect sperm function over time. Smoking and a few medications may decrease male fertility.

fertilized by your partner's sperm. However, some research suggests that when fertilization occurs, an older egg is less likely than a younger one to develop into a blastocyst — the ball of cells that becomes implanted into the uterus, causing pregnancy.

One possible reason for this is that older eggs are more likely than younger ones to have chromosome problems — both abnormalities and more mild degenerative changes. When conception occurs, these problems may prevent the fertilized egg from implanting and developing normally inside your uterus or they may even result in early miscarriage. The group of chromosomal abnormalities called aneuploidy is the most common cause of miscarriage early in pregnancy. In fact, aneuploidy often causes a miscarriage even before a woman knows she's pregnant.

Egg quantity

Scientists think that some women may use up their eggs more quickly than others, thereby reducing their chances of conceiving. When the pool of available eggs drops below a certain minimum level, fertility may be compromised.

Women typically start losing more eggs per menstrual cycle around ages 35 to 40, when fertility also begins declining more rapidly. Doctors and scientists hope to someday develop therapies to slow accelerated egg loss, thus prolonging women's reproductive lives.

Uterine receptivity

Some studies have found that women in their mid- to late 30s tend to have a decline in uterine receptivity, which can prevent an embryo from implanting properly. However, other studies have found just the opposite, showing no evidence of decreased receptiveness with increasing age.

Changing hormone levels

As you reach your mid-30s, your body produces more follicle-stimulating hormone (FSH) and estradiol and less of a hormone called inhibin B. Scientists think these changes may indirectly compromise the formation of follicles — tiny sacs that each contain a single, immature egg — in your ovaries and the growing and thickening of your uterine lining in preparation for pregnancy, as well as the development of the growing embryo. More research is needed.

Tests to detect these hormonal changes have been shown to be valid predictors of whether you'll be able to get pregnant through the use of assisted reproductive technologies, such as in vitro fertilization (IVF). But they've never been studied outside this context, so they may not be useful for gauging whether you'll be able to get pregnant the "old-fashioned" way.

Pregnancy complications and age

If you're in your 30s or 40s and planning to get pregnant, you may be worried about the risk of miscarriage or health problems for yourself. You may also be concerned that your baby will be at increased risk of chromosome abnormalities or birth defects.

The risk of certain complications does increase with age. American obstetrical practice has evolved to consider age 35 the threshold for concern. In fact, the change in risk is gradual over time; there's no "light switch effect" at age 35.

In addition, the older mother of today is at significantly lower risk of problems than the older mother of 20 years ago. In the past, women giving birth over age 35 were typically having the last of several children, which in itself posed the risk of complications. These women also often received inadequate prenatal care. Today, more women giving birth over age 35 are having their first or second child, and they're more likely to receive good prenatal care.

If you start your pregnancy in good health, get regular prenatal care and adopt a healthy lifestyle, it's very likely things will progress normally, with few or no complications. In fact, a growing body of research suggests that although there are risks with having a baby after age 35, these risks are manageable and positive outcomes are likely. It's a good idea, though, to educate yourself about the potential risks of pregnancy at different ages. That way, you'll be prepared, no matter what happens.

Risks for you

Pregnant women over age 35 face the following increased risks:

- **Pregnancy loss.** The risk of miscarriage goes up after age 35, increasing even further after age 40. For women at age 40, the risk of miscarriage is about 25 percent, or one in four pregnancies. This increased risk of pregnancy loss is primarily caused by chromosome abnormalities in the baby.
- **Multiple pregnancy.** Women over age 35 are more likely than younger women to become pregnant through assisted reproductive technologies, such as in vitro fertilization (IVF). Because these procedures typically involve implanting two to three fertilized eggs in the uterus, they're more likely to result in twins or other multiples.

    Even without IVF, the risk of having twins goes up with a mother's increasing age. Hormonal changes can make it more likely for a woman to release more than one egg at a time, boosting her chances of conceiving nonidentical (fraternal) twins.
- **High blood pressure.** As you age, you're more likely to get high blood pressure for the first time during pregnancy. You're also more likely to develop preeclampsia — a condition marked by high blood pressure, swelling of your face and hands, and protein in your urine after your 20th week of pregnancy.
- **Gestational diabetes.** As you age, you're more likely to develop diabetes during pregnancy, when you've never had it before. This is called gestational diabetes. If it's untreated, your baby can grow too large during your pregnancy, making Caesarean birth more likely. It also increases your newborn's chances of having yellowing of the skin caused by a buildup of a substance called bilirubin (jaundice) and difficulty controlling his or her blood sugar (hypoglycemia).
- **Placenta previa.** If you're over age 35, you have a somewhat higher risk of developing placenta previa during pregnancy. Placenta previa is a condition in which your placenta is in the wrong position, either partially or completely covering your cervix. It may cause bleeding in the last trimester of pregnancy, which could mean you'll have to be hospitalized. It typically requires that your baby be born by Caesarean birth.
- **Abnormal fetal position.** Research shows that women over age 35 are more likely to have a baby in the rump- or feet-first position (breech

position) or other position making vaginal delivery difficult. This makes delivery by Caesarean birth much more likely.

- **Preterm labor.** Women over age 35 are more likely to have contractions that begin opening the cervix before the end of the 37th week. To reduce your risk of preterm labor, don't smoke while you're pregnant.
- **Caesarean birth.** Because pregnant women over age 35 tend to have more complications as a rule, more of them have Caesarean births. Other factors may be at work. Researchers suggest that because women over age 35 are more likely than are younger women to become pregnant through the use of assisted reproductive technologies, they're more likely to be carrying twins or triplets, making Caesarean birth more likely. Plus, health care providers may tend to manage these pregnancies very closely — and perhaps be more willing to resort to Caesarean birth at the first sign of trouble. For example, when the baby is monitored electronically during labor, there's a greater likelihood of worrisome signs such as a slowed heart rate. This may lead to a Caesarean birth.

Women over age 35 are also more likely than are younger women to have their labor started by medical means (induced), often by choice. This, too, increases the likelihood of Caesarean birth. Some research shows that older women are more apt to gain excessive weight during pregnancy, which increases their risk of labor difficulties and, as a result, a Caesarean birth.

Risks for your baby

Babies born to women over age 35 have the following increased risks:

- **Stillbirth.** For reasons not well understood, women over age 35 have a higher risk of giving birth to a stillborn baby.
- **Birth before 32 weeks.** Research suggests that babies born to women over age 35 are more likely than others to arrive before 32 weeks' gestation, when there's a greater risk of complications and death.
- **Low birth weight.** Doctors define a low-birth-weight baby as one born at term weighing less than 5 1/2 pounds. These babies tend to grow more slowly at first, although most tend to catch up with their normal-weight counterparts by the time they turn 1 1/2 or 2 years old. At birth, low-birth-weight babies are more likely to have hypoglycemia and trouble maintaining their body temperature (hypothermia). To reduce your risk of having a low-birth-weight baby, don't smoke during pregnancy.
- **Macrosomia.** This condition, in which your baby weighs 9 pounds, 14 ounces or more at birth, is more common among women after age 30. If your baby is overly big, delivery may be more difficult for both of you. You may be more likely to have a Caesarean birth, and your baby may be more likely to suffer a birth injury, such as a fractured collarbone. Large newborns may also have trouble with hypoglycemia and jaundice.

- **Chromosome abnormalities.** Babies born to women over age 35 are at increased risk of being born with a chromosome problem, particularly trisomy 21, 18 or 13. A trisomy is the most common type of chromosome abnormality. It means the baby has three copies of a chromosome instead of two. Down syndrome, one of the most common chromosome abnormalities, is also known as trisomy 21, meaning the baby has three copies of chromosome 21. Trisomies 13 and 18 are usually much more severe than Down syndrome, but they're also less common.

   If you're under 30, your risk of having a live-born baby with Down syndrome is less than one in 1,000. At age 30, your risk is about one in 1,000. At 35, it's about one in 400 (one-quarter of 1 percent) and at age 40, it's about 1 in 100 (1 percent).

   If you're in your 30s or 40s, you may choose to have a prenatal test such as amniocentesis to check for chromosome abnormalities such as Down syndrome. However, these tests have risks. If you're worried about the possibility of chromosome abnormalities in your baby, talk with your health care provider about the best plan of action for you.
- **Birth defects (nonchromosomal abnormalities).** Some studies suggest that the risk of giving birth to a baby with a nonchromosomal abnormality, such as a congenital heart defect, clubfoot or a diaphragmatic hernia, increases as a woman gets older. However, other studies have reported opposite results. More research is needed.

This month, you may also be interested in:
- **"Decision Guide: Understanding genetic carrier screening," page 269**
- **"Decision Guide: Understanding prenatal testing," page 289**
- **"Complications: Maternal health problems and pregnancy," page 507**

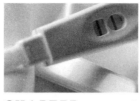

month 1: weeks 1 to 4

My husband and I had been trying to conceive for almost a year. I was delighted when my menstrual cycle was late. My husband, ever cautious, took a wait-and-see attitude.

After a few days had passed without my menstrual cycle starting, I bought a home pregnancy test. My husband waited in the living room while I took the test that would tell us whether we were parents-to-be. Sure enough, a faint blue line appeared on the test. I showed it to my husband, who said excitedly, "It's a maybe?"

No maybe about it. We were expecting our first child.

— One couple's experience

Your baby's growth during weeks 1 to 4

If you're like most expectant parents, your mind is full of questions. What does my baby look like right now? How big is he or she? How is she or he changing this week? Becoming familiar with how your baby develops, week by week, will help you answer some of those questions. It may also help you understand some of the changes taking place in your body.

Weeks 1 and 2: Preconception and fertilization

Preconception
It may seem a bit strange, but the first week of your pregnancy is actually your last menstrual period before becoming pregnant. Why is that? Doctors and other health care professionals calculate your due date by counting 40 weeks from the start of your last cycle. That means they count your period as part of your pregnancy, even though your baby hasn't been conceived yet.

Conception typically occurs about two weeks after the start of your last menstrual period. When your baby arrives, it will have been about 38 weeks since he or she was conceived, but your pregnancy will have "officially" lasted 40 weeks.

Even while menstruation is happening, your body begins producing a hormone called follicle-stimulating hormone, which fosters development of an egg in your ovary. The egg matures within a small cavity in your ovary called a follicle. A few days later, your body produces a hormone called luteinizing hormone. It causes the follicle to swell and burst through the wall of your ovary, releasing the egg. This is called ovulation. You have two ovaries, but in any given cycle, ovulation occurs from just one of them.

The egg moves slowly into your fallopian tube, which connects your ovary and uterus. There it awaits a fertilizing sperm. Finger-like structures at the junction between your ovary and fallopian tube, called fimbriae, catch the egg when ovulation occurs, keeping it on the right course.

If you have intercourse before or during this time, you can become pregnant. If fertilization doesn't occur, for whatever reason, the egg and the lining of your uterus will be shed through your menstrual period.

Fertilization

This is when it all begins. Your egg and your partner's sperm unite to form a single cell — the starting point for an extraordinary chain of events. That microscopic cell will divide again and again. In about 38 weeks, it will have grown into a new person made up of more than 2 trillion cells — your beautiful new baby girl or boy.

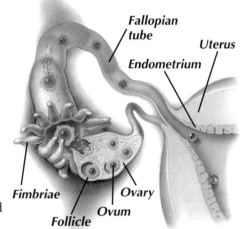

The process begins when you and your partner have sexual intercourse. When he ejaculates, your partner releases into your vagina semen containing up to 1 billion sperm cells. Each sperm has a long, whip-like tail that propels it toward your egg.

Hundreds of millions of these sperm swim up through your reproductive system. With the help of your uterus and fallopian tubes, they travel from your vagina, up through the lower opening of your uterus (cervix), through your uterus and into your fallopian tube. Many sperm are lost along the way. Only a fraction of the sperm reach the egg's position in the fallopian tube. Fertilization occurs when a single sperm makes this journey successfully and penetrates the wall of your egg.

Your egg has a covering of nutrient cells called the corona radiata and a gelatinous shell called the zona pellucida. To fertilize your egg, your partner's sperm must penetrate this covering. At this point, your egg is about $1/200$ of an inch in diameter, too small to be seen.

Up to 100 sperm may try to penetrate the wall of your egg, and several may begin to enter the outer egg capsule. But in the end, only one succeeds and enters the egg itself. After that, the membrane of the egg changes and all other sperm are locked out.

Occasionally, more than one follicle matures and more than one egg is released. This can result in multiple births if each of the eggs is fertilized by a sperm.

As the sperm penetrates to the center of your egg, the two cells merge to become a one-celled entity called a zygote. The zygote has 46 chromosomes — 23 from you and 23 from your partner. These chromosomes contain thousands and thousands of genes. This genetic material will determine your baby's sex, eye color, hair color, body size, facial features and — at least to some extent — intelligence and personality. Fertilization is now complete.

BOY OR GIRL?

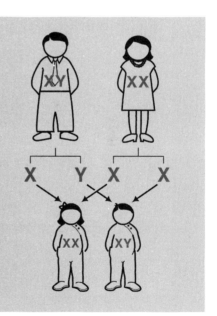

Your baby's sex is determined at the moment he or she is conceived. Of the 46 chromosomes that make up your baby's genetic material, two chromosomes called sex chromosomes — one from your egg and one from your partner's sperm — determine your baby's sex. A woman's egg contains only X sex chromosomes. A man's sperm, however, may contain either an X or Y sex chromosome.

If, at the instant of fertilization, a sperm with an X sex chromosome meets your egg, which also has an X sex chromosome, your baby will be a girl (XX). If a sperm containing a Y sex chromosome joins up with your egg, your baby will be a boy (XY). It's always the father's genetic contribution that determines the sex of the baby.

Weeks 3 and 4: Implantation and early development

Although your baby was just conceived, he or she gets to work right away. The next step in the process is cell division. Within about 12 hours, your one-celled zygote divides into two cells and then those two each split into two, and so on, with the number of cells doubling every 12 hours. The cells continue to divide as the zygote moves through your fallopian tube to your uterus. Within about three days after fertilization, it becomes a cluster of 13 to 32 cells resembling a tiny raspberry. At this stage, your developing baby is called a morula. It now leaves the fallopian tube to enter your uterus.

ESTIMATING YOUR DUE DATE

Use this chart to determine milestones during your pregnancy. For example, if the first day of your last menstrual period was March 27, your estimated due date is Jan. 1.

If the first day of your last menstrual period isn't listed, use the closest listed date and adjust the other dates accordingly. For example, if the first day of your last menstrual period was April 4 (one day past the listed date of April 3), your estimated due date is Jan. 9 (one day past the listed date of Jan. 8).

Week 1 If the first day of your last menstrual period was:	Week 3 Conception likely occurred around:	Weeks 5-10 Period of greatest risk of birth defects		Week 12 Risk of miscar-riage decreases	Week 23 Some preemies can now survive	Week 40 (full term) Estimated due date
		Beginning of organ formation	Major organs have formed			
Jan 2	Jan 16	Feb 6	Mar 13	Mar 27	Jun 12	Oct 9
Jan 9	Jan 23	Feb 13	Mar 20	Apr 3	Jun 19	Oct 16
Jan 16	Jan 30	Feb 20	Mar 27	Apr 10	Jun 26	Oct 23
Jan 23	Feb 6	Feb 27	Apr 3	Apr 17	Jul 3	Oct 30
Jan 30	Feb 13	Mar 6	Apr 10	Apr 24	Jul 10	Nov 6
Feb 6	Feb 20	Mar 13	Apr 17	May 1	Jul 17	Nov 13
Feb 13	Feb 27	Mar 20	Apr 24	May 8	Jul 24	Nov 20
Feb 20	Mar 6	Mar 27	May 1	May 15	Jul 31	Nov 27
Feb 27	Mar 13	Apr 3	May 8	May 22	Aug 7	Dec 4
Mar 6	Mar 20	Apr 10	May 15	May 29	Aug 14	Dec 11
Mar 13	Mar 27	Apr 17	May 22	Jun 5	Aug 21	Dec 18
Mar 20	Apr 3	Apr 24	May 29	Jun 12	Aug 28	Dec 25
Mar 27	Apr 10	May 1	Jun 5	Jun 19	Sep 4	Jan 1
Apr 3	Apr 17	May 8	Jun 12	Jun 26	Sep 11	Jan 8
Apr 10	Apr 24	May 15	Jun 19	Jul 3	Sep 18	Jan 15
Apr 17	May 1	May 22	Jun 26	Jul 10	Sep 25	Jan 22
Apr 24	May 8	May 29	Jul 3	Jul 17	Oct 2	Jan 29
May 1	May 15	Jun 5	Jul 10	Jul 24	Oct 9	Feb 5
May 8	May 22	Jun 12	Jul 17	Jul 31	Oct 16	Feb 12
May 15	May 29	Jun 19	Jul 24	Aug 7	Oct 23	Feb 19
May 22	Jun 5	Jun 26	Jul 31	Aug 14	Oct 30	Feb 26
May 29	Jun 12	Jul 3	Aug 7	Aug 21	Nov 6	Mar 5

Within four to five days after fertilization, your developing baby — by this time made up of about 500 cells — reaches its destination inside your uterus. It has changed from a solid mass of cells to a group of cells arranged around a fluid-filled cavity. At this stage, it's called a blastocyst. The inner section of the blastocyst is a compact mass of cells that will develop into your baby. The outer layer of cells, called the trophoblast,

Week 1 If the first day of your last menstrual period was:	**Week 3** Conception likely occurred around:	**Weeks 5-10** Period of greatest risk of birth defects		**Week 12** Risk of miscarriage decreases	**Week 23** Some preemies can now survive	**Week 40 (full term)** Estimated due date
		Beginning of organ formation	Major organs have formed			
Jun 5	Jun 19	Jul 10	Aug 14	Aug 28	Nov 13	Mar 12
Jun 12	Jun 26	Jul 17	Aug 21	Sep 4	Nov 20	Mar 19
Jun 19	Jul 3	Jul 24	Aug 28	Sep 11	Nov 27	Mar 26
Jun 26	Jul 10	Jul 31	Sep 4	Sep 18	Dec 4	Apr 2
Jul 3	Jul 17	Aug 7	Sep 11	Sep 26	Dec 11	Apr 9
Jul 10	Jul 24	Aug 14	Sep 18	Oct 2	Dec 18	Apr 16
Jul 17	Jul 31	Aug 21	Sep 25	Oct 9	Dec 25	Apr 23
Jul 24	Aug 7	Aug 28	Oct 2	Oct 16	Jan 1	Apr 30
Jul 31	Aug 14	Sep 4	Oct 9	Oct 23	Jan 8	May 7
Aug 7	Aug 21	Sep 11	Oct 16	Oct 30	Jan 15	May 14
Aug 14	Aug 28	Sep 18	Oct 23	Nov 6	Jan 22	May 21
Aug 21	Sep 4	Sep 25	Oct 30	Nov 13	Jan 29	May 28
Aug 28	Sep 11	Oct 2	Nov 6	Nov 20	Feb 5	Jun 4
Sep 4	Sep 18	Oct 9	Nov 13	Nov 27	Feb 12	Jun 11
Sep 11	Sep 25	Oct 16	Nov 20	Dec 4	Feb 19	Jun 18
Sep 18	Oct 2	Oct 23	Nov 27	Dec 11	Feb 26	Jun 25
Sep 25	Oct 9	Oct 30	Dec 4	Dec 18	Mar 5	Jul 2
Oct 2	Oct 16	Nov 6	Dec 11	Dec 25	Mar 12	Jul 9
Oct 9	Oct 23	Nov 13	Dec 18	Jan 1	Mar 19	Jul 16
Oct 16	Oct 30	Nov 20	Dec 25	Jan 8	Mar 26	Jul 23
Oct 23	Nov 6	Nov 27	Jan 1	Jan 15	Apr 2	Jul 30
Oct 30	Nov 13	Dec 4	Jan 8	Jan 22	Apr 9	Aug 6
Nov 6	Nov 20	Dec 11	Jan 15	Jan 29	Apr 16	Aug 13
Nov 13	Nov 27	Dec 18	Jan 22	Feb 5	Apr 23	Aug 20
Nov 20	Dec 4	Dec 25	Jan 29	Feb 12	Apr 30	Aug 27
Nov 27	Dec 11	Jan 1	Feb 5	Feb 19	May 7	Sep 3
Dec 4	Dec 18	Jan 8	Feb 12	Feb 26	May 14	Sep 10
Dec 11	Dec 25	Jan 15	Feb 19	Mar 5	May 21	Sep 17
Dec 18	Jan 1	Jan 22	Feb 26	Mar 12	May 28	Sep 24
Dec 25	Jan 8	Jan 29	Mar 5	Mar 19	Jun 4	Oct 1

will become the placenta, which will provide nourishment to your baby as it grows.

After arriving in your uterus, the blastocyst clings to its surface for a time. It then releases enzymes that eat away at the lining of your uterus, allowing it to embed itself there. This typically happens about a week after fertilization. By the 12th day after fertilization, the blastocyst is firmly embedded in its new home. It adheres tightly to the lining of your uterus, called the endometrium, where it receives nourishment from your bloodstream.

Also within about 12 days after fertilization, the placenta begins to form. At first, tiny projections sprout from the wall of the blastocyst. From these sprouts, wavy masses of tiny blood-vessel-filled tissue develop. Called chorionic villi, they grow amid the capillaries of your uterus and ultimately cover most of the placenta.

At 14 days after conception, four weeks since your last menstrual period, your baby is about 1/25 of an inch long. It's divided into three different layers, from which all tissues and organs will eventually develop:

- The top layer is called the ectoderm. It will give rise to a groove along the midline of your baby's body, called the neural tube. Your baby's brain, spinal cord, spinal nerves and backbone will develop here.
- The middle layer of cells is called the mesoderm. It will form the beginnings of your baby's heart and a primitive circulatory system — blood vessels, blood cells and lymph vessels. The foundations for bones, muscles, kidneys, and ovaries or testicles also will develop here.
- The inner layer of cells is known as the endoderm. It will become a simple tube lined with mucous membranes, from which your baby's lungs, intestines and urinary bladder will develop.

Your body during weeks 1 to 4

During pregnancy, it's natural to be curious about how your baby is developing. But it's also natural to want to know more about the changes taking place in your own body. The changes are significant. In the time your tiny zygote grows into a full-sized infant, your body prepares itself to provide the nourishment your baby will need to grow and develop properly, as well as for labor and delivery.

Week 1: Preconception

In the time leading up to conception, it's important to make lifestyle choices that prepare your body for pregnancy and motherhood. These choices will also give your baby-to-be the best possible start in life. Don't smoke, drink alcohol or use drugs. If you're taking a prescription medication, ask your health care provider for advice regarding its use during pregnancy. And be sure to take a daily vitamin supplement containing at least 400 micrograms of folic acid.

Getting adequate folic acid will reduce your baby's risk of developing defects in the neural tube. This component of the embryo gives rise to the brain, spinal cord, spinal nerves and backbone. Spina bifida, a defect in the spine that results in failure of your baby's vertebrae to fuse together, is one example of a neural tube defect that can be largely avoided if you get enough folic acid.

Weeks 2 and 3: Ovulation, fertilization and implantation

The lining of your uterus, which will nourish your baby, is developing. Your body is secreting follicle-stimulating hormone, which will cause an egg in your ovary to mature. As you ovulate and the egg is released into your fallopian tube, the hormones involved in the process — estrogen and progesterone — cause a slight increase in your body temperature and a change in secretions from your cervical glands.

When fertilization occurs, the corpus luteum — a small structure that surrounds your developing baby — starts to grow and produce small amounts of progesterone. This helps support your pregnancy. Progesterone keeps your uterus from contracting. It also promotes growth of blood vessels in your uterine wall, essential for your baby's nourishment.

Roughly four days after fertilization, your developing baby is at the blastocyst stage. At about this time, your placenta begins producing a hormone called human chorionic gonadotropin (HCG). This hormone can be first detected in your blood and shortly later in your urine. Home pregnancy tests can detect HCG in a sample of your urine about six to 12 days after fertilization.

By the time your developing baby travels through your fallopian tube and implants itself in the lining of your uterus — about a week after fertilization — your endometrium has grown thick enough to support it.

As your baby implants, you may notice spotting, a scanty menstrual flow or yellowish vaginal discharge. You may mistake it for the start of your normal menstrual period. This spotting may in fact be a first sign of pregnancy. It comes from the small amount of bleeding that can occur when your developing baby implants itself into the lining of your uterus.

Also around the time of implantation, finger-like projections that will become your placenta begin producing large amounts of the hormones estrogen and progesterone. These hormones ultimately cause growth and changes in your uterus, endometrium, cervix, vagina and breasts.

At this point, you are pregnant, although it's too early for you to have missed a period or to have any other symptoms of pregnancy. In these first days after fertilization, miscarriage is common, often before you know you're pregnant. Scientists estimate that three of every four lost pregnancies are the result of a failure of implantation. In the first week to 10 days after conception, infections or exposure to harmful environmental factors, such as drugs, cigarettes, alcohol, medications and chemicals, can interfere with your baby implanting in your uterus. At this stage of the pregnancy, such exposures can result in pregnancy loss, but not birth defects. Most of the

WHEN TO TAKE A HOME PREGNANCY TEST

I think I'm pregnant. When can I take a home pregnancy test?

You'll want to wait at least until the first day of your missed cycle — and perhaps a bit longer. Here's why. Home pregnancy tests measure a hormone produced after the fertilized egg attaches in the wall of the uterus. This hormone, called HCG, isn't present until six to 12 days after fertilization. The timing varies, so testing when your menstrual cycle is only a day late might miss a developing pregnancy.

How accurate are the tests?

The tests are quite good. A recent study showed that the tests are capable of diagnosing 90 percent of pregnancies on the first day of the missed period. By one week after the first day of the missed period, that rises to as much as 97 percent.

For the most accurate test results:
- Follow the specific directions of your home pregnancy test exactly.
- Test using your first urine of the morning, which has the highest concentration of HCG.

How does the pregnancy test work?

After your developing baby prompts the production of HCG, this hormone can be detected in your blood and shortly later in your urine. Home pregnancy tests can detect HCG in your urine. The tests usually require that you place a pregnancy test stick in a sample of your urine. Within a few minutes, the presence of a dot or line on the test stick indicates whether HCG is present in your urine. If it is, the test is positive, meaning you are pregnant.

What if the test says I'm pregnant?

If the test result is positive, make plans to see your health care provider to begin prenatal care. Ask him or her to prescribe prenatal vitamins.

What if the test says I'm not pregnant?

If your result is negative, but you still have the signs and symptoms of pregnancy, wait a few days and then take a second test. Or ask to have a pregnancy test done at your health care provider's office.

time, however, pregnancy losses result from mistakes in the process of development that aren't under anyone's control.

Week 4: Early pregnancy

Even this early in your pregnancy, your body is undergoing significant physical changes.

Your heart and circulatory system

During the first weeks of pregnancy, your body begins producing more blood to carry oxygen and nutrients to your baby. The increase is greatest in the first 12 weeks, when pregnancy makes enormous demands on your circulation. By the end of your pregnancy, your blood volume will have increased by 30 percent to 50 percent. Increasing your fluid intake at this stage of your pregnancy can help your body adjust to this change.

To accommodate this increased blood flow, your heart is starting to pump harder and faster. Your pulse may quicken by as much as 15 beats a minute.

These dramatic changes in your body may already give you symptoms of pregnancy. For example, you may be so tired that you're ready for bed right after the evening meal. Or you may want to nap more often. Try to rest when you feel fatigued.

Your breasts

One of the first physical changes of pregnancy is a change in the way your breasts feel. They may feel tender, tingly or sore, or they may feel fuller and heavier. You may think that your breasts and nipples are already starting to enlarge. That may be the case, even this early in your pregnancy.

Stimulated by increased production of estrogen and progesterone, your breasts will enlarge throughout your pregnancy as the milk-producing glands inside them grow in size. You may also notice that the rings of brown or reddish-brown skin around your nipples (areolas) are starting to enlarge and darken. This is the result of increased blood circulation and growth of pigmented cells. It may be a permanent change to your body.

Your uterus

At four weeks into your pregnancy, your uterus is also beginning to change. Its lining is thickening, and the blood vessels in the lining are starting to enlarge to nourish your growing baby.

Your cervix

Your cervix, the opening in your uterus through which your baby will emerge, is beginning to soften and change color. Your health care provider may look for this change during your first examination as confirmation of your pregnancy.

Self-care resources

The changes in your body during the first month of pregnancy can produce some uncomfortable signs and symptoms. For more information on dealing with common complaints such as breast tenderness, fatigue, headaches and increased urination, see Part 3, "Pregnancy Reference Guide" on page 413.

Your emotions during weeks 1 to 4

Pregnancy can be exciting, boring, anxiety producing and deeply satisfying — sometimes all at once. You're probably experiencing some new, unexpected emotions, some comforting and others unsettling.

Your reaction to your pregnancy

Whether your pregnancy was planned or unplanned, you may have conflicting feelings about it. Even if you're thrilled at being pregnant, you probably have extra emotional stress in your life right now. You may worry about whether your baby will be healthy and how you'll adjust to motherhood. You may also have concerns about the increased financial demands of raising a child. If you work outside the home, you may worry about being able to sustain your productivity throughout pregnancy, especially if your work is very demanding. Don't berate yourself for feeling this way. These concerns are natural and normal.

Mood swings

Adjusting to being pregnant and preparing for new responsibilities may leave you feeling up one day and down the next. Your emotions may range from exhilaration to exhaustion, delight to depression. Your moods can also change considerably over the course of a single day.

Some of these mood swings may result from the physical stresses your growing baby is placing on your body. Some may be the result of fatigue, pure and simple. Mood changes may also be caused by the release of certain hormones and changes in your metabolism.

To meet the demands of your growing baby, different hormones are produced at different levels throughout your pregnancy. Though the mechanisms aren't well understood, doctors believe these hormonal changes contribute to mood swings during pregnancy. Sudden fluctuations in progesterone, estrogen and other hormones likely play some role in mood swings. The effects of hormones from the thyroid and adrenal glands also are receiving considerable scientific attention.

Your moods are likely to be strongly influenced by the nurturing and support you receive from your partner and family. Perhaps now as never before, you need understanding, support and encouragement as you progress through pregnancy and develop your identity as a mother.

Your partner's reaction to your pregnancy

If you have mixed feelings about being pregnant, chances are your partner does too. He may be thrilled with the prospect of fatherhood. It offers new possibilities in the role of father. He may be exhilarated by the anticipation of sharing a loving relationship with a daughter or son.

On the other hand, he may have doubts and concerns. He may doubt whether he can meet the financial challenges of fatherhood. He may wonder if it's the right thing to do to bring a child into a world with so many problems. He may fear that a baby will forever change your lifestyle.

These feelings are normal. Few fathers-to-be ever feel fully prepared for what's ahead. In fact, the reality of your partner's impending fatherhood probably won't set in right away. It may not be until about your 24th week of pregnancy, when your partner places his hand on your abdomen and can feel the baby kicking, that it really hits him that he's going to be a dad.

Encourage your partner to identify his doubts and worries and be honest about what he's feeling, both the good and the bad. You do the same. Discussing your feelings honestly and openly will strengthen your relationship with your partner and help the two of you start the important work of preparing a home for your baby.

Your relationship with your partner

Becoming a mother-to-be can take time away from your other roles and relationships. Maybe you already see yourself as a parent. As a result, you may lose some of your psychological identity as a partner and lover.

There may be times when your partner is interested in having sexual intercourse and you aren't. If you reject his overtures in the bedroom, he may think you're rejecting him. In truth, you're probably just tired, sad or worried. Let your partner know that you need his presence, support and tenderness, but, perhaps right now, without sexual overtones.

Misunderstanding and conflicts between you and your partner are inevitable and normal during pregnancy. You may view your partner's increased focus on work, for example, as a form of withdrawal from the relationship, which makes you feel hurt and rejected. Your partner, on the other hand, may simply be trying to provide more security for your family.

Understanding and communication are the keys to preventing or minimizing conflicts. Talk openly and honestly with your partner so that you can anticipate the stress points in your relationship and take steps to minimize or avoid them.

Appointments with your health care provider

You've taken a home pregnancy test, and it says you're pregnant. Now's the time to set up your first appointment with the person you've chosen as your obstetrical health care provider. Whether you've chosen a family physician, obstetrician-gynecologist or nurse-midwife, that person will treat, educate and reassure you throughout your pregnancy. Developing a strong relationship with your health care provider starts now, at the very beginning of your pregnancy. Health care providers enjoy the celebration inherent in pregnancy and birth and want to enhance your celebration of it, too.

Your first visit to your health care provider after you've learned you're pregnant will focus mainly on assessing your overall health, identifying any risk factors for your pregnancy and determining your baby's gestational age.

For more information on choosing the health care provider who's right for you, see "Decision Guide: Choosing your health care provider for pregnancy" on page 277.

Preparing for the appointment

At your first appointment, your health care provider will review your past and current health, including any chronic medical conditions you have and problems you've had during past pregnancies, if any. Gathering as much information as possible about your past and present health is one of your health care provider's biggest goals at your first visit. The answers you give have an impact on the care you receive.

Some health care providers make the first part of this appointment a one-on-one conversation with just you — the mom-to-be — and later invite your partner to join you. This gives you a chance to privately discuss any health and social issues from your past that you may not want to share with your partner. In the time before your first appointment, you may want to write down details on your menstrual cycles, your contraceptive use, your and your partner's family medical history, your work environment and your lifestyle.

Your first visit with your health care provider will also give you a chance to ask the many questions you may have. Make it easy on yourself by starting to jot your questions down as they occur to you. It's easier to collect your thoughts before your appointment than to do so during a short visit.

When to call a health care professional during weeks 1 to 4

It's normal to have fears and worries about the physical changes you're experiencing with your pregnancy. Things aren't always clear-cut. Is a little spotting normal for early pregnancy, or is it a sign of an early miscarriage? Is a nagging headache just the result of increased blood circulation, or is it something more serious? It can be difficult to tell when you should grin and bear it and when you should take action. If this is your first pregnancy, you may be even more uncertain.

In making these judgments, look to your doctor, nurse-midwife or other health care provider as your primary resource. When you have your first office visit, ask for a list of the signs and symptoms he or she wants to hear about right away. That will give you a good idea of what your health care provider considers to be an emergency.

The bottom line? When in doubt, call. It's better to be safe than sorry.

This month, you may also be interested in:
- **"Decision guide: Choosing your health care provider for pregnancy," page 277**
- **"Complications: Maternal health problems and pregnancy," page 507**

When to call

Here's a guide to possibly troublesome signs and symptoms and when you should notify your health care provider in the first month.

Signs or symptoms	When to tell your health care provider
Vaginal bleeding or spotting	
Slight spotting that goes away within a day	Next visit
Any spotting or bleeding lasting longer than a day	Within 24 hours
Moderate to heavy bleeding	Immediately
Any amount of bleeding accompanied by pain, cramping, fever or chills	Immediately
Passing of tissue	Immediately
Pain	
Occasional pulling, twinging or pinching sensation on one or both sides of your abdomen	Next visit
Occasional mild headaches	Next visit
A moderate, bothersome headache that doesn't go away after treatment with acetaminophen (Tylenol, others)	Within 24 hours
A severe or persistent headache, especially with dizziness, faintness, nausea or vomiting, or visual disturbances	Immediately
Moderate or severe pelvic pain	Immediately
Any degree of pelvic pain that doesn't subside within four hours	Immediately
Pain with fever or bleeding	Immediately
Vomiting	
Occasional	Next visit
Once every day	Next visit
More than three times a day or with inability to eat or drink between vomiting episodes	Within 24 hours
With pain or fever	Immediately
Other	
Chills or fever (102 F or higher)	Immediately
Painful urination	Same day
Increased frequency of urination	Next visit
Inability to urinate	Same day
Mild constipation	Next visit
Severe constipation, no bowel movement for three days	Same day

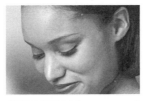

CHAPTER   2

month 2: weeks 5 to 8

Your baby's growth during weeks 5 to 8

Your baby is growing and changing. During weeks five through eight of your pregnancy, your baby's cells multiply rapidly and begin to perform specific functions. This process of specialization is called differentiation. It's necessary to produce all the different cells that make up a human being. As a result of differentiation, your baby's main external features also begin to take shape.

Week 5

No longer just a mass of cells, your baby — officially called an embryo — is beginning to take on a distinct form.

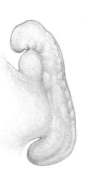

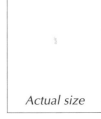

Actual size

The embryo has divided into three layers. From these layers, all tissues and organs will develop. In the top layer, a groove develops and then closes to form the neural tube, which will eventually develop into your baby's brain, spinal cord, spinal nerves and backbone. It runs along the midline of the body, from the top to the bottom of the embryo. The closure of the neural tube begins in the embryo's midsection. It proceeds upward and downward from there, like a double zipper. The top portion thickens to begin forming the brain.

From the embryo's middle layer of cells, the heart and the circulatory system are taking shape. A bulge at the center of the embryo will develop into your baby's heart. By week's end, the earliest blood elements and blood vessels have formed, both in the embryo and the developing placenta.

57

Your baby's first heartbeats occur at 21 to 22 days after conception, although you and your health care provider can't hear them yet. It may be possible to see this motion on an ultrasound, however. With these changes, circulation begins, making the circulatory system the first functioning organ system.

Your baby also has an inner layer of cells, from which lungs, intestines and the urinary bladder will develop. This week, not much is happening in the inner layer. It will be awhile yet before those areas take shape.

At the moment of conception, your baby was a single-celled zygote and was microscopic in size. By the fifth week of your pregnancy, three weeks after conception, your baby is about 1/17 of an inch long, about the size of the tip of a pen.

Week 6

Growth is rapid during the sixth week. Your baby triples in size. He or she starts to show basic facial features. Optic vesicles, which later form the eyes, are beginning to develop. Passageways that will make up the inner ear also are beginning to form. An opening for the mouth is formed by the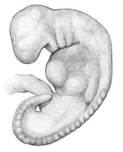

Actual size

ingrowth of tissue from above and from the sides of the face. Below the mouth, where the neck will develop, are small folds that ultimately will become your baby's neck and lower jaw.

By the sixth week of your pregnancy, the neural tube along your baby's back has closed over. The brain is growing rapidly to fill the now-formed, enlarging head. Your baby's brain is also developing distinct regions. Some cranial nerves are visible.

In the front of the chest, your baby's heart is pumping rudimentary blood through the main blood vessels and beating at a regular rhythm. The beginnings of the digestive and respiratory systems are forming, too. In addition, 40 small blocks of tissue are developing along your baby's midline. These will form the connective tissue, ribs and muscles of your baby's back and sides. Small buds that will grow into your baby's arms and legs are now visible.

By the sixth week of your pregnancy, four weeks after conception, your baby is about 1/8 of an inch long.

Week 7

This week the umbilical cord, the vital link between your baby and your placenta, is clearly visible at the site where your baby implanted in your uterus.

The umbilical cord contains two arteries and one large vein. Nutrients and oxygen-rich blood pass from your placenta to your baby by way of the single vein and then back to your placenta through the two arteries. It takes about 30 seconds for a blood cell to make the entire trip.

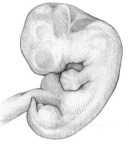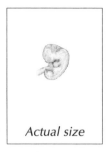

Actual size

In addition, your baby's brain is continuing to become more complex. Cavities and passages necessary for circulation of spinal fluid have formed. Your baby's growing skull is still transparent. If you were able to get a look at it under a magnifying glass, you might see the smooth surface of your baby's tiny, developing brain.

Your baby's face is taking on more definition this week. A mouth perforation, tiny nostrils, ear indentations and color in the irises of the eyes are now visible. The lenses of your baby's eyes are forming. The middle portions of the ears are connecting the inner ear to the outer world.

Your baby's arms, legs, hands and feet are taking shape, though the beginnings of fingers and toes are about a week away. The arm bud that sprouted just last week has already developed into a shoulder portion and a hand portion, which looks like a tiny paddle.

At seven weeks into your pregnancy, your baby is 1/3 of an inch long, a little bigger than the top of a pencil eraser.

Week 8

Your baby's fingers and toes begin to form this week, although they are still webbed. Your baby's tiny arms and legs are growing longer and more defined. Paddle-shaped foot and hand areas are evident. Wrists, elbows and ankles are clearly visi-

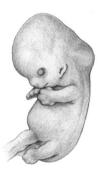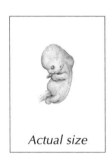

Actual size

ble. Your baby may even be able to flex at the elbows and wrists.

Your baby's eyelids also are beginning to form. Until the eyelids are done growing, your baby's eyes will appear open. In addition, this week your baby's ears, upper lip and tip of the nose begin taking on recognizable form.

Your baby's digestive tract is continuing to grow, especially the intestines. Heart function and circulation are now more fully developed. Your baby's heart is pumping at about 150 beats a minute, about twice the adult rate.

At the eighth week of your pregnancy, your baby is just over 1/2 of an inch long.

EARLY HAZARDS TO YOUR BABY'S HEALTH

Your developing baby is most vulnerable during the period from three to eight weeks after conception. That is weeks five through 10 of your pregnancy. All major organs are forming during this time, and injury to the embryo can result in a major birth defect, such as spina bifida.

Things that can cause damage to your baby include:

- **Teratogens.** These are substances that cause physical defects in your developing baby. Examples include alcohol, certain medications and recreational drugs. Avoid them.
- **Infections.** Viruses and bacteria can potentially harm your baby in early pregnancy. A baby can only acquire one of these infections through the mother, but you may not even feel very ill with some of the conditions that can cause serious defects. Fortunately, you will have been immunized against many of these infections. You may have a natural immunity against others. Still, it makes sense to take appropriate precautions to avoid exposure to illnesses such as chickenpox, measles, mumps, German measles (rubella) or cytomegalovirus (CMV).
- **Radiation.** High doses of ionizing radiation, such as radiation therapy for cancer, can harm your baby. But the low doses in a diagnostic X-ray pose no significant increase in the risk of birth defects. However, when you're pregnant it's best not to have an X-ray unless it's necessary, just as you wouldn't undergo any medical procedure or take medications unless it's necessary at any other time. If you may have a serious health problem where an X-ray can provide important information, it's probably best to do it. Unless it's very extensive, diagnostic X-rays may be more helpful than harmful, even in early pregnancy. If you had an X-ray before you knew you were pregnant, don't be alarmed. Talk with your health care provider.
- **Poor nutrition.** Extremely poor eating habits during pregnancy can harm your baby. Eating too little of a specific nutrient can cause cell development to be less than ideal. However, the early embryo isn't likely to be harmed by a lack of calories, even if nausea and vomiting limit the calories you can take in.

Be sure to take a daily vitamin supplement containing at least 400 micrograms of folic acid. This will reduce your baby's risk of developing spina bifida or other neural tube defects.

Your body during weeks 5 to 8

The second month of pregnancy brings enormous changes for your body. It's the time you're likely to begin experiencing most of the major discomforts and annoyances of early pregnancy, such as nausea, heartburn, fatigue, insomnia and frequent urination. But don't let these get you down. Consider them as signs that your pregnancy is proceeding smoothly. A recent study, in fact, found that women who experience pregnancy-related signs and symptoms by their eighth week were less likely to have a miscarriage.

The importance of hormones

Hormones are the chemical messengers that regulate many aspects of your pregnancy. The hormone progesterone is produced first by your ovaries and then by your placenta. It keeps your uterus from contracting. It also promotes growth of blood vessels in the walls of your uterus, essential for your baby's nourishment. Your ovaries and placenta also produce estrogen. It causes growth and changes in your uterus, endometrium, cervix, vagina and breasts. Estrogen also influences many key body processes, such as the amount of insulin you produce.

Your placenta produces two other important hormones: human chorionic gonadotropin (HCG) and human placental lactogen (HPL). HCG helps maintain the corpus luteum, which is the mass of cells that remain in the ovary after the egg's release from a mature follicle. HPL is the hormone most involved in your baby's growth. It alters your metabolism to make sugars and proteins more available to your baby. It also stimulates your breasts to develop and prepare to produce milk.

How your body is changing

Hormones released throughout your pregnancy do two things. They influence the growth of your baby, and they send signals that change the way your own organs function. In fact, the hormonal changes of pregnancy affect nearly every part of your body.

Here's an overview of what's happening, and where:

Your hormones

Hormone production is continuing to increase this month. This increase is likely resulting in some unpleasant signs and symptoms. You might be experiencing nausea and vomiting, breast soreness, headaches, dizziness, increased urination, insomnia and vivid dreams. Nausea and vomiting may be the most significant hormone-related change you've experienced since last month.

Scientists aren't quite sure why hormonal changes cause nausea and vomiting. Changes in your gastrointestinal system in response to high hormone levels almost certainly play a role. Increased progesterone slows down the pace at which your food passes through your digestive tract. Therefore, your stomach empties somewhat more slowly, which may make you more likely to have nausea and vomiting. Estrogen may have a direct effect on the brain that triggers nausea.

Nausea and vomiting affect up to 70 percent of pregnant women. These uncomfortable problems typically begin between the fourth and eighth weeks of pregnancy. They usually subside by 14 weeks. Even though it's commonly called morning sickness, it can occur at any time of day.

For some women, nausea and vomiting in early pregnancy are accompanied by excessive salivation — an uncommon condition called ptyalism. It may be that women with ptyalism aren't producing any more saliva than usual, but that they're having trouble swallowing it because of their nausea.

Your heart and circulatory system

Your body is continuing to produce more blood to carry oxygen and nutrients to your baby. Increased blood production will continue throughout your pregnancy. It will be especially high this month and next, while pregnancy is making enormous demands on your circulation.

Despite this effort, your blood vessels are dilating even more quickly and your circulation is just a bit short of blood volume. To accommodate these changes, your heart is continuing to pump harder and faster. These changes in your circulatory system may be causing fatigue, dizziness and headaches.

Your breasts

Stimulated by increased production of estrogen and progesterone, your breasts are continuing to enlarge as the milk-producing glands inside them grow in size. You may also notice that your areolas, the rings of brown or reddish-brown skin around your nipples, are starting to enlarge and darken. This is the result of increased blood circulation. Your breasts may feel tender, tingly or sore. Or they may feel fuller and heavier.

Your uterus

If this is your first pregnancy, your uterus used to be about the size of a pear. Now it's starting to expand. By the time you deliver your baby, it will have expanded to about 1,000 times its original size.

To house your growing baby, your uterus expands from an area within your pelvis to just below your rib cage. Through this month and the next, your uterus will fit inside your pelvis. However, its increasing size may cause you to feel the need to urinate more often. You may also leak urine when you sneeze, cough or laugh. This is a simple matter of geography. During the first few months of pregnancy, your bladder lies directly in front and slightly under your uterus. As your uterus grows, your bladder gets crowded out.

Throughout these weeks, the placenta is continuing to grow and secure its attachment to the uterus. Sometimes this results in minor bleeding, which usually is normal. But if this does happen, let your health care provider know about it.

Your cervix

This month, your cervix becomes bluish tinged and continues to soften. Over the course of your pregnancy, your cervix will become softer and softer. This prepares it for thinning (effacement) and opening (dilation), necessary parts of childbirth.

By the seventh week of pregnancy, the mucous plug is well established in your cervix. This structure blocks the cervical canal during pregnancy, to prevent germs from getting into your uterus. The plug loosens and passes late in pregnancy, typically when your cervix starts to thin out and open in preparation for labor.

Your vagina

You may experience some vaginal bleeding during the first 12 weeks of your pregnancy. Statistics indicate that as many as 40 percent of pregnant women may have some bleeding. However, statistics also indicate that fewer than half these women will have miscarriages.

THE 'WARMED-UP' EFFECT

If you've been pregnant once before, you may notice that you're bigger than you were at the same time during your last pregnancy. You may also notice that side effects seem to be happening earlier this time.

You could call this the "warmed-up" effect. Like a balloon that's easier to blow up the second or third time around, your uterus may expand more quickly and easily once it has been through one pregnancy. Your abdominal muscles and ligaments have already been stretched once, so they give more easily as your uterus expands on the second go-round.

The downside is that because your uterus is getting bigger, faster, you may experience symptoms such as pelvic pressure and back pain sooner in this pregnancy than you did in your first pregnancy.

Self-care resources

The changes in your body during weeks five to eight of pregnancy can produce some uncomfortable signs and symptoms. For more information on dealing with common complaints such as breast tenderness, fatigue, faintness and vomiting, see Part 3, "Pregnancy Reference Guide" on page 413.

Your emotions during weeks 5 to 8

Pregnancy is a psychological journey as well as a biological one. You're still the daughter of your parents. Yet soon you'll be the mother of your own child. You'll have a new role to play and a new identity. The emotions you're feeling in the face of this reality can be both overwhelmingly positive and distressingly negative.

Anticipation

Anticipation is a normal part of making the transition to parenthood. It's a time for collecting information about how to be a good mother. It begins early in pregnancy.

It has its foundations in the parenting you received as a child and your observations of other families you've encountered. The memories of how you were raised, along with your personal ideals of parenting, serve as a bank of images you can draw from as you think about what your own parenting style will be.

During this time of anticipation, you'll probably have dreams and fantasies about what your baby will be like. These imaginings aren't a waste of time. They're the beginnings of your emotional bond with your baby.

Worries and fears

During your second month of pregnancy, the excitement you felt when you learned you were pregnant may be dampened by fear. What if you might have done something to harm your baby — before you knew you were pregnant? What about that aspirin you took for a headache? Or that glass of wine you had with dinner? Or that bout of the flu?

It's important to realize that you can't plan or control everything about your pregnancy. But it's also important to make lifestyle choices that give you the best chance of having a healthy pregnancy. If you have concerns, share them with your health care provider. Doing so may put your mind at ease.

You may also be worried about other things. How will you cope with the pain of labor and delivery? Will you be a good mother? Discuss these worries with your partner. If you hide them, worries can cause tension in your relationship. They can create a sense of distance between you and your partner at a time when you both need the warmth of a close, loving relationship.

Some women experience disturbing, anxiety-provoking dreams or feelings during early pregnancy. These thoughts may seem senseless or irrational, yet they are normal and very common. For most new parents, such thoughts usually pass. However, if troubling thoughts and feelings persist and are disturbing to you, consider talking to your health care provider, who may refer you to a therapist or counselor to help you manage such thoughts.

Appointments with your health care provider

What to expect at your first appointment

When the day of your first appointment arrives, allow plenty of time in your schedule, up to two or three hours so that you won't feel rushed. You'll probably be meeting several different people, including nurses and office staff who work with your health care provider.

After discussing your medical history with you, your health care provider will perform a physical exam and calculate your due date. During or just after your first prenatal visit, you can also expect to have several lab tests.

Assessing your medical history

At your first appointment, your health care provider will review your past and current health, including any chronic medical conditions you have and problems you've had during past pregnancies, if any. Gathering as much

FIRST-APPOINTMENT CHECKLIST

✓ Discussion of your medical history at your first appointment with your health care provider will likely cover the following topics:

❑ Details of any previous pregnancies

❑ The typical length of time between your periods

❑ The first day of your last period

❑ Your use of contraceptives

❑ Prescription or over-the-counter medications you're taking

❑ Allergies you have

❑ Medical conditions or diseases you have had or now have

❑ Past surgeries, if any

❑ Your work environment

❑ Your lifestyle behaviors, such as exercise, diet, smoking or exposure to secondhand smoke, and the use of alcoholic beverages or recreational drugs

❑ Risk factors for sexually transmitted diseases — such as you or your partner having more than one sexual partner

❑ Past or present medical problems, such as diabetes, high blood pressure (hypertension), lupus or depression, in your or your partner's immediate family — father, mother, siblings

❑ Family histories, on both sides, of babies with congenital abnormalities or genetic diseases

❑ Details on your home environment, such as whether you feel safe and supported at home

information as possible about your past and present health is one of your health care provider's biggest goals at your first visit. The answers you give will have an impact on the care you receive.

Come to your appointment prepared to answer questions about these topics, your pregnancy to date and your insurance coverage.

While you're discussing your medical history with your health care provider, you'll also have a chance to ask the many questions you may have about your pregnancy. If you've been keeping a running list of questions, bring it to your first appointment so that you won't forget anything.

The physical exam

During the physical exam on your first prenatal visit, your health care provider will probably check your weight, height and blood pressure and assess your general health. The pelvic exam is an important part of this evaluation.

During the exam, your health care provider may look in your vagina using a device called a speculum. This device allows for a clear view of your cervix, the opening to your uterus. Changes in your cervix and in the size of your uterus help your health care provider tell how far along you are.

While the speculum is still in place, your health care provider may gently collect some cells and mucus from your cervix for a Pap test and to screen for infections. The Pap test helps detect abnormalities that indicate precancer or cancer of the cervix. Infections of the cervix such as the sexually transmitted diseases gonorrhea and chlamydia can affect your pregnancy and the health of your baby.

After removing the speculum, your health care provider may insert two gloved fingers into your vagina to check your cervix and, with the other hand on top of your abdomen, check the size of your uterus and ovaries. Many health care providers evaluate the size of your birth canal during this exam. These measurements may help predict whether you might have problems during labor and delivery, though it's difficult to make an accurate prediction about it this early in the pregnancy. But if your pelvis seems too narrow for a baby's head to easily pass through the birth canal, your health care provider may make a note of this in your file as something to reevaluate later.

You may be apprehensive about having a pelvic exam. Many women are. During the exam, try to relax as much as you can. Breathe slowly and deeply. If you tense up, your muscles can tighten, which can make the exam more uncomfortable. Remember, a typical pelvic exam takes only a couple of minutes.

You may have some vaginal bleeding after your pelvic exam and Pap test, especially within 24 hours of your visit. The bleeding may be just some light spotting, or it may be a little heavier. It usually goes away within a day. This occurs often because the softened cervix of pregnancy bleeds a bit after a

Pap test. The bleeding is from the outside of your cervix and isn't a risk to your baby. If you're concerned about it, call your health care provider.

Calculating your due date

Your health care provider is just as interested in your due date as you are. Why is that? Establishing the due date early in pregnancy allows your health care provider to monitor your baby's growth as accurately and precisely as possible. It's more difficult to provide an accurate due date if your health care provider doesn't see you early in your pregnancy. A firm idea about when your baby is due helps your health care provider interpret lab results. Certain lab test results change over the course of your pregnancy. As a result, a test result might be mistakenly interpreted as abnormal if the estimate of your baby's age is off. Knowing the due date also significantly affects how your health care provider might manage preterm labor, if it occurs.

PRETERM LABOR: ARE YOU AT RISK?

Your health care provider will want to assess your risk of preterm labor — that is, labor and delivery that occurs before the end of the 37th week of pregnancy. The exact causes of preterm birth aren't known. But some factors seem to increase a woman's risk of preterm labor, including:
- A previous preterm birth
- A pregnancy with twins, triplets or more
- Several previous miscarriages or abortions
- An infection of the amniotic fluid or the fetal membranes
- An excess of amniotic fluid (hydramnios)
- Abnormalities of the uterus
- Problems with the placenta
- A serious illness or disease in the mother
- Cigarette smoking
- The use of illicit drugs
- Advanced maternal age

In the United States, black women are at higher risk of preterm labor than are American Indian, Hispanic, white, Asian or Pacific Island women.

To estimate a due date, most health care providers take the date when your last period began, add seven days and then subtract three months. For example, if your last period started on Nov. 20, adding seven days (Nov. 27) and subtracting three months gives you a due date of Aug. 27.

Laboratory tests

Routine lab tests during your first prenatal visit include blood tests to determine your blood type (A, B, AB or O) and rhesus factor (for example, Rh positive or Rh negative), and determine whether you've been exposed to syphilis, German measles (rubella) or hepatitis B. Most Americans were vaccinated against German measles as children and are still immune. But if you aren't, you must avoid contact with anyone who has German measles while you're pregnant. Exposure to German measles can have serious consequences for your growing baby.

Your blood is also screened for red blood cell antibodies — most commonly, Rh antibodies. These types of antibodies can increase your baby's risk of developing anemia and jaundice after birth. You'll also be offered a test for human immunodeficiency virus (HIV), the virus that causes AIDS. Tests for immunity to chickenpox, measles, mumps and toxoplasmosis may be done as well. Some women may be screened for thyroid problems. It typically takes just one needle stick and one blood sample to run all these tests.

You'll probably be asked to provide a urine sample. An analysis of your urine can determine whether you have a bladder or kidney infection, which would require treatment. The urine sample can also be tested for increased sugar, indicating diabetes, and protein, indicating possible kidney disease.

Getting the most from your first visit

Whether this is your first pregnancy or not, your first prenatal visit with your health care provider gives you a chance to review your health and lifestyle and talk honestly about being pregnant and giving birth. To get the most out of your first visit, keep the following tips in mind:

- Spend some time during the visit talking with your health care provider about your general lifestyle and how you might improve it to have the healthiest possible pregnancy. Possible topics to cover include nutrition, exercise, smoking, alcohol use and how you'll handle your pregnancy in your workplace.
- Raise any concerns or fears you may have about your pregnancy and childbirth. The sooner these fears and concerns are addressed, the sooner you can have peace of mind.
- Be assertive and persistent. If your health care provider doesn't answer your questions to your satisfaction or uses words you don't understand, ask again until you do understand.
- Be honest and accurate when talking with your health care provider. The quality of care you receive depends in large part on the quality of the information you provide.

Setting up your next visit

Your health determines how many follow-up visits your health care provider will recommend. Most women have visits every four to six weeks until their eighth month. Then the visits become more frequent: every two weeks until the start of the ninth month, then weekly until the baby arrives. If you have a chronic health problem, such as diabetes or high blood pressure (hypertension), you'll probably need to have more frequent visits with your health care provider. If you're in good health and have previously been pregnant and gone through labor, you may be able to schedule fewer visits. If any problems or concerns arise between visits, contact your health care provider.

When to call a health care professional during weeks 5 to 8

When in doubt, call. It's always better to be safe than sorry.

This month, you may also be interested in:
- **"Decision Guide: Managing travel during pregnancy," page 321**
- **"Complications: Hyperemesis gravidarum," page 550**

When to call

Here's a guide to possibly troublesome signs and symptoms and when you should notify your health care provider in the second month.

Signs or symptoms	When to tell your health care provider
Vaginal bleeding or spotting	
Slight spotting that goes away within a day	Next visit
Any spotting or bleeding lasting longer than a day	Within 24 hours
Moderate to heavy bleeding	Immediately
Any amount of bleeding accompanied by pain, cramping, fever or chills	Immediately
Passing of tissue	Immediately
Pain	
Occasional pulling, twinging or pinching sensation on one or both sides of your abdomen	Next visit
Occasional mild headaches	Next visit
A moderate, bothersome headache that doesn't go away after treatment with acetaminophen (Tylenol, others)	Within 24 hours
A severe or persistent headache, especially with dizziness, faintness, nausea or vomiting, or visual disturbances	Immediately
Moderate or severe pelvic pain	Immediately
Any degree of pelvic pain that doesn't subside within four hours	Immediately
Pain with fever or bleeding	Immediately
Vomiting	
Occasional	Next visit
Once every day	Next visit
More than three times a day or with inability to eat or drink between vomiting episodes	Within 24 hours
With pain or fever	Immediately
Other	
Chills or fever (102 F or higher)	Immediately
Painful urination	Same day
Increased frequency of urination	Next visit
Inability to urinate	Same day
Mild constipation	Next visit
Severe constipation, no bowel movement for three days	Same day

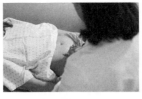

CHAPTER   3

month 3: weeks 9 to 12

Your baby's growth during weeks 9 to 12

Week 9

This week your baby is becoming distinctly human in shape, looking less like a tadpole and more like a person. The embryonic tail at the bottom of your baby's spinal cord is shrinking and disappearing, and the face is more rounded.

Your baby's head is quite large compared with the rest of the body

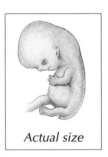

Actual size

and is tucked down onto the chest. Hands and feet are continuing to form fingers and toes, and elbows are more pronounced. Nipples and hair follicles are forming.

Your baby's pancreas, bile ducts, gallbladder and anus have formed, and the intestines are growing longer. Internal reproductive organs, such as testes or ovaries, are starting to develop this week, but your baby's external genitals don't yet have noticeable male or female characteristics.

Your baby may start making some movements this week, but you won't be able to feel them for several more weeks.

At nine weeks into your pregnancy, seven weeks since conception, your baby is almost 1 inch long and weighs a bit less than ⅛ of an ounce.

Week 10

By week 10 the beginnings of all of your baby's vital organs have formed. The embryonic tail has disappeared completely, and fully separated fingers and

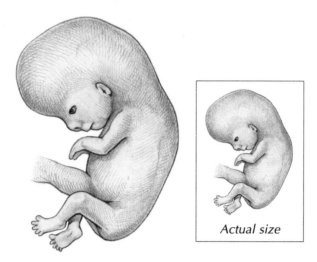

Actual size

toes have formed. The bones of the skeleton are now forming. Your baby's eyelids are more developed, and the eyes look closed. The outer ears are starting to assume their final form. Your baby is also starting to develop buds for teeth.

Your baby's brain is now starting to grow more quickly. This week almost 250,000 new neurons are being produced in his or her brain every minute.

If your baby is a boy, his testes will start producing the male hormone testosterone this week.

Week 11

At 11 weeks and one day of your pregnancy to the time your baby is full term, he or she is officially described as a fetus. With all organ systems in place, week 11 begins a time of rapid growth. From now until your 20th week of pregnancy — the halfway mark — your baby will increase his or her weight 30-fold and will about triple in length. To accommodate all this growth, blood vessels in your placenta are growing larger and more numerous to keep up the supply of nutrients to your baby.

Your baby's ears are moving up and to the side of the head this week, and his or her reproductive organs are developing quickly, too. By the end of the week, what was a tiny tissue bud of external genitalia has developed into either a recognizable penis or a clitoris and labia majora.

Week 12

Your baby's face takes on further definition this week, as the chin and nose become more refined. This week also marks the arrival of fingernails and toenails. Your baby's heart rate may speed up by a few beats per minute.

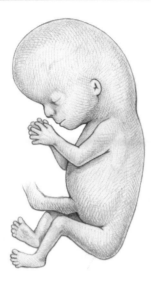

Eighty percent of actual size

By the 12th week of your pregnancy, your baby is nearing 3 inches long and weighs about 4/5 of an ounce. The end of the 12th week marks the end of your first trimester.

Your body during weeks 9 to 12

The third month of pregnancy is the last month in your first trimester. Some of the first discomforts and annoyances of pregnancy, such as morning sickness and frequent urination, may be particularly troublesome this month. But the end is in sight — at least for a while. For most women, the side effects of early pregnancy greatly diminish in the second trimester.

Your hormones
Hormone production is continuing to increase this month, but a shift is going on. By the end of your 12th week of pregnancy, your baby and placenta will be producing more estrogen and progesterone than your ovaries do.

Your body's increased hormone production is likely continuing to cause unpleasant signs and symptoms, such as nausea and vomiting, breast soreness, headaches, dizziness, increased urination, insomnia and vivid dreams. Nausea and vomiting may be especially bothersome. If you have morning sickness, it may last this entire month. It will likely subside midway into next month. It almost always subsides by the end of next month.

On the upside, your increased blood volume and increased production of the hormone human chorionic gonadotropin (HCG) are working together this month to give you that pregnant "glow." Greater blood volume is bringing more blood to your blood vessels, resulting in skin that looks slightly flushed and plump. The final part of the glow comes from the hormones HCG and progesterone, which are increasing the amount of oil secreted by the oil glands in your face, causing your skin to look smoother and slightly shinier.

One possible downside: If you commonly experienced acne breakouts during your menstrual period before you were pregnant, this extra oil may be making you more prone to acne.

Your heart and circulatory system

Your body's increased blood production will continue throughout your pregnancy, but this month marks the end of the time of greatest increase. To accommodate this change, your heart is continuing to pump harder. It's also pumping faster. These changes in your circulatory system may be continuing to cause unwelcome physical signs and symptoms, such as fatigue, dizziness and headaches.

Your eyes

While you're pregnant, your body retains extra fluid. This causes the outer layer of your eye, called the cornea, to get about 3 percent thicker. This change typically becomes obvious by about the 10th week of your pregnancy, lasting until about six weeks after your baby is born. At the same time, the pressure of fluid within your eyes, called intraocular pressure, decreases about 10 percent during pregnancy.

As a result of these two events, you may begin to have slightly blurred vision this month. If you wear contact lenses, particularly hard lenses, you may find them uncomfortable to wear. Still, there's no need to change your contact lenses. Your eyes will return to normal after you give birth.

Your breasts

Your breasts and the milk-producing glands inside them are continuing to grow, stimulated by increased production of estrogen and progesterone. The areolas, the rings of brown or reddish-brown skin around your nipples, may also be larger and darker. Your breasts may continue to feel tender or sore, though the soreness is probably easing a bit. Your breasts may feel fuller and heavier as well.

Your uterus

Up to your 12th week of pregnancy, your uterus fits inside your pelvis. It's probably hard for anyone to tell you're pregnant just by looking at you. Even so, you'll likely have pregnancy-related signs and symptoms. Throughout this month, because of your uterus' increasing size and proximity to your bladder, you'll probably continue to feel the need to urinate more often. By the end of the month, your uterus will have expanded up out of your pelvic cavity, so the pressure on your bladder won't be as great.

Your bones, muscles and joints

You may be continuing to feel some twinges, cramps or pulling in your lower abdomen. The ligaments supporting your uterus are stretching to accommodate its growth. Early in the second trimester, it's common to have sharp pain on one side or the other, usually provoked by a sudden movement. This pain is the result of a hard stretch of the round ligament that tethers the uterus to the abdominal wall. It isn't harmful, but it can hurt.

Weight gain

When you add up your baby's weight, your placenta, the amniotic fluid, the increased amount of blood your body has produced, the fluid accumulated in your own body tissues and your bigger uterus and breasts, you'll probably have gained about 2 pounds by the end of your 12th week of pregnancy. If your pre-pregnancy weight is in the normal range, you'll probably gain about 25 to 35 pounds during your pregnancy. Most of your weight gain will occur in the second half of your pregnancy and after your 33rd or 34th week, when you'll probably gain about a pound a week.

Self-care resources

The changes in your body during the third month of pregnancy can produce some unpleasant signs and symptoms. For more information on dealing with common complaints such as abdominal pain or cramping, acne, fatigue, frequent urination, and vomiting, see Part 3, "Pregnancy Reference Guide" on page 413.

Your emotions during weeks 9 to 12

Body image

In the early months of your pregnancy, you may be preoccupied with the physical changes occurring in your body. Given the emphasis our culture puts on being slim, you may be upset about these changes. Simply put, you may feel fat and unattractive. These feelings may be especially strong this month, as you start developing a small potbelly.

Changes in your body's shape and function can affect the way you feel. You may feel less attractive in general and to your partner in particular. You may be especially bothered by body image concerns if this is your first pregnancy.

If you have a negative body image, you may be having trouble enjoying or even wanting to have sex with your partner. You may not be able to imagine why your partner would even want to make love.

If you're feeling this way, keep a couple of things in mind. For most women, interest in intercourse continues during pregnancy, but it may decrease a bit. This is normal. Also, though it may be hard for you to believe, you partner is probably proud of the physical changes in your body that come with pregnancy. Ask him about it.

There's more to a sexual relationship than intercourse. Massage can heighten sensuality and intimacy and lead comfortably to intercourse. Or it can be an enjoyable end in itself. Find the balance that works best for you and your partner.

Appointments with your health care provider

You'll likely have your second prenatal visit with your health care provider this month. Your second visit to your health care provider will probably be briefer than your first, but it will probably include many of the same things. Your health care provider may check your weight and blood pressure. Rarely will you need another pelvic exam unless something unusual was discovered at your first visit.

One thing to look forward to during your second visit: If the visit occurs around the 12th week of your pregnancy, your health care provider may use a special listening device called a Doppler, which may allow you to hear your baby's heartbeat for the first time.

When to call a health care professional during weeks 9 to 12

When in doubt, call. It's always better to be safe than sorry.

When to call

Here's a guide to possibly troublesome signs and symptoms and when you should notify your health care provider in the third month.

Signs or symptoms	When to tell your health care provider
Vaginal bleeding or spotting	
Slight spotting that goes away within a day	Next visit
Any spotting or bleeding lasting longer than a day	Within 24 hours
Moderate to heavy bleeding	Immediately
Any amount of bleeding accompanied by pain, cramping, fever or chills	Immediately
Passing of tissue	Immediately
Pain	
Occasional pulling, twinging or pinching sensation on one or both sides of your abdomen	Next visit
Occasional mild headaches	Next visit
A moderate, bothersome headache that doesn't go away after treatment with acetaminophen (Tylenol, others)	Within 24 hours
A severe or persistent headache, especially with dizziness, faintness, nausea or vomiting, or visual disturbances	Immediately
Moderate or severe pelvic pain	Immediately
Any degree of pelvic pain that doesn't subside within four hours	Immediately
Pain with fever or bleeding	Immediately
Vomiting	
Occasional	Next visit
Once every day	Next visit
More than three times a day or with inability to eat or drink between vomiting episodes	Within 24 hours
With pain or fever	Immediately
Other	
Chills or fever (102 F or higher)	Immediately
Painful urination	Same day
Increased frequency of urination	Next visit
Inability to urinate	Same day
Mild constipation	Next visit
Severe constipation, no bowel movement for three days	Same day

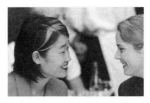

CHAPTER   4

month 4: weeks 13 to 16

*W*hew! We're through the first trimester. My husband and I now feel more comfortable telling people that we're expecting a baby. My tummy is starting to "pop" just a little, which is both fun and a bit frightening. I'm feeling better, too, not quite so nauseated and tired. Thank goodness for the second trimester!

— One mother's experience

Your baby's growth during weeks 13 to 16

Week 13

As you enter the second trimester, all of your baby's organs, nerves and muscles are formed and just beginning to function together. Your baby's eyes and ears are now clearly identifiable, although the eyelids are fused together to protect the developing eyes. They won't reopen until about your 30th week. Tissue that will become bone is developing around your baby's head and within the arms and legs. If you were able to sneak a peek at your baby this week, you might see some tiny ribs.

Your baby is now able to move his or her body in a jerky fashion, flexing the arms and kicking the legs. But you won't be able to feel these movements until your baby grows a bit larger. Your baby might even be able to put a thumb in his or her mouth this week. Sucking will come later.

Week 14

Your baby's reproductive system is the site of most of the action this week. If you're having a boy, his prostate gland is developing. If you're having a girl, her ovaries are moving down from her abdomen into her pelvis. In addition, because the thyroid gland is now functioning, your baby starts producing hormones this week. By the end of this week, the roof of your baby's mouth (palate) will be completely formed.

Week 15

Eyebrows and hairs on your baby's scalp are starting to appear this week. If your baby is going to have dark hair, the hair follicles may begin making the pigment that will give the hair its color.

Your baby's eyes and ears now have a baby-like appearance, and the ears have almost reached their final position, although they're still riding a little low on the head. In addition, your baby is developing skin so thin that you can see the blood vessels through it.

The bone and marrow that make up your baby's skeletal system are continuing to develop this week. Muscle development is continuing, too. By the end of this week, your baby will be able to make a fist.

Week 16

The skeletal system and nervous system have made enough connections to coordinate limb and body movement. In addition, your baby's facial muscles are now developed well enough to allow for a variety of expressions. Inside your uterus, your baby may be squinting or frowning at you, although these movements aren't conscious expressions of emotions.

Your baby's skeletal system is continuing to develop as more calcium is deposited on the bones. If you're having a girl, millions of eggs are forming in her ovaries this week. Beginning at 16 weeks, your baby's eyes are sensitive to light.

Eighty percent of actual size

Although you probably don't even know it, your baby may be having frequent bouts of the hiccups. Hiccups often develop before a baby's breathing movements become common. Because your baby's trachea is filled with fluid rather than air, the hiccups don't make that characteristic hiccup sound.

At 16 weeks into your pregnancy, your baby is between 4 and 5 inches long and weighs a bit less than 3 ounces.

Your body during weeks 13 to 16

This month begins your second trimester, what's sometimes called the golden period of pregnancy. The name is apt. The side effects of early pregnancy taper off, but the discomforts of the third trimester haven't yet begun. Plus, your risk of miscarriage is now greatly reduced. New sensations are common during this time.

The changes that began in your first weeks of pregnancy are increasing and accelerating — and becoming more obvious to others. Here's an overview of what's happening and where.

Your hormones

Throughout your pregnancy, hormones are released by your placenta, ovaries, adrenal glands and pituitary gland. Your hormone levels are continuing to increase this month, influencing the growth of your baby and affecting every organ system in your body.

Your heart and circulatory system

Your circulatory system is continuing to expand rapidly. This expansion may be tending to lower your blood pressure. In fact, during the first 24 weeks of your pregnancy, your systolic blood pressure (the top number) will probably drop by five to 10 points, and your diastolic blood pressure (the bottom number) by 10 to 15 points. After that they'll gradually return to pre-pregnancy levels.

You may be experiencing dizziness or faintness during hot weather or when you're taking a hot bath or shower. This occurs because heat makes the tiny blood vessels in your skin dilate, temporarily reducing the amount of blood returning to your heart.

Your body is continuing to make more blood this month. Right now, the extra blood you're producing is mostly plasma, the fluid portion of blood. During the first 20 weeks of pregnancy, you produce more plasma, more quickly, than you produce red blood cells. Until your red blood cells have a chance to catch up, they're outnumbered, resulting in lower concentrations.

If you don't get the iron you need this month to help your body make more red blood cells, you may become anemic. Anemia results when you don't have enough red blood cells in your blood, and therefore not enough of the protein hemoglobin to carry oxygen to your body's tissues. Anemia can make you tired and more susceptible to illness, but unless the anemia is severe, it's unlikely to hurt your baby. Pregnancy is designed so that even if you're not getting enough iron, your baby is.

Increased blood flow throughout your body may be causing some new unpleasant signs and symptoms this month. Your nasal tissues may be swollen and fragile. You may be producing more mucus, resulting in nasal stuffiness and congestion. You may also have nosebleeds or bleeding gums when you brush your teeth, even if you never did before. About 80 percent of pregnant women experience gum softening or bleeding. None of these problems will harm you or your baby, but they can be disconcerting and annoying.

Your respiratory system

Stimulated by progesterone, your lung capacity is increasing this month. With each breath, your lungs are inhaling and exhaling up to 30 percent to 40 percent more air than they did before. These changes in your respiratory system are allowing your blood to carry large quantities of oxygen to your placenta and baby. In addition, they're allowing your blood to remove more carbon dioxide from your body than it does normally.

You may notice that you're breathing slightly faster this month. You may also be experiencing shortness of breath. Two-thirds of all pregnant women do, usually beginning around the 13th week of pregnancy. This is because your brain is decreasing the carbon dioxide level in your blood in order to make it easier to transfer more carbon dioxide from your baby to you. To do this, the brain adjusts your breathing volume and rate. As a result, many women feel short of breath.

To accommodate your increased lung capacity, your rib cage will enlarge over the course of your pregnancy, by two to three inches in circumference.

Your digestive system

Increased amounts of the hormones progesterone and estrogen during pregnancy tend to relax every smooth muscle in your body, including your digestive tract. Under the influence of these hormones, your digestive system has slowed down. The movements that push swallowed food from your esophagus down into your stomach are slower, and your stomach also is taking longer to empty.

This slowdown is designed to allow nutrients more time to be absorbed into your bloodstream and reach your baby. Unfortunately, when you combine it with an expanding uterus crowding out other organs in your abdomen, this slowdown may also be causing heartburn and constipation, two of the most common and uncomfortable side effects of pregnancy. You may be experiencing these unpleasant side effects this month.

About half of all pregnant women experience heartburn. It results when digestive acid backs up into the esophagus, the tube that leads from your throat to your stomach. When this happens, stomach acids irritate the lining of the esophagus, causing the telltale burning sensation.

The story is much the same with constipation, which also affects at least half of all pregnant women. It's caused or at least encouraged by a slowed digestive system and pressure from the ever-expanding uterus on the lower bowel. In addition, your colon absorbs more water during pregnancy, which tends to make stools harder and bowel movements more difficult.

Your breasts

Your breasts and the milk-producing glands inside them are continuing to grow in size this month, stimulated by increased production of estrogen and progesterone. Skin darkening around the rings of brown or reddish-brown skin around your nipples (areolas) may be especially noticeable now. Although some of this increased pigmentation will fade after you've given birth, these areas are likely to remain darker than they were before you were pregnant. Your breasts are likely continuing to feel tender or sore, or they may feel fuller and heavier.

Your uterus

As your uterus is expanding to make room for your growing baby, so too is your abdomen. This will begin to be much more noticeable this month.

Now that you're in your second trimester, your uterus is heavier. It's also higher and more forward, which is changing your center of gravity. Without even knowing it, you may be starting to adjust your posture and the ways you stand, move and walk. You may at times feel as if you're going to tip over. This is normal. You'll return to your more graceful self after your baby is born.

As your uterus is becoming too big to fit within your pelvis, your internal organs are being pushed out of their usual places. Plus, greater tension is being placed on your surrounding muscles and ligaments. All this growth is likely causing some aches and pains this month.

Pressure from your uterus on the veins returning blood from your legs may be causing leg cramps, especially at night. You may also notice that your navel is starting to protrude. This, too, is the result of pressure from your growing uterus. After you deliver your baby, your navel will almost certainly return to normal.

You may be experiencing some pain in your lower abdomen this month. This is probably related to the stretching of ligaments and muscles around your expanding uterus, which doesn't pose a threat to you or your baby. However, if you're having abdominal pain, tell your health care provider about it.

Your urinary tract

The hormone progesterone is relaxing the muscles of your ureters, the tubes that carry urine from your kidneys to your bladder, slowing your flow of urine. In addition, your expanding uterus is further impeding your urine flow. These changes, combined with a tendency to excrete more glucose in your urine, may be making you more prone to bladder and kidney infections this month.

If you're urinating even more often than normal, feeling burning on urination or experiencing a fever, you may have a urinary tract infection. Report these signs and symptoms to your health care provider. Abdominal pain and backache also may signal a urinary tract infection. Recognizing and treating urinary tract infections are especially important during pregnancy. When left untreated, these infections are a common cause of preterm labor later in pregnancy.

Your bones, muscles and joints

This month your bones, joints and muscles are continuing to adapt to the stresses of carrying your baby. The ligaments supporting your abdomen are becoming more elastic, and the joints between your pelvic bones are beginning to soften and loosen. Ultimately, these changes will make it easier for your pelvis to expand during childbirth so that your baby can pass through. For now, these changes may be causing some back pain.

The lower portion of your spine may be starting to curve backward to compensate for the shift in your center of gravity caused by your growing baby. Without this change, you'd probably fall over. But this change in your posture may be putting a strain on your back muscles and ligaments and may be causing some back pain.

Your vagina

You may notice that you have more vaginal discharge this month. That's normal. It's caused by the effects of hormones on the cells that line your vagina. Pregnancy hormones stimulate mucus production, but most of this normal discharge is turnover of the rapidly growing cells from the vagina. These cells combine with normal vaginal moisture to form a thin, white discharge. Its high acidity is thought to play a role in suppressing the growth of potentially harmful bacteria.

The hormone changes of pregnancy can disrupt the balance of your vaginal environment. When this happens, one type of organism living there may grow faster than the others, causing a vaginal infection. If you have vaginal discharge that's greenish or yellowish, strong smelling or accompanied by redness, itching and irritation of the vulva, contact your health care provider. But don't be too alarmed. Vaginal infections are common in pregnancy and can be treated successfully.

Over-the-counter medications for yeast infections are available, but don't use one while you're pregnant without talking to your health care provider first. Because other types of vaginal infections can cause signs and symptoms similar to those caused by yeast infections, it's best for your health care provider to exactly determine what type of vaginal infection you have before you start treatment.

Your skin

The pregnancy hormones at work in your body may be starting to cause changes in your skin this month. One of the most common — skin darkening — occurs in 90 percent of all pregnant women. You may be noticing darker areas of skin on or around your nipples, in the area between your vulva and anus (perineum), around your navel, and on your armpits and inner thighs. These changes will be more pronounced if you have dark skin. Skin darkening almost always fades after delivery, but some areas are likely to remain darker than before you were pregnant.

You may also be noticing mild skin darkening on your face. This condition, called chloasma or the mask of pregnancy, affects about half of all pregnant women, mostly those who have dark hair and fair skin. It usually appears on the forehead, temples, cheeks, chin and nose. It may not be as intense as other increases in pigmentation and generally fades completely after delivery.

Other changes may include:
- Darkening of the white line running from your navel to your pubic hair.
- Darkening of existing moles, freckles and skin blemishes.
- Redness and itching on the palms of your hands and soles of your feet. Thought to be caused by increased estrogen production, this skin change affects two-thirds of pregnant women.
- Bluish, blotchy patches on your legs and feet, especially when you're cold. This skin change, caused by increased estrogen, will disappear after your baby is born.
- New, more numerous moles.
- Faster-growing fingernails and toenails, or nails that are brittle or soft and grooved.
- Increased perspiration and heat rash. Pregnant women often perspire more as a result of the action of hormones and the need to control the heat produced by the developing baby. This skin dampness makes heat rashes more common.

Most of these skin changes are nothing to worry about. They usually disappear after your baby is born. Changes in moles or new moles are the exception. The moles that appear during pregnancy are usually not the types that are linked to skin cancer. However, it's still a good idea to show any new moles to your health care provider.

Weight gain

You'll probably gain about a pound a week this month, for a total of about 4 pounds. It's typical for your weekly weight gain to vary somewhat —

gaining a pound and a half one week and only half a pound the next. Unless a very dramatic change in weight occurs, health care providers tend to look at long-term trends rather than changes over just one month.

Self-care resources

The changes in your body during the fourth month of pregnancy can produce some unpleasant signs and symptoms. For more information on dealing with common complaints such as back pain, constipation, heartburn and leg cramps, see Part 3, "Pregnancy Reference Guide" on page 413.

Your emotions during weeks 13 to 16

Your baby is probably starting to seem more real to you this month, especially now that you're growing out of your jeans and you've been able to hear your baby's heartbeat during visits to your health care provider. You're likely also finding that your nausea is easing off, you're sleeping better, and your energy is returning. As a result, you're probably feeling less moody and more up to the challenge of preparing a home for your baby.

Strike while the iron is hot. While your mood and energy are up, start taking care of the "housekeeping" details of pregnancy. If you're interested in childbirth classes for you and your partner, investigate the options and get signed up. Ask friends and family to recommend pediatricians or other health care providers for your baby. Once you've identified a few candidates, schedule meetings with them so that you can discuss philosophy and office procedures (see "Decision Guide: Choosing your baby's health care provider" on page 359). Now is also a good time to familiarize yourself with maternity and paternity leave policies and to investigate child-care options if both you and your partner will be returning to work after your baby is born.

As you take care of these details, you may find it a little difficult to concentrate. You may even feel a little scatterbrained or forgetful. This is normal, no matter how organized you were (or weren't) before pregnancy. Take these foggy moments in stride. You'll be back to your usual self in a few months.

Appointments with your health care provider

Your visit to your health care provider this month may focus on tracking your baby's growth, confirming your due date and watching for any problems with your health.

At this visit, your health care provider may measure the size of your uterus to help determine the baby's age. This is done by checking what's called the fundal height — the distance from the top (fundus) of your uterus to your pubic bone.

After you've emptied your bladder, your health care provider can find the top of your uterus by gently tapping and pressing on your abdomen and measuring from that point down along the front of your abdomen to your pubic bone.

In addition to performing the fundal height check, your health care provider may check your weight and blood pressure and ask you about any signs and symptoms you've been experiencing. If you haven't done so already, you may get to hear your baby's heartbeat using a special listening device called a Doppler.

If you haven't decided about prenatal diagnostic testing, now is a good time to review these tests with your health care provider and make a plan (see "Decision Guide: Understanding prenatal testing" on page 289, for help in making those decisions).

When to call a health care professional during weeks 13 to 16

You're probably finding your fourth month of pregnancy to be easier than your first three. Even so, knowing about potential problems and when to contact your health care provider are just as important now as they were during the first trimester.

This month, you may be interested in:
- **"Decision Guide: Understanding prenatal testing," page 289**
- **"Complications: Preterm labor," page 533**
- **"Complications: Depression during pregnancy," page 545**

WHEN TO CALL

Here's a guide to possibly troublesome signs and symptoms and when you should notify your health care provider in the fourth month.

Signs or symptoms	When to tell your health care provider
Vaginal bleeding, spotting or discharge	
Slight spotting	Same day
Any spotting or bleeding lasting longer than a day	Immediately
Moderate to heavy bleeding	Immediately
Any amount of bleeding accompanied by pain, cramping, fever or chills	Immediately
Passing of tissue	Immediately
Persistent vaginal discharge that's greenish or yellowish, strong-smelling or accompanied by redness, itching and irritation around the vulva throughout the day	Within 24 hours
Pain	
Occasional pulling, twinging or pinching sensation on one or both sides of your abdomen	Next visit
Occasional mild headaches	Next visit
A moderate, bothersome headache that doesn't go away after treatment with acetaminophen (Tylenol, others)	Within 24 hours
A severe or persistent headache, especially with dizziness, faintness, nausea or vomiting, or visual disturbances	Immediately
Moderate or severe pelvic pain	Immediately
Any degree of pelvic pain that doesn't subside within four hours	Within 24 hours
Leg cramp that awakens you from sleep	Next visit
Leg pain with redness and swelling	Immediately
Pain with fever or bleeding	Immediately
Vomiting	
Occasional	Next visit
Once every day	Next visit
More than three times a day or with inability to eat or drink between vomiting episodes	Within 24 hours
With pain or fever	Immediately

Signs or symptoms	When to tell your health care provider
Other	
Chills or fever (102 F or higher)	Immediately
Painful urination	Same day
Cravings for nonfood substances, such as clay, dirt and laundry starch	Next visit
Consistently low mood, loss of pleasure in things you normally enjoy	Next visit
Above signs and symptoms along with thoughts of harming yourself or others	Immediately

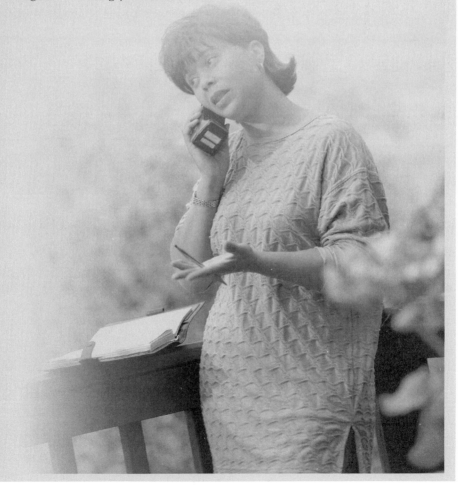

Twins, triplets and quads — Oh, my!

For about three in every 100 pregnant women, this month's visit to their health care provider will bring the surprising news that they're expecting twins, triplets or more, called multiple gestations.

The number of women having multiples is on the rise. Two factors help explain the increase. First, more women over 30 are having babies, and multiple gestations occur more frequently in women over 30. Second, the use of fertility drugs and assisted reproductive technologies results in more multiples. Physical signs of a multiple pregnancy, such as a uterus that's larger than normal or more than one fetal heartbeat, are easily detected during a routine physical exam. The results of a "triple screen" test also can suggest twins or other multiples.

If your health care provider suspects that you're carrying multiple babies, he or she will probably perform an ultrasound exam to confirm these suspicions. During an ultrasound exam, sound waves are used to create a television-like picture of your uterus and your baby — or babies. Because of today's widespread use of ultrasound, more than 90 percent of twin pregnancies are diagnosed before delivery.

How multiples are made

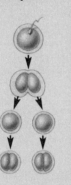 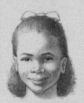

Identical twins occur when a single fertilized egg splits and develops into two fetuses that have identical genetic makeups.

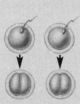

Fraternal twins, the most common kind, occur when two different eggs are fertilized by two different sperm.

Twins come in two types: identical and fraternal. Identical twins occur when a single fertilized egg splits and develops into two fetuses. Genetically, the two babies are identical. They will be the same sex and look exactly alike.

Fraternal twins occur when two separate eggs are fertilized by two different sperm. In this case, the twins can be two girls, two boys or a boy and a girl. Genetically, the twins are no more alike than are any other siblings.

It may be possible to determine whether twins are identical or fraternal with an ultrasound. For instance, if one is a boy and one is a girl, they're fraternal. In addition, the membranes around the fetuses may or may not suggest identical twins. Additional testing may be needed after the babies are born to determine if they're identical.

Triplets can occur in several ways. In most cases, three separate eggs produced by the mother are fertilized by three separate sperm. Another possibility is for a single fertilized egg to divide two ways, creating identical twins, with a second egg fertilized by a second sperm resulting in a fraternal third baby. It's also possible for a single fertilized egg to divide three ways, resulting in three identical babies, although this is very rare.

What multiples mean for mom

If you're carrying twins, triplets or other multiples, some of the side effects of pregnancy may be particularly unpleasant. Nausea and vomiting, heartburn, insomnia and fatigue may be especially troublesome. Because of the increased space required by your growing babies, you may also have abdominal pain and shortness of breath. Later in your pregnancy, you may feel pressure on your pubic bone, the structure located over the lowest part of the front of your pelvis.

Carrying multiple babies means you'll probably be seeing your health care provider more often. Special care is essential in multiple pregnancies. It allows your health care provider to track the growth of your babies and closely monitor your health, anticipating potential problems before they occur.

With more than one baby to nourish, your nutrition and weight gain become even more important. You'll likely have to eat more, gain more weight and get more iron. If you're carrying twins, your health care provider may recommend that you take in about 300 more calories a day, for a total of 2,700 to 2,800 calories. With twins, the American Dietetic Association recommends a weight gain of 34 to 45 pounds. With triplets, it recommends a weight gain of 50 pounds.

A lowered blood cell count (anemia) is more likely with multiples. Thus, your health care provider may recommend that you take a supplement with 60 to 100 milligrams of elemental iron. You may also be asked to limit some of your activities, such as work, travel and exercise. Work with your health care provider to develop a list of recommendations.

Possible complications of multiples

Carrying more than one baby increases your chances of some pregnancy complications. The more babies you're carrying, the greater your chances of having problems. These can include:

- **Preterm labor.** Preterm labor occurs when contractions begin to open the cervix before the 37th week of pregnancy. It happens more often in multiple pregnancies than in pregnancies involving just one baby.

  Preterm labor can result in the early birth of one or more of the babies. Nearly 60 percent of twins and more than 90 percent of triplets are born before 37 weeks' gestation. The average gestational age of twins is 37 weeks. Triplets frequently arrive by 35 weeks, sometimes earlier. Almost all quadruplets and higher-order multiples come early.

  Babies that arrive early have a greater chance of being low birth weight (under 5½ pounds) and having other health complications. For that reason, your health care provider will likely monitor you closely for signs of preterm labor. You'll want to do the same. If you start having contractions that are more frequent or are becoming stronger, contact your health care provider immediately.

Depending on the age of your babies, preterm labor can sometimes be managed with careful observation and bed rest. For more on preterm labor, see page 533.

- **Preeclampsia.** High blood pressure caused by pregnancy (preeclampsia) also is more common in mothers of multiples. It tends to occur earlier in those carrying more than one child. Signs and symptoms of preeclampsia include rapid weight gain, headaches, abdominal pain, vision problems, and swelling of your hands and feet. Contact your health care provider if you experience these problems.

- **Higher risk of Caesarean birth.** The chance of having a Caesarean birth is higher with twins and other multiples. However, about half of women carrying twins can expect to have a vaginal birth. If you're carrying more than two babies, your health care provider may recommend a Caesarean birth as the safest delivery method for the babies.

- **Twin-twin transfusion.** Twin-twin transfusion occurs only in identical twins. It can happen when a blood vessel in the placenta connects the circulatory systems of the two babies. It's possible that one twin may receive too much blood flow and the other too little. A baby receiving too much may grow larger and develop an overload of blood in its circulatory system. The other twin may be smaller, grow more slowly and become anemic. The situation can put one or both babies in jeopardy. At times, early delivery of the twins may be necessary.

Some new treatments may help. Studies suggest that use of amniocentesis to drain off excess fluid can help. At some specialized hospitals, laser surgery is used to seal off the connection between the blood vessels. Generally, a team of high-risk-care obstetricians and neonatologists care for these babies. The babies are usually delivered as soon as the benefits of early birth outweigh the potential problems of prematurity.

- **Vanishing twin syndrome.** At times, an early ultrasound may show twins. But later ultrasounds may show little or no evidence of one of the twins. This is called the vanishing twin syndrome. Experts aren't sure why it happens. It may be frustrating or confusing, but don't blame yourself for it. Moms-to-be don't have any control over this outcome.

- **Conjoined twins.** Conjoined twins can result from an incomplete division of identical twins. In the past, babies with this condition were commonly referred to as Siamese twins. This occurs very rarely, only in one in 100,000 births. Conjoined twins may be joined at the chest, head or pelvis. In some cases, the twins may share one or more internal organs. At times, surgery is used to separate conjoined twins. The success of the operation depends in part on where the twins are joined and how many organs are shared.

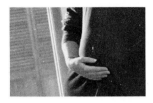

month 5: weeks 17 to 20

It starts with these tiny little flutters, as if someone is tickling me lightly from the inside. It takes me by surprise, then disappears before I can put my hand on my abdomen. Now these unexpected touches are the joy of my day. I'm feeling my baby move.

— *One mother's experience*

Your baby's growth during weeks 17 to 20

Week 17

Eyebrows and hairs on your baby's scalp are continuing to appear this week. Your baby is probably continuing to have bouts of the hiccups. Although you aren't able to hear them, you may begin to feel them, especially if this is your second baby.

This week, brown fat is beginning to develop under your baby's skin. This will help keep your baby warm after birth, when the temperature change from your uterus to the outside world will be quite noticeable, to say the least. Your baby will add more layers of fat in the later months of your pregnancy.

Week 18

This week your baby's bones are beginning to harden, a process called ossification.

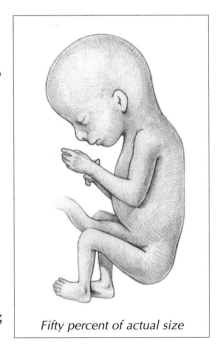

Fifty percent of actual size

Bones in your baby's legs and inner ear are among the first to ossify. With the bones in the inner ear now well developed enough to function and the nerve endings from your baby's brain now "hooked up" to the ears, your baby can hear sounds. He or she may hear your heart beating, your stomach rumbling or blood moving through the umbilical cord. Your baby may even become startled by loud noises.

Your baby can also now swallow. Inside your uterus, your baby may be swallowing a good dose of amniotic fluid every day. Scientists think this may have something to do with keeping your amniotic fluid at the appropriate, constant level.

Week 19

This week your baby's skin becomes covered with a slippery, white, fatty coating called vernix caseosa, or vernix for short. Vernix helps protect your baby's delicate skin, keeping it from becoming chapped or scratched. Under the vernix, a fine, down-like hair called lanugo covers your baby's skin.

Your baby's kidneys are developed enough to make urine this week. Your baby's urine is excreted into your amniotic sac, the bag of waters inside your uterus that contains your baby and your amniotic fluid.

Your baby's hearing is now well-developed. He or she is probably hearing lots of different sounds, maybe even your conversations. Mom's voice is by far the most prominent in any conversation. If you sing or talk to your baby, it's reasonable to think he or she might notice. It's less clear whether your baby is currently able to recognize particular sounds.

Your baby's brain is developing millions of motor neurons, nerves that help the muscles and brain communicate. As a result, your baby probably is now making conscious muscle movements, such as sucking a thumb or moving his or her head, as well as involuntary movements. You may or may not be able to feel these movements yet. If you haven't, you will soon.

Week 20

Your baby's skin is thickening and developing layers this week, under the protection of the vernix. Skin layers include the epidermis, the outermost layer of skin; the dermis, a middle layer, which makes up 90 percent of the skin; and the subcutis, the deepest layer of skin, made up mostly of fat.

Your baby's hair and nails are continuing to grow. If you could sneak a peek at your baby this week, you would see a fetus remarkably baby-like in appearance, with thin eyebrows, hair on the scalp and rather well-developed limbs.

At the halfway point of your pregnancy, 20 weeks, you've probably begun to feel your baby's movements. Make a note of the date, and tell your health care provider at your next visit. Your baby is now about 6 inches long and weighs about 9 ounces — a little over half a pound.

Your body during weeks 17 to 20

This month you'll reach the midway point of pregnancy — 20 weeks. Your uterus will expand to your navel.

Sometime during this month, you'll have a very special experience. You'll feel your baby's first fluttering movements, what doctors and other health care professionals call quickening.

These movements may feel like butterflies in your stomach or a growling stomach. These early movements may be somewhat erratic. They'll become more regular later in your pregnancy. The most active time for many babies is the second half of the seventh month and the entire eighth month.

The many changes that began in your first weeks of pregnancy are continuing to increase and accelerate. Your pregnancy is now probably obvious to everyone.

Your hormones

Your hormone levels are continuing to increase this month, influencing the growth of your baby and affecting all of your organ systems.

Your heart and circulatory system

Your circulatory system is continuing to expand rapidly. As a result, your blood pressure will probably stay lower than normal this month and next. After that, it will likely return to where it was before you were pregnant. You may feel lightheaded, dizzy, nauseated or faint when you stand up after lying down or after a hot shower.

Your body is also continuing to make more blood. Through this month, the extra blood you're producing is mostly plasma, the fluid portion of blood. After that, your body will increase production of red blood cells — if you're getting enough iron.

Iron deficiency anemia, a condition marked by a decline in red blood cells, may result if you're not getting the 30 milligrams of iron you need each day to fuel increased production of red blood cells. This condition develops most often after 20 weeks of pregnancy. It can make you tired and more susceptible to illness. But unless it's severe, it's unlikely to hurt your baby.

You may be continuing to experience some annoying side effects of pregnancy this month, such as nasal congestion, nosebleeds and bleeding gums when you brush your teeth. These changes are the result of increased blood flow to your nasal passages and gums.

Your respiratory system
Stimulated by the hormone progesterone, your lung capacity is continuing to increase this month. With each breath, your lungs are continuing to inhale and exhale up to 40 percent more air than they did before. You also may be continuing to breathe slightly faster. Many women become aware of some shortness of breath.

Your digestive system
Under the influence of pregnancy hormones, your digestive system remains sluggish. Owing to this and your expanding uterus, you may continue to experience heartburn and constipation. You're not alone, if that helps. Half of all women experience heartburn or constipation during pregnancy.

Your breasts
Changes in your breasts may be especially noticeable this month. With more blood flowing to them and the milk-producing glands inside growing in size, they now may be almost two cup sizes larger than before you were pregnant. Veins in your breasts may be more visible now, too.

Your uterus
It goes without saying — your uterus is continuing to expand. By your 20th week, it will reach your navel. When it reaches its full size, it will extend from your pubic area to the bottom of your rib cage.

As your baby is growing within your uterus, so, too, is your placenta. By 17 weeks into your pregnancy, your placenta is more than an inch thick, containing thousands of blood vessels to carry oxygen and nutrients to your baby.

Your larger uterus is now almost certainly affecting your center of gravity and, therefore, how you stand, move and walk. As you adjust to this new reality, you may feel especially clumsy. You may also experience continued aches and pains, especially in your back and lower abdomen.

Around the 20th week of pregnancy, you may feel a pulling or stabbing pain in your groin or a sharp cramp down your side, especially after making a sudden move or reaching for something. This pain results from stretching your round ligament, one of several ligaments that hold your uterus. The pain associated with stretching your round ligament usually lasts several minutes and then goes away. Although it can be painful, it isn't harmful.

However, it's a good idea to discuss any continuous abdominal pain with your health care provider. Abdominal pain can be a symptom of preterm labor or other problems.

Your urinary tract

Slowed urine flow is continuing this month, the result of your expanding uterus and relaxed muscles in the tubes carrying urine from your kidneys to your bladder. As a result, you're at continued risk for developing a urinary tract infection.

Signs and symptoms of a urinary tract infection include urinating more often than normal, burning on urination, fever, abdominal pain and backache. If you have any of these problems, contact your health care provider. Even if you don't have a urinary tract infection, it's better to be safe than sorry. These infections are a common cause of preterm labor.

Your bones, muscles and joints

The ligaments supporting your abdomen are continuing to become more elastic, and the joints between your pelvic bones are continuing to soften and loosen. In addition, your lower spine is probably now curving backward to help keep you from falling forward. Together, these changes in your bones, joints and ligaments may now be causing you some back pain.

Back pain affects half of all pregnant women. It can begin at any time during pregnancy, but it most commonly starts between the fifth and seventh months. You may find back pain to be merely an annoyance. If it was a problem for you before you were pregnant, you may find that back pain significantly interferes with your daily activities.

If you have back pain that doesn't go away or occurs along with lower abdominal cramping, contact your health care provider immediately.

Your vagina

You may be continuing to notice more vaginal discharge this month. Thin, white discharge with a mild odor is caused by the effects of pregnancy hormones on the glands in your cervix and the skin of your vagina. It's normal in pregnancy and it isn't cause for concern.

Do call your health care provider, though, if you have vaginal discharge that's greenish or yellowish, strong-smelling or accompanied by redness, itching and irritation of the vulva. These are signs and symptoms of a vaginal infection, which are common in pregnancy and can be treated successfully.

Your skin

If changes in your skin appeared last month, they are likely still apparent this month and may be for the rest of your pregnancy. In addition to the skin changes that are typical during month four, this month you may have mild skin darkening on your face. You may also have darkening around your nipples, navel, armpits, inner thighs and perineum — the area between the anus and the vulva.

Most of these changes are nothing to worry about. They usually fade after your baby is born. Changes in moles or new moles are the exception. If you have a new mole or a mole that has changed a lot in size or appearance, contact your health care provider.

Weight gain

You'll probably gain about a pound a week this month, for a total of about 4 pounds. By the time you reach your 20th week, you'll probably have gained about 10 pounds.

Self-care resources

The changes in your body during the fifth month of pregnancy can produce some unpleasant signs and symptoms. For more information on dealing with common complaints such as nosebleeds, skin darkening and shortness of breath, see Part 3, "Pregnancy Reference Guide" on page 413.

Your emotions during weeks 17 to 20

Feeling your baby move

By your 20th week of pregnancy — or earlier if this is at least your second pregnancy — you've probably begun to feel your baby move. These early movements are called quickening, and they're a great source of amusement and reassurance for most women. These early movements remind you of the reality that your baby is a separate, unique individual, allowing you to begin imagining what your baby will be like. They're also a much more pleasant and exciting reminder of being pregnant than are nausea and other signs and symptoms.

The process of becoming emotionally attached to your baby is probably in full swing now. As your pregnancy progresses, you and your partner will both be able to feel your baby's movements — he by placing his hand on your abdomen. This increases your emotional involvement with your baby.

You may be wondering whether you can communicate with or positively influence your baby at this point in your pregnancy. That's hard to know. The abilities of babies in the womb have only recently begun to be studied. But it certainly can't hurt to play soft music or talk soothingly and lovingly to your baby. Besides, it may make you feel good and help you become sensitive to your baby's needs, an important part of becoming a parent.

Having an ultrasound

If you have an ultrasound exam this month, you're in for an extraordinary experience. Ultrasound allows you to see your baby's shape and form, including the tiny heart beating in the tiny chest.

Most of the time, babies are completely healthy, and an ultrasound exam is an exciting and rewarding experience. For many moms-to-be, it's as thrilling as first feeling the baby move. Ultrasound also provides fathers with a more direct means of experiencing pregnancy.

Invite your partner to accompany you to your ultrasound exam. This tangible image can strengthen his emotional involvement in your pregnancy and foster his attachment to your baby.

For more details on how an ultrasound exam is performed and what it can show, see "Decision Guide: Understanding prenatal testing" on page 289.

Appointments with your health care provider

Your visit to your health care provider this month will again focus on tracking the growth of your baby, confirming your due date and watching for any problems with your own health. If you remember the date when you first felt your baby move, tell your health care provider. This date will be one more piece of the puzzle in determining your baby's age most accurately.

As during your visit last month, your health care provider will probably also measure the size of your uterus by checking the fundal height — the distance from the top (fundus) of your uterus to your pubic bone. This measurement will help your health care provider be more certain about your baby's age and growth. From your 18th to 34th weeks of pregnancy, your fundal height, in centimeters, will probably equal the number of weeks of your pregnancy.

In addition to performing the fundal height test, your health care provider will probably check your weight and blood pressure and ask you about any signs and symptoms you've been experiencing. During your visit to your health care provider this month, you may have an ultrasound exam. This is also the month when a genetic amniocentesis is done if that is desired. With amniocentesis, a sample of the amniotic fluid is taken from the sac surrounding the baby. This sample can be tested to see if the baby has certain abnormalities, such as Down syndrome.

This month, you may be interested in:
- **"Decision Guide: Understanding prenatal testing," page 289**
- **"Complications: Iron deficiency anemia," page 553**

When to call a health care professional during weeks 17 to 20

Knowing about potential problems and when to contact your health care provider are just as important now as ever before.

WHEN TO CALL

 Here's a guide to possibly troublesome signs and symptoms and when you should notify your health care provider in the fifth month.

Signs or symptoms	When to tell your health care provider
Vaginal bleeding or spotting	
Slight spotting	Same day
Any spotting or bleeding lasting longer than a day	Immediately
Moderate to heavy bleeding	Immediately
Any amount of bleeding accompanied by pain, cramping, fever or chills	Immediately
Passing of tissue	Immediately
Persistent vaginal discharge that is greenish or yellowish, strong smelling or accompanied by redness, itching and irritation around the vulva throughout the day	Within 24 hours
Pain	
Occasional pulling, twinging or pinching sensation on one or both sides of your abdomen	Next visit
Occasional mild headaches	Next visit
A moderate, bothersome headache that doesn't go away after treatment with acetaminophen (Tylenol, others)	Within 24 hours
A severe or persistent headache, especially with dizziness, faintness, nausea or vomiting, or visual disturbances	Immediately
Moderate or severe pelvic pain	Immediately
Any degree of abdominal or pelvic pain that doesn't subside within four hours	Within 24 hours
Leg cramp that awakens you from sleep	Next visit
Leg pain with redness and swelling	Immediately
Pain with fever or bleeding	Immediately

Signs or symptoms	When to tell your health care provider
Vomiting	
Occasional	Next visit
Once every day	Next visit
More than three times a day or with inability to eat or drink between vomiting episodes	Within 24 hours
With pain or fever	Immediately
Other	
Chills or fever (102 F or higher)	Immediately
Painful urination	Same day
Steady or heavy discharge of watery fluid from your vagina	Immediately
Cravings for nonfood substances, such as clay, dirt and laundry starch	Next visit
Consistently low mood, loss of pleasure in things you normally enjoy	Next visit
Above signs and symptoms along with thoughts of harming yourself or others	Immediately
Fatigue and weakness, shortness of breath, heart palpitations, dizziness or lightheadedness	Next visit if occurring occasionally Same day if occurring often

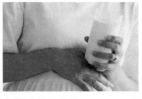

CHAPTER   6

month 6: weeks 21 to 24

Your baby's growth during weeks 21 to 24

Week 21

This week your baby will begin absorbing small amounts of sugars from the amniotic fluid he or she swallows throughout the day. These sugars will pass through your baby's digestive system, which is now developed enough to handle them. Sugars from your amniotic fluid, however, make up only a tiny portion of your baby's nourishment. Most of what your baby needs is still being delivered through your placenta.

Also this week, your baby's bone marrow is starting to make blood cells. The bone marrow works along with the liver and spleen, which have been responsible for making blood cells up to this point.

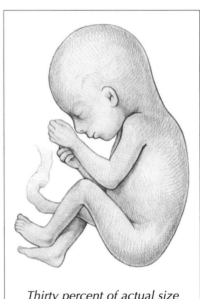

Thirty percent of actual size

Week 22

The senses of taste and touch are making good progress this week. Taste buds are starting to form on your baby's tongue, and your baby's brain and nerve endings are now mature enough to process the sensation of touch. If you could sneak a peek at your baby this week, you might see him or her experimenting with this newfound sense of touch — feeling his or her face, sucking a thumb or touching other body parts. At this point your baby isn't looking for anything in particular but rather is touching whatever comes to hand.

Your baby's reproductive system is continuing to develop, too. If you're having a boy, his testes are beginning to descend from his abdomen this week. If you're having a girl, her uterus and ovaries are now in place, and her vagina is developed. Your baby girl has already made all the eggs she'll need for her own reproductive life.

By 22 weeks into your pregnancy, your baby is about 7½ inches long, head to rump, and weighs about 1 pound.

Week 23

Your baby's lungs are developing rapidly this week, just starting preparation for life on the outside. The lungs are beginning to produce the substance that lines the air sacs in the lungs (surfactant). This substance allows the air sacs to inflate easily. It also keeps them from collapsing and sticking together when they deflate.

If your baby was born before this time, the lungs would have had no chance of working. But now it's possible that the lungs could function outside the womb. However, your baby would need a lot more surfactant to handle breathing air without help.

In addition, the blood vessels in your baby's lungs are growing and developing in preparation for breathing. Your baby is making breathing movements, but these are just trial runs. He or she moves amniotic fluid in and out of the lungs. Your baby is still receiving oxygen through your placenta. There's no air in the lungs until after birth.

Although your baby now looks like a baby, he or she is still slender and delicate looking, with little body fat and thin, wrinkled, loose-hanging skin. When fat production catches up to skin production, your baby will grow into this skin. He or she will look less like a senior citizen and more like an infant.

Babies born at 23 weeks can sometimes survive if they receive the appropriate medical care in a neonatal intensive care unit (NICU). But complications are common and usually serious. The blood vessels in the brain are delicate and immature at 23 weeks, especially in the rapidly growing regions deep in the middle of the brain, called the germinal matrix. The immaturity of these blood vessels increases the risk of spontaneous bleeding in the brain after birth, called intracranial hemorrhage (ICH) or intraventricular hemorrhage (IVH). If this bleeding is severe, it can put babies at risk of developmental problems. In addition, because the retinas of the eyes aren't fully formed until near the end of pregnancy, babies born at 23 weeks can develop an eye problem called retinopathy of prematurity, which can cause impaired vision.

On the bright side, the long-term outlook for premature babies is improving each year as knowledge in the field of fetal medicine continues to grow. As a result, a baby born even as early as 23 weeks can grow up to be a healthy, normal child — if he or she receives top-quality care and is fortunate enough not to develop complications. There's no doubt, though, that the baby is better off staying in the uterus at this age.

Week 24

This week your baby is probably starting to get a sense of whether he or she is upside-down or right side up inside your amniotic sac. That's because your baby's inner ear, which controls balance in the body, is now developed.

Babies born at 24 weeks have a greater than 50-50 chance of survival. The odds get better with every passing week. Still, complications are frequent and serious.

By the 24th week of your pregnancy, your baby is 15 inches long and weighs about 1½ pounds.

Your body during weeks 21 to 24

This month you're starting the second half of your pregnancy. Your uterus will expand beyond your navel, and you'll probably feel your baby's first kicks. These are a far cry from the fluttery, butterflies-in-the-stomach movements of last month. Here's an overview of what's happening and where.

Your hormones
Different hormones are being produced at varying rates to meet the demands of your growing baby. As you move through your pregnancy, your levels of estrogen and progesterone increase to amounts 10 times greater than those of a woman who isn't pregnant.

Throughout the first five months of your pregnancy, your level of progesterone was slightly higher than your level of estrogen. This month your estrogen level is catching up. At 21 or 22 weeks, the two hormones will be at about the same level. By your 24th week, your estrogen level will be slightly higher than your progesterone level.

Your heart and circulatory system
Your blood pressure will probably continue to stay lower than normal this month. After your 24th week, it will likely return to where it was before you were pregnant. Your body is also continuing to make more blood this month. By this time, production of red blood cells should be catching up to

production of plasma — if you're getting enough iron. If you're not getting the 30 milligrams of iron you need each day, you may be at risk of developing iron deficiency anemia.

You may be continuing to experience nasal congestion, nosebleeds and bleeding gums when you brush your teeth. These changes are the result of continued increased blood flow to your nasal passages and gums.

Your respiratory system

To accommodate your increasing lung capacity, your rib cage is enlarging. By the time your baby is born, the distance around your rib cage will have expanded by two to three inches. After your child is born, it will return to its pre-pregnancy size.

Changes in your respiratory system are likely continuing to cause you to breathe slightly faster, but any shortness of breath has probably lessened. Sometimes your breathing will become even easier late in your pregnancy, when your baby begins to move down into your pelvis in preparation for birth.

Your breasts

Your breasts are continuing to grow larger this month and are now probably ready to produce milk. You may see tiny droplets of watery or yellowish fluid appearing on your nipples, even this early. This is early milk (colostrum). It's loaded with active, infection-fighting antibodies from your body. If you breast-feed, colostrum will be your baby's food for the first few days after birth.

Blood vessels in your breasts are continuing to be more visible, too, showing through your skin as pink or blue lines.

Your uterus

This month, perhaps around your 22nd week of pregnancy, your uterus may begin practicing for labor and delivery. It starts exercising its muscle mass to build strength for the big job ahead. These warm-up contractions are called Braxton-Hicks contractions. They're occasional, painless contractions that feel like a squeezing sensation near the top of your uterus or in your lower abdomen and groin.

Braxton-Hicks contractions are also called false labor. That's because they're very different from the contractions involved in true labor. Braxton-Hicks contractions occur on an irregular schedule and vary in length and intensity. True labor contractions follow a pattern, growing longer, stronger and closer together. Braxton-Hicks contractions tend to be concentrated in one area. True labor contractions tend to radiate throughout your abdomen and lower back.

That said, it can be easy to mistake Braxton-Hicks contractions for the real thing. Contact your health care provider if you're having contractions that concern you, especially if they become painful or if you have more than six in an hour. Painful, regular contractions at this stage of your pregnancy may be a sign of preterm labor.

The biggest difference between true labor and Braxton-Hicks contractions is the effect on your cervix. With Braxton-Hicks, your cervix doesn't change. With true labor the cervix begins to open (dilate). You may need to see your health care provider to determine whether the contractions are the real thing.

Your urinary tract

You continue to be at risk of developing a urinary tract infection this month. This is a result of the normal body changes of pregnancy. Slowed urine flow is caused by your growing uterus and "flabbier," progesterone-induced muscle tone in the ureters, which carry urine from your kidneys to your bladder.

If you're urinating even more often than usual, feeling burning on urination or experiencing a fever, abdominal pain or backache, contact your health care provider. These are signs and symptoms of a urinary tract infection, which is a common cause of preterm labor.

Your bones, muscles and joints

The ligaments supporting your abdomen are continuing to stretch this month, and the joints between your pelvic bones are continuing to soften and loosen in preparation for childbirth. In addition, your lower spine is likely continuing to curve backward to help keep you from falling forward from the weight of your growing baby. Together, these changes in your bones, joints and ligaments may be continuing to cause back pain.

Your vagina

You're probably continuing to have thin, white vaginal discharge with little or no odor. It's normal. Many women have increased vaginal discharge during pregnancy.

If, however, your vaginal discharge is greenish or yellowish, strong-smelling or accompanied by redness, itching or irritation of the vulva, there may be cause for concern. These are signs and symptoms of a vaginal infection, also one of the side effects of pregnancy hormones. Call your health care provider if you experience any of these problems.

Weight gain

Once again, you'll probably gain about a pound a week this month, for a total of about 4 pounds. You may gain 1½ pounds one week and only half a pound the next, but that's not cause for concern. As long as your weight gain is remaining relatively stable, without any sudden increases or decreases, you're doing great.

Self-care resources

The changes in your body during the sixth month of pregnancy can produce some unpleasant signs and symptoms. For more information on dealing with common complaints such as back pain, clumsiness, leg cramps and rashes, see Part 3, "Pregnancy Reference Guide" on page 413.

Your emotions during weeks 21 to 24

Confronting your fears

This month you may be starting to have some fears about the process of giving birth. In fact, you may have been having them for a while: "What if I don't make it to the hospital in time? How will I cope with baring myself in front of strangers? What if I lose control during labor? What if there's something wrong with the baby?"

Your partner is probably pondering some of these same questions. Often, parents-to-be have the same concerns as their partners but don't admit it. Each may think he or she must be "strong" for the other. Your partner is probably also worried about something happening to you during labor and delivery.

Childbirth preparation classes are a great place to address these fears. They typically begin between the sixth and seventh months of pregnancy and involve weekly sessions over six to eight weeks. These classes are a unique opportunity. They allow you to talk about your fears with other couples who probably share the same concerns. Plus, they provide you with access to a trained childbirth educator who can address your fears point by point, dispelling myths and providing helpful information. This can lighten your emotional load.

Take time to sit down and make a list of your fears, and ask your partner to do the same. Then compare lists. Share those concerns with your childbirth educator, with the other couples in your class and with your health care provider. Sharing helps. When you share your fears, they have less power over you.

Being intimate with your partner

If you're like many women, you may be more interested in sex now than you were earlier in your pregnancy. You may even be more interested in sex now than you were before you became pregnant. Enjoy this feeling while it lasts — and before your baby arrives to put a significant crimp in your style.

This heightened sexuality is by no means universal, and it's possible you may not feel it at all. As you enter the final months of pregnancy, you may find your desire waning again or waning even further.

Appointments with your health care provider

Your visit to your health care provider this month may focus on tracking the growth of your baby and watching for any problems with your own health.

As during your visit last month, your health care provider can gauge the size of your uterus by checking the fundal height — the distance from the top (fundus) of your uterus to your pubic bone. This month your fundal height will probably be about 21 to 24 centimeters — roughly equal to the number of weeks of your pregnancy.

In addition to performing the fundal height test, your health care provider may check your weight and blood pressure and evaluate your baby's heart rate. Your health care provider may also ask you about any signs and symptoms you may be experiencing.

When to call a health care professional during weeks 21 to 24

Knowing about potential problems and when to contact your health care provider are just as important now as ever before. As always, when in doubt, call.

This month you may be interested in:
- **"Decision Guide: Considering vaginal birth after Caesarean birth,"** **page 345**
- **"Decision Guide: Exploring elective Caesarean birth,"** **page 351**

WHEN TO CALL

Here's a guide to possibly troublesome signs and symptoms and when you should notify your health care provider in the sixth month.

Signs or symptoms	When to tell your health care provider
Vaginal bleeding, spotting or discharge	
Slight spotting	Same day
Any spotting or bleeding lasting longer than a day	Immediately
Moderate to heavy bleeding	Immediately
Any amount of bleeding accompanied by pain, cramping, fever or chills	Immediately
Passing of tissue	Immediately
Persistent vaginal discharge that is greenish or yellowish, strong smelling or accompanied by redness, itching and irritation around the vulva throughout the day	Within 24 hours
Pain	
Occasional pulling, twinging or pinching sensation on one or both sides of your abdomen	Next visit
Occasional mild headaches	Next visit
A moderate, bothersome headache that doesn't go away after treatment with acetaminophen (Tylenol, others)	Within 24 hours
A severe or persistent headache, especially with dizziness, faintness, nausea or vomiting, or visual disturbances	Immediately
Moderate or severe abdominal or pelvic pain	Immediately
Leg cramp that awakens you from sleep	Next visit
Leg cramp with swelling and redness	Immediately
Pain with fever or bleeding	Immediately

Signs or symptoms	When to tell your health care provider
Vomiting	
Occasional	Next visit
Once every day	Next visit
More than three times a day or with inability to eat or drink between vomiting episodes	Within 24 hours
With pain or fever	Immediately
Other	
Chills or fever (102 F or higher)	Immediately
Steady or heavy discharge of watery fluid from your vagina	Immediately
Sudden swelling of your face, hands or feet	Immediately
Visual disturbances (dimness, blurring)	Immediately
Cravings for nonfood substances, such as clay, dirt and laundry starch	Next visit
Consistently low mood, loss of pleasure in things you normally enjoy	Next visit
Above signs and symptoms along with thoughts of harming yourself or others	Immediately
Fatigue and weakness, shortness of breath, heart palpitations, dizziness or lightheadedness	Next visit if occurring occasionally Same day if occurring often
Fainting	Immediately
More frequent urination with pain or burning on urination, fever, abdominal pain or back pain	Same day

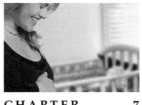

month 7: weeks 25 to 28

Your baby's growth during weeks 25 to 28

Week 25

Your baby's hands are now fully developed, complete with miniature fingernails and the ability to curl his or her fingers into a tiny fist. Your baby is probably using these hands this week to discover different body parts. He or she is exploring the environment and structures inside your uterus, including the umbilical cord. The nerve connections to your baby's hands have a long way to go, though. If she or he wants to grasp a big toe, it won't be an easy task.

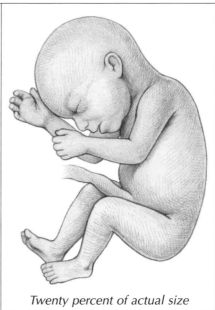

Twenty percent of actual size

Week 26

Your baby's eyebrows and eyelashes are now well formed. The hair on his or her head is longer and more plentiful. Your baby still looks red and wrinkled, but more fat is accumulating under the skin with each passing day. As your baby continues to gain weight over the next 14 weeks until birth, this wrinkly suit of skin will become a better fit.

Your baby's footprints and fingerprints also are formed. All the components that make up the eyes have developed, but your baby probably won't open his or her eyes for about two more weeks. By 26 weeks, your baby weighs between 1 1/2 and 2 pounds.

Week 27

By your 27th week, your baby looks like a thinner, smaller, redder version of what he or she will look like at birth. Your baby's lungs, liver and immune system aren't yet fully mature. If birth were to occur this week, your baby's chances of survival would be at least 85 percent.

Your baby may be starting to recognize your voice this week, as well as your partner's. But it's probably a little hard to hear clearly, given that his or her ears are covered with vernix, the thick, fatty coating that protects the skin from becoming chapped or scratched. It's also hard for your baby to hear through the amniotic fluid in your uterus — similar to how hard it is to hear under water.

At 27 weeks, your baby is three to four times as long as he or she was at 12 weeks.

Week 28

Your baby's eyes, which have been sealed shut for the last few months to allow the retinas to develop, are probably beginning to open and close this week. If you could sneak a peek at your baby this week, you might be able to determine the color of his or her eyes. But this may not be the final word on the subject. Your baby's eye color may change in the first six months of life, especially if his or her eyes are blue or gray-blue at birth.

Your baby's brain also is continuing to develop and expand rapidly this week. In addition, your baby is continuing to accumulate layers of fat underneath the skin.

Your baby is now sleeping and waking on a regular schedule. But this schedule isn't like that of an adult or even of a newborn. At this size, your baby probably sleeps for only 20 to 30 minutes at a time. You probably notice your baby's movements most readily when you're sitting or lying down.

By the 28th week of your pregnancy, the end of your seventh month, your baby is about 10 inches long, crown to rump, and weighs about 2 pounds.

Your body during weeks 25 to 28

This month your uterus will expand to midway between your navel and breasts. Your baby will become increasingly active, especially in the second half of the month. By the end of your 28th week, you'll have completed 70 percent of your pregnancy. The homestretch is near!

Here's an overview of what's happening and where.

Your heart and circulatory system

This month your blood pressure will probably go up, returning to roughly where it was before you were pregnant. In addition, you may feel a fluttering or pounding sensation around your heart. It may feel as if your heart has skipped a beat. This feeling may worry you, but it usually doesn't signify anything serious. This sensation often lessens in the later months of pregnancy.

Still, if you have this feeling, tell your health care provider about it, especially if you're also having chest pain or shortness of breath. Your health care provider may want to run some tests to further evaluate your condition.

Your respiratory system

Stimulated by the hormone progesterone, your lung capacity is continuing to increase this month. This change in your respiratory system allows your blood to carry oxygen in and carbon dioxide out at an increased rate. As a result, you may be continuing to breathe slightly faster and experiencing some shortness of breath.

Your digestive system

Progesterone is continuing to slow the movement of food through your digestive system this month, and your expanding uterus is continuing to crowd and press on your intestines. As a result, you're likely to continue experiencing heartburn or constipation, or both.

Your breasts

The milk-producing glands inside your breasts are continuing to grow larger this month, in preparation for breast-feeding. You may notice that the tiny, bump-like skin glands encircling your areolas are more prominent now, too. This is another way your body is preparing for breast-feeding. When the time comes, these glands will secrete oils to moisturize and soften the skin around your nipples and areolas. This will help keep your nipples from cracking and chafing from the demands of breast-feeding.

Your uterus

This month your uterus will reach roughly the midway point between your navel and breasts. By the time everything is said and done, it will occupy the area from your pubic area to the bottom of your rib cage.

Your baby will probably be increasingly active this month, particularly in the second half of the month. For many babies, the most active time is between 27 and 32 weeks. With this increased activity, you may have trouble telling the difference between practice contractions, true contractions and your baby's kicks or punches.

If you're concerned, remember a couple of things. False labor contractions (Braxton-Hicks) seem to have no rhyme or reason. They vary in length and strength and occur on an irregular schedule, if you can even call it that. True labor contractions follow a pattern. They get longer, stronger and closer together. Plus, true contractions tend to radiate throughout your abdomen and lower back. False contractions tend to be concentrated in one area, usually the top of your uterus or your lower abdomen and groin.

If you're having contractions that concern you, contact your health care provider. This is especially important if your contractions become painful or if you have more than six in an hour. Regular contractions at this stage of your pregnancy may be a sign of preterm labor.

Your urinary tract

Your urine flow is continuing to be slow this month, due to your expanding uterus and relaxed muscles in the tubes carrying urine from the kidneys to the bladder. As a result, you're at continued risk of developing a urinary tract infection. If you're urinating more frequently and also experiencing burning, pain, fever or a change in the odor or color of your urine, you may have an infection. Contact your health care provider. Urinary tract infections are a common cause of preterm labor.

Your bones, muscles and joints

The ligaments supporting your pelvic bones are continuing to become more elastic this month. Ultimately, this will make it easier for your pelvis to expand during childbirth so that your baby can pass through. Now, however, lack of the usual support from these ligaments increases your risk of back strain.

The joints in the pelvis commonly hurt with this newfound flexibility as well. This pain is in the middle-front of your pelvis or on either side of the midline of your back.

If you haven't had back pain up to this point, you may start to have it this month. Back pain affects half of all pregnant women and typically begins between the fifth and seventh months of pregnancy.

You're probably continuing to curve your lower spine backward to compensate for how your center of gravity has shifted under the weight of your baby. If you didn't do this, you might fall over. This change in posture puts a strain on your back muscles and ligaments, and it may be causing back pain.

Your vagina

You may be continuing to notice increased vaginal discharge this month, a side effect of pregnancy hormones on the cells in your vagina. If it's thin and white with little or no odor, there's no cause for concern. If it's greenish or yellowish, strong smelling or accompanied by redness, itching or irritation of the vulva, see your health care provider. You may have a vaginal infection, also one of the side effects of pregnancy hormones. But don't be alarmed. Vaginal infections are common in pregnancy and can be treated.

Weight gain

This month you'll probably continue to gain around a pound a week, for a total of about 4 pounds. If you're concerned about your weight gain, remember this: Most of the weight you're gaining is not fat. It's mostly the weight of your baby, your placenta, your amniotic fluid and the fluid accumulating in your own body tissues.

Self-care resources

The changes in your body during the seventh month of pregnancy can produce some unpleasant signs and symptoms. For more information on dealing with common concerns such as constipation and itchiness, see Part 3, "Pregnancy Reference Guide" on page 413.

Your emotions during weeks 25 to 28

Enjoying pregnancy

This month marks the end of the second trimester of pregnancy. Things will undoubtedly be exciting during the last three months until your baby arrives, but they'll also likely be a bit stressful. You'll be busy buying final supplies, finishing your baby's room, attending childbirth classes and making more frequent visits to your health care provider. Plus, the last three months of pregnancy will bring new physical demands on your body.

Make an effort to really enjoy this month of your pregnancy — before the craziness and discomforts of the final months begin. Take some time to think about your pregnancy thus far and write down your thoughts in a journal. Play soft music or talk soothingly and lovingly to your baby. Take photos so that you can show your baby what you looked like when he or she was "under construction." Do whatever works for you to revel in the emotions and sensations of being pregnant. They'll be gone in just a few short months.

Appointments with your health care provider

During this month's visit, your health care provider may again track the growth of your baby by measuring the size of your uterus. Your fundal height this month — the distance from the top (fundus) of your uterus to your pubic bone — will probably fall between 25 and 28 centimeters — roughly equal to the number of weeks of your pregnancy.

At this month's visit, your health care provider may be able to tell you whether your baby is positioned headfirst or feet- or rump-first in your uterus. Babies in the feet- or rump-first position are in what's known as the breech position. In most cases, these babies need to be delivered by Caesarean birth. Your baby still has lots of time to change position, though, and probably will. So don't be worried if your baby is in the breech position this month.

In addition to checking your baby's size, position and heart rate, your health care provider may again monitor your own health at this month's prenatal visit. He or she can check your weight and blood pressure and ask you about any signs and symptoms you may be experiencing.

You'll also likely have a glucose challenge test to check for gestational diabetes, a temporary form of diabetes that develops in some women who didn't have the condition before they were pregnant. In addition, if you have a rhesus (Rh) factor of Rh negative, you'll probably be tested for Rh antibodies this month. You also may receive your first injection of Rh immunoglobulin (RhIg). A blood test to check for anemia likely will be done as well.

Glucose challenge testing

Glucose challenge testing is usually done between your 26th and 28th weeks of pregnancy, although your health care provider may perform the test earlier if the risk factors warrant it. To complete the test, you'll first drink one full glass of a glucose solution. After about an hour, your health care provider or other health care professional will draw a blood sample from a vein in your arm so that your blood glucose level can be checked. If the results are abnormal, you'll have to come back for a second test called an oral glucose tolerance test.

If you need the second test, you'll be asked to fast overnight. When you arrive at your health care provider's office, you'll then drink another, more concentrated glucose solution. Over the next three hours, your blood will be drawn several times, yielding several different blood glucose measurements. Among women whose first glucose test result was abnormal, studies show that only about 15 percent will be diagnosed with gestational diabetes with this follow-up test.

If you're diagnosed with gestational diabetes, you'll have to work to carefully control your blood glucose for the rest of your pregnancy so that your baby doesn't become too large. You'll also need to have your blood glucose level checked regularly until you give birth. Your health care provider can recommend a treatment plan that's right for you.

Rh antibodies testing

Rh factor is a type of protein found on the surface of red blood cells in most people. More than 85 percent of people have it; they're said to be Rh positive. Those who don't have it are said to be Rh negative.

When you're not pregnant, your Rh status has no effect on your health, and if you're Rh positive, you have no cause for concern during pregnancy either. But if you're Rh negative and your baby is Rh positive — which can happen if your partner is Rh positive — a problem called Rh incompatibility may result.

If you tested Rh negative early in your pregnancy, you can have a blood test for Rh antibodies this month, probably near the end of the month. If results show that you're not producing Rh antibodies, your health care provider can give you an injection of RhIg into a muscle, just as an insurance policy. The RhIg injection will coat any Rh-positive cells that may be floating around in your bloodstream, preventing them from being recognized as foreign. With no Rh factor to fight, antibodies won't form. Think of it as a pre-emptive strike against the formation of Rh antibodies.

When to call a health care professional during weeks 25 to 28

At this point in your pregnancy, you need to be alert to the possibility of preterm labor. Preterm labor means contractions that begin opening (dilating) your cervix before the end of the 37th week. Babies born early usually have a low birth weight, which is defined as less than 5½ pounds. Their low weight and other problems associated with preterm birth put them at risk of several health problems.

Be vigilant for these signs and symptoms of preterm labor:
- Uterine contractions, possibly painless, that feel like abdominal tightening
- Contractions accompanied by low back pain or a feeling of heaviness in your lower pelvis and upper thighs
- Changes in vaginal discharge, such as light spotting or bleeding, watery fluid leaking from your vagina or thick discharge tinged with blood

If you notice more than five uterine contractions in an hour, even if they're not painful, take these steps: Drink a large glass of water and lie down. If you experience six or more contractions in the next hour, contact your health care provider or your hospital or go in. This is especially important if you have bleeding along with cramps or pain. Any vaginal bleeding at this stage of pregnancy may be a warning of preterm labor and needs to be evaluated.

This month you may be interested in:
- "Complications: Preterm labor," page 533
- "Complications: Gestational diabetes," page 547
- "Complications: Rhesus factor incompatibility," page 559

WHEN TO CALL

Here's a guide to possibly troublesome signs and symptoms and when you should notify your health care provider in the seventh month.

Signs or symptoms	When to tell your health care provider
Vaginal bleeding, spotting or discharge	
Slight spotting	Same day
Any spotting or bleeding lasting longer than a day	Immediately
Moderate to heavy bleeding	Immediately
Any amount of bleeding accompanied by pain, cramping, fever or chills	Immediately
Persistent vaginal discharge that's greenish or yellowish, strong smelling, or accompanied by redness, itching and irritation around the vulva throughout the day	Within 24 hours
Pain	
Uterine contractions, more than six each hour for two or more hours	Immediately
Occasional pulling, twinging or pinching sensation on one or both sides of your abdomen	Next visit
Occasional mild headaches	Next visit
A moderate, bothersome headache that doesn't go away after treatment with acetaminophen (Tylenol, others)	Within 24 hours
A severe or persistent headache, especially with dizziness, faintness, nausea or vomiting, or visual disturbances	Immediately
Moderate or severe abdominal or pelvic pain	Immediately
Leg cramp that awakens you from sleep	Next visit
Leg cramp with swelling and redness	Immediately
Pain with fever or bleeding	Immediately

Signs or symptoms	When to tell your health care provider
Vomiting	
Occasional	Next visit*
Once every day	Next visit
More than three times a day or with inability to eat or drink between vomiting episodes	Within 24 hours
With pain or fever	Immediately
Other	
Chills or fever (102 F or higher)	Immediately
Steady or heavy discharge of watery fluid from your vagina	Immediately
Sudden swelling of your face, hands or feet	Same day
Visual disturbances (dimness, blurring)	Immediately
Cravings for nonfood substances, such as clay, dirt and laundry starch	Next visit
Consistently low mood, loss of pleasure in things you normally enjoy	Next visit
Above signs and symptoms along with thoughts of harming yourself or others	Immediately
Fatigue and weakness, shortness of breath, heart palpitations, dizziness or lightheadedness	Next visit if occurring occasionally Same day if occurring often
Fainting	Immediately
More frequent urination with pain or burning on urination, fever, abdominal pain or back pain	Same day

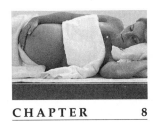

CHAPTER 8

month 8: weeks 29 to 32

Your baby's growth during weeks 29 to 32

Week 29

Your baby's weight and size are continuing to increase this week. As a result, you're probably feeling increased activity inside your uterus, with your baby's movements more frequent and vigorous. Some of your baby's jabs and punches may even take your breath away.

Week 30

Your baby is continuing to steadily add weight and layers of fat. From now until about your 37th week of pregnancy, your baby will gain about a half-pound a week.

Your baby may be practicing breathing movements this week by moving his or her diaphragm in a repeating rhythm. These movements may even give your baby a case of hiccups. As your baby continues making these movements, you may occasionally notice a slight twitching in your uterus, like little spasms.

At 30 weeks into your pregnancy, your baby weighs about 3 pounds and is about 10½ inches long, crown to rump.

Week 31

Your baby's reproductive system is continuing to develop this week. If your baby is a boy, his testicles are moving from their location near the kidneys through the groin on their way into the scrotum. If your baby is a girl, her clitoris is now relatively prominent. However, her labia are still small and don't yet cover it.

Your baby's lungs are now more developed, but they're not yet fully mature. If your baby is born this week, he or she will probably need to stay six weeks or more in a neonatal intensive care unit (NICU) and will need the help of a ventilator to breathe. However, because your baby's brain is more mature than it was several weeks ago, he or she will be at reduced risk of having bleeding in the brain.

Week 32

Lanugo, the layer of soft, downy hair that has grown on your baby's skin for the past few months, is starting to fall off this week. Your baby will probably lose most of his or her lanugo over the next few weeks. Right after your baby's birth, you may see some remnants of it on his or her shoulders or back.

You may notice a change in your baby's movements this week, now that he or she has grown to the point of being crowded inside your uterus. Although your baby is probably moving around just as much, kicks and other movements may seem less forceful.

You may want to check on your baby's movements from time to time, especially if you think you've noticed decreased activity. To do this, lie on your left side for 30 to 60 minutes and keep a tally of how often you feel your baby move. Your baby's kicks or movements may seem a little muffled, given the space constraints inside your uterus. If you notice fewer than 10 movements in two hours, contact your health care provider. A sudden decrease in movement could signal a problem.

By 32 weeks, your baby weighs about 4 pounds and is almost 11½ inches long, crown to rump. Although no one would welcome the early arrival of your baby, it's comforting to know that almost all babies born at this age will survive and have a normal life.

Your body during weeks 29 to 32

This month, your uterus will continue its expansion toward the bottom of your rib cage, creating a new set of physical changes and signs and symptoms. Nearly all of the signs and symptoms of late pregnancy are caused by the expansion of your uterus. Plus, you'll probably start to feel tired again much of the time. Here's an overview of what's happening and where.

Your heart and circulatory system
Your heart and circulatory system are continuing to work overtime to carry oxygen and nutrients to your baby. To meet the demands of your pregnancy, your body is making more blood than it does normally, and your heart is

pumping it faster. As of the beginning of this month, your heart may be beating 20 percent faster than it did before you were pregnant.

Unfortunately, the changes in your circulatory system that support your growing baby may be causing some new and unpleasant side effects for you. As your veins are becoming larger to accommodate your increased blood flow and the baby compresses some of your pelvic veins, you may notice that they're beginning to protrude and become visible as bluish or reddish lines beneath the surface of your skin, particularly on your legs and ankles.

If so, you're not alone. About 20 percent of pregnant women develop varicose veins. They're caused by weaknesses in the valves within the veins that carry blood back to your heart. They typically show up in the later months of pregnancy, when the veins in your legs have expanded and your uterus has grown to the point that it's putting increased pressure on them.

You may also be developing spider veins (vascular spiders). These tiny reddish spots with raised lines branching out from the center, like spider legs, are another consequence of increased blood circulation. You may notice them on your face, neck, upper chest or arms. They'll probably disappear a few weeks after your baby is born.

If you're really unlucky, you may also have hemorrhoids. These are varicose veins in your rectum. They're caused by increased blood volume and increased pressure from your growing uterus on your pelvic veins, which return blood to your heart from your legs and organs of the pelvis. Constipation increases the risk. Some women develop hemorrhoids for the first time during pregnancy. For others, who've had them before, pregnancy makes them larger and more troublesome.

You may also notice that your eyelids and face are becoming puffy, mostly in the morning. This, too, is the result of increased blood circulation. About half of all pregnant women experience this change during the last three months of pregnancy.

Your respiratory system

Your diaphragm — the broad, flat muscle that lies under your lungs — is continuing to be pushed up out of its normal place by your expanding uterus. By the time your baby is born, your diaphragm will have risen about 1 1/2 inches from its normal position.

This month your uterus is pushing up enough that you may feel it's more work to move your diaphragm. As a result, you're probably feeling short of breath, as if you just can't get enough air. This may be a bit disconcerting for you, but there's no need to worry about your baby. Your lung capacities may be rearranged, but because of the effect of progesterone on the respiratory center in your brain, you're breathing more deeply. With each breath, you're taking more air into your lungs than you did before you were pregnant.

Your breasts

Your breasts are continuing to grow this month. Although you may feel at times as if you're carrying all of your extra weight in your breasts, that's not the case. Over the course of your pregnancy, your growing breasts will account for about 1 to 3 pounds of the weight you gain. Only a small portion of this extra weight will be from fat. The majority of the weight you gain in your breasts will come from enlarged milk-producing glands and increased blood circulation.

Since the beginning of the pregnancy, your pituitary gland has been making prolactin, one of the hormones that prepares and stimulates the production of milk from the glands of your breasts.

Over the next couple of weeks, this and other changes will likely cause you to begin making colostrum. Colostrum is the protein-laden substance that will nourish your baby during his or her first few days of life. If you haven't yet started to leak colostrum from your breasts, you may this month.

Your uterus

Your uterus is continuing to expand, causing many of the unpleasant side effects noted above. You may have varicose veins, hemorrhoids, shortness of breath, heartburn and constipation, maybe all in the same week.

Your uterus may be continuing to practice for labor and delivery by producing false labor (Braxton-Hicks contractions). Remember, false labor contractions are a sporadic phenomenon. True labor contractions follow a pattern. They get longer, stronger and closer together. If you're having contractions that concern you, contact your health care provider, especially if they're painful or if you have more than five in an hour. Painful, regular contractions may be a sign of preterm (before the 37th week) labor.

Your urinary tract

Given the increased pressure of your growing uterus on your bladder, you may start leaking urine this month, especially when you laugh, cough or sneeze. This is one of the most annoying side effects of pregnancy, but it won't last forever. It will likely disappear after your baby is born.

You continue to be at risk of developing a urinary tract infection this month, a consequence of slowed urine flow caused by your expanding uterus and relaxed muscles in the ureters that carry urine from your kidneys to your bladder.

If you are urinating more often than normal, are experiencing burning on urination, or have a fever, abdominal pain or backache, contact your health care provider. These are signs and symptoms of urinary tract infection and shouldn't be ignored. Urinary infections can damage your kidneys and provoke preterm labor.

Your vagina

If you have bright red bleeding from your vagina at any time this month, call your health care provider. The bleeding could be a sign of placenta previa, a condition in which the placenta partially or completely covers the inside opening of the cervix and tears away from the cervix as your uterus expands. This condition, which occurs in one in 200 pregnancies, is a medical emergency.

Your bones, muscles and joints

The increased hormones of pregnancy are continuing to soften and loosen the connective tissues in your body. In your pelvic area, the joints between the bones are becoming more relaxed. This is a necessary preparation for childbirth, but it may be causing hip pain, probably just on one side. Low back pain caused by your growing uterus may be adding to your discomfort.

Your growing uterus may also be putting pressure on your two sciatic nerves, which run from your lower back down your legs to your feet. This may be causing pain, tingling or numbness running down your buttocks, hips or thighs — a condition called sciatica. Sciatica is unpleasant, but it's temporary and generally not serious. When your baby changes position closer to the time of delivery, your sciatic pain will likely lessen.

Your skin

In addition to varicose veins and vascular spiders, some other skin changes may begin to appear this month. The skin across your abdomen may be dry and itchy from all of the stretching and tightening. About 20 percent of pregnant women have itchiness on their abdomen or all over their bodies.

If your itching is severe and you have reddish, raised patches on your skin, you may have a condition called PUPPP, which stands for pruritic urticarial papules and plaques of pregnancy. PUPPP affects about one out of every 150 pregnant women. It usually appears first on the abdomen and then spreads to the arms, legs, buttocks or thighs. Scientists aren't sure what causes PUPPP, but it tends to run in families. It's also more common among women who are pregnant for the first time and among women carrying twins or other multiples. PUPPP can be treated with prescription medications.

You may also be starting to notice pink, reddish or purplish indented streaks on the skin covering your breasts, abdomen, or perhaps even upper arms, buttocks or thighs. These are stretch marks, and up to half of all pregnant women get them. Contrary to popular belief, stretch marks aren't necessarily related to weight gain. They seem to be caused, quite literally, by a stretching of the skin, coupled with a normal increase in the hormone cortisol, which may weaken the elastic fibers of your skin. Scientists think your genes play the biggest role in determining whether you'll get stretch marks.

There's nothing you can do to prevent stretch marks. Because they develop from deep within the connective tissue under your skin, applying creams or ointments to your skin will have no effect. With time, they'll fade to light pink or grayish stripes. But they won't completely disappear.

Your hair

You may notice this month that your hair seems fuller and more luxuriant. This is the result of a pregnancy-induced change in your hair's growth cycle.

Normally, hair grows about a half-inch each month for two to eight years. It then goes into a resting phase, stops growing and eventually falls out. During pregnancy, hairs tend to remain in the resting phase longer. Because fewer hairs fall out each day, you have a fuller head of hair.

If this is happening to you, enjoy it while it lasts. Once your baby is born, your hair's resting phase will shorten, and you'll lose more hairs each day. For a few months, your hair may even feel thinner. Your hair will then return to normal, typically within six months to a year.

Weight gain

You'll probably gain about a pound a week this month, for a total of about 4 pounds. As the month progresses, you may notice some burning, numbness, tingling or pain in your hands. These are symptoms of carpal tunnel syndrome, a consequence of weight gain and swelling in pregnancy that affects up to 25 percent of pregnant women.

With the extra weight and fluid in your body, the nerve inside the carpal tunnel in your wrist can become compressed, causing the telltale carpal tunnel symptoms. The effects of carpal tunnel syndrome may be disturbing, but they'll probably disappear after your baby is born.

Self-care resources

The changes in your body during the eighth month of pregnancy can produce some unpleasant signs and symptoms. For more information on dealing with common complaints such as carpal tunnel, sciatica, skin changes, or varicose veins, see Part 3, "Pregnancy Reference Guide" on page 413.

Your emotions during weeks 29 to 32

Conquering anxiety

In just a few weeks, you'll be responsible for a new human being. That fact is probably really starting to sink in this month. As a result, you may be feeling anxious and overwhelmed, especially if this is your first baby. To help keep anxiety at bay, review the decisions that need to be made before your baby is born. Is your baby going to see a pediatrician or a family doctor? Are you going to breast-feed or use formula? If your baby is a boy, are you going to have him circumcised? Taking stock of where you stand on these issues will help you feel more in control of the situation now. Plus, it will make your new responsibilities seem less daunting once your baby arrives.

The anxiety or even the natural anticipation you're feeling about your baby's arrival may be making it difficult for you to get to sleep or sleep through the night. If you're feeling restless or anxious at night, try some of the relaxation exercises you've learned in childbirth classes. They may help you get some rest, and doing them now will be good practice for the big event.

Appointments with your health care provider

This month's visit to your health care provider will likely be your last once-a-month visit. Next month, you'll probably see your health care provider every two weeks and then once a week until your baby is born. During your visit this month, your health care provider can again check your blood pressure and weight and ask you about any signs and symptoms you may be having. You'll probably also be asked to describe your baby's activity "schedule" and movements.

As during other visits, your health care provider can also track the growth of your baby by measuring the size of your uterus. Your fundal height measurements this month — the distance from the top (fundus) of your uterus to your pubic bone — will probably measure between 29 and 32 centimeters — roughly equal to the number of weeks of your pregnancy.

REMEMBER THE SIGNS AND SYMPTOMS OF PRETERM LABOR

The risk of preterm labor continues this month. Here's a reminder of the signs and symptoms to watch for:
- Uterine contractions — possibly painless — that feel like a tightening in your abdomen
- Contractions accompanied by low back pain or a feeling of heaviness in your lower pelvis and upper thighs
- Changes in vaginal discharge, such as light spotting or bleeding, watery fluid leaking from your vagina or thick discharge tinged with blood

If you notice more than six contractions in an hour, even if they're not painful, contact your health care provider or your hospital. This is especially important if you have vaginal bleeding along with abdominal cramps or pain.

This month, you may also be interested in:
- "Decision Guide: Considering circumcision for your son," page 355
- "Decision Guide: Choosing your baby's health care provider," page 359
- "Decision Guide: The breast or the bottle?" page 363

WHEN TO CALL

Here's a guide to possibly troublesome signs and symptoms and when you should notify your health care provider in the eighth month.

Signs or symptoms	When to tell your health care provider
Vaginal bleeding, spotting or discharge	
Any amount of bleeding	Immediately
Persistent vaginal discharge that's greenish or yellowish, strong smelling, or accompanied by redness, itching and irritation around the vulva throughout the day	Within 24 hours
Pain	
Uterine contractions, more than six each hour for two or more hours	Immediately
Occasional pulling, twinging or pinching sensation on one or both sides of your abdomen	Next visit
Occasional mild headaches	Next visit
A moderate, bothersome headache that doesn't go away after treatment with acetaminophen (Tylenol, others)	Within 24 hours
A severe or persistent headache, especially with dizziness, faintness, nausea or vomiting, or visual disturbances	Immediately
Moderate or severe abdominal or pelvic pain	Immediately
Leg cramp that awakens you from sleep	Next visit
Leg cramp with swelling and redness	Immediately
Pain with fever or bleeding	Immediately
Vomiting	
Occasional	Next visit
Once every day	Next visit
More than three times a day or with inability to eat or drink between vomiting episodes	Within 24 hours
With pain or fever	Immediately

Signs or symptoms	When to tell your health care provider
Other	
Chills or fever (102 F or higher)	Immediately
Steady or heavy discharge of watery fluid from your vagina	Immediately
Sudden swelling of your face, hands or feet	Same day
Visual disturbances (dimness, blurring)	Immediately
Cravings for nonfood substances, such as clay, dirt and laundry starch	Next visit
Consistently low mood, loss of pleasure in things you normally enjoy	Next visit
Above signs and symptoms along with thoughts of harming yourself or others	Immediately
Fatigue and weakness, shortness of breath, heart palpitations, dizziness or lightheadedness	Next visit if occurring occasionally Same day if occurring often
Fainting	Immediately
More frequent urination with pain or burning on urination, fever, abdominal pain or back pain	Same day

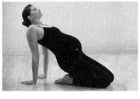

CHAPTER   9

month 9: weeks 33 to 36

Your baby's growth during weeks 33 to 36

Week 33

Your baby is continuing to gain weight at a fairly rapid rate, putting on about a half-pound a week. In fact, the next four weeks will be a period of extraordinary growth. As your pregnancy approaches term next month, your baby will begin to gain weight a bit more slowly.

The pupils of your baby's eyes are now well developed enough to constrict, dilate and detect light. Your baby's lungs are much more completely developed, which allows for some optimism if he or she is born this week. Babies born at this stage need extra care, but almost all will be healthy.

Week 34

The white, waxy coating protecting your baby's skin (vernix) is becoming thicker this week. When your baby is born, you may see traces of vernix first-hand, especially under your baby's arms, behind the ears and in the groin area.

At the same time, the soft, downy hair that has grown on the skin for the past several months (lanugo) is now almost completely gone.

At 34 weeks into your pregnancy, your baby weighs about 5 1/2 pounds and is about 12 1/2 inches long, crown to rump.

Week 35

Your baby is continuing to pack on the pounds, accumulating fat all over his or her body, especially around the shoulders. In fact, the next three weeks will likely be your baby's most rapid period of weight gain, with weekly gains of up to a half-pound.

Given the crowded conditions inside your uterus, you may feel fewer of your baby's movements this week. Crowding may make it harder for this bigger, stronger baby to give you a punch, but you'll probably feel lots of stretches, rolls and wiggles.

Week 36

By this week, your baby has almost completely grown into that once-wrinkly skin. If you could sneak a peek at your baby this week, you'd see an infant you could almost describe as plump, with a little but fully rounded face. The fullness of your baby's face is the result of recent fat deposits and powerful sucking muscles that are fully developed and ready for action.

At 36 weeks into your pregnancy, the end of your ninth month, your baby weighs about 6 pounds or a little more.

Your body during weeks 33 to 36

Your body is working hard this month to prepare for labor and delivery. Your baby is big and may be disturbing your sleep. Your muscles are sore from carrying this large bundle. Put it all together, and you're probably feeling tired most of the time. If you're worn out, take a break. Rest with your feet up. Fatigue is your body's way of telling you to slow down.

Here's an overview of what's happening and where.

Your respiratory system
Pushed up by your expanding uterus, your diaphragm is continuing to occupy part of the space normally reserved for your lungs, altering the way you breathe. As a result, you're probably continuing to feel as if you can't get enough air. If your baby drops lower into your uterus and pelvis this month, as some do, this will probably change. With some of the upward pressure on your diaphragm relieved, you may be able to breathe a little more easily.

Your breasts
The milk-producing glands inside your breasts are continuing to grow larger this month, increasing your breast size overall. The tiny oil-producing glands that moisturize the skin around your nipples and areolas may be more noticeable now, too.

Your uterus
This month, your baby is settling into position inside your uterus, getting ready to make his or her grand entrance. If your baby is in the proper posi-

tion, as most are, his or her head is down, with arms and legs pulled up tightly against the chest.

You may feel your baby drop this month, settling deeper into your pelvis in preparation for delivery. This is what's known as lightening, although that's a somewhat misleading term. Although your upper abdomen may feel relief, that's usually more than compensated for by increased pressure in the pelvis, hips and bladder.

Some women, especially first-time moms, experience lightening several weeks before delivery. Others experience it the day labor begins. It's hard to say when your baby will drop in the pelvis or if you'll notice it when it happens.

Your digestive system

If your baby drops this month, you may notice a change in some of your gastrointestinal problems such as heartburn or constipation. You may feel more like eating because your baby is no longer putting as much pressure on your stomach and intestines. If you've been having heartburn, it may become less frequent or less severe.

Your urinary tract

You're probably continuing to leak urine this month, especially when you laugh, cough or sneeze. This problem is the result of your growing baby pressing on your bladder.

The bad news? If your baby drops this month, your urinary problems are likely to intensify. As your baby moves deeper into your pelvis, you'll feel more pressure on your bladder. Suffice it to say that you'll become very familiar with the bathroom. In the final weeks of your pregnancy, you may wake up several times a night just to urinate. This all will most likely disappear after your baby is born.

Your bones, muscles and joints

The connective tissues in your body are continuing to soften and loosen this month in preparation for labor and delivery. This may be especially noticeable now in your pelvic area. You may feel as if your legs are becoming detached from the rest of your body — for the record, they're not.

Don't give up your exercise program, but be careful about exercising this month. Given all the softening and loosening going on, it's easy to suffer a muscle or joint injury.

You may be continuing to have hip pain on one side or low back pain caused by your growing uterus. You may also be having sciatic pain — tingling or numbness in your buttocks, hips or thighs caused by the pressure of your uterus on your two sciatic nerves. If your baby drops this month, though, this pain may let up.

Your vagina

Your cervix may begin to dilate this month. About the time that begins, you may feel a sharp, stabbing pain in your vagina. This doesn't mean you're in labor. The cause of this pain isn't well understood, but it doesn't pose a threat to you or your baby.

Your cervix can start to dilate weeks, days or hours before labor begins. Especially if you've had a baby before, it might not dilate at all before labor. Every woman is different.

Vaginal pain late in pregnancy usually isn't anything to be concerned about, but tell your health care provider about it if it causes a lot of discomfort. One caution: Don't mistake vaginal pain for abdominal pain. If pain in your lower abdomen is accompanied by fever, chills, diarrhea or bleeding, call your health care provider.

Remember, you'll almost certainly have some contractions (labor pains) this month. It's possible they won't bother you at all, and you may not even notice them. If you do feel cramps at the same time as the uterus seems to ball up and get hard, pay attention to how regular and frequent the contractions are. Practice contractions are unpredictable and, even when frequent, they don't settle into a regular rhythm. The contractions of true labor are frequent — five minutes apart or closer — and are repeated at regular intervals.

Your skin

Pregnancy-induced skin changes that may be apparent this month include:
- Varicose veins, particularly on your legs and ankles
- Vascular spiders, especially on your face, neck, upper chest or arms
- Dryness and itching on your abdomen or all over your body
- Stretch marks on the skin covering your breasts, abdomen, upper arms, buttocks or thighs

Many of these changes will fade or disappear after your baby is born. Some evidence of stretch marks will likely remain, although they usually fade to light pink or grayish stripes.

Weight gain

You'll probably gain about a pound a week this month, for a total of about 4 pounds. When you reach term next month, you'll probably have gained a total of about 25 to 35 pounds.

Self-care resources

The changes in your body during the ninth month of pregnancy can produce some unpleasant signs and symptoms. For more information on dealing with common complaints such as heartburn, clumsiness, sciatica and shortness of breath, see Part 3, "Pregnancy Reference Guide" on page 413.

Preparing your body for labor

You can do certain exercises this month and next that may help make your body ready for labor. These exercises, described below, concentrate on the muscles that will receive the most stress during labor and delivery.

Kegel exercises

Why do them?

The muscles in your pelvic floor help support your uterus, bladder and bowel. Toning them by doing Kegel exercises will help ease your discomfort during the last months of your pregnancy and may help minimize two common problems that can begin during pregnancy and continue afterward: leakage of urine and hemorrhoids. In fact, a recent study found that strengthening your pelvic floor muscles during pregnancy appears to reduce your risk of developing urinary incontinence, both during and after pregnancy.

How to do them

Identify your pelvic floor muscles — the muscles around your vagina and anus. To make sure you've found the right muscles, try to stop the flow of urine while you're going to the bathroom. If you stop it, you've found the right muscles. Don't make this a habit, though. Doing Kegel exercises while urinating or when your bladder is full can actually weaken the muscles. It can also lead to incomplete emptying of the bladder, which can increase your risk of developing a urinary tract infection.

If you're having trouble finding the right muscles, try a different technique. Place a finger inside your vagina and feel your vagina tighten when you squeeze. The muscles you squeezed are your pelvic floor muscles.

Once you've identified your pelvic floor muscles, empty your bladder and get into a sitting or standing position. Then firmly tense your pelvic floor muscles. Try it at frequent intervals for five seconds at a time, four or five times in a row. Work up to where you can keep the muscles contracted for 10 seconds at a time, relaxing for 10 seconds between contractions. Do three sets of 10 Kegel exercises throughout the day, and also do three sets of mini-Kegels. Count quickly to 10 or 20, contracting and relaxing your pelvic floor muscles each time you say a number.

While you're doing Kegel exercises, don't flex the muscles in your abdomen, thighs or buttocks. This can actually worsen the muscle tone of your pelvic floor muscles. And don't hold your breath. Just relax and focus on contracting the muscles around your vagina and anus.

Tailor sitting

Why do it?

Tailor sitting improves your posture and strengthens and stretches the muscles in your back, thighs and pelvis. It can help keep your pelvic joints flexible, improve blood flow to your lower body and may make for an easier delivery.

How to do it

Sit on the floor with your back straight and bring the bottoms of your feet together, your heels in toward your groin area. Let your knees drop comfortably out to the side so that you feel a stretch in your inner thighs. Don't bounce your knees up and down.

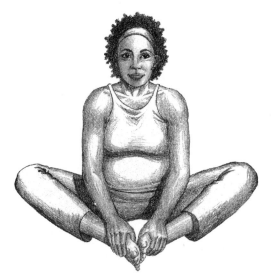

This exercise isn't as hard as it sounds. Pregnancy tends to make your joints more flexible. But if it's too hard for you, try sitting against a wall to support your back, putting cushions under each thigh or just sitting with your legs crossed and changing the front leg from time to time. Keep your back straight.

Squat and wall slide

Why do them?

If you're able to squat every few minutes or so during labor, it may help open your pelvic outlet, allowing more room for your baby to descend. Squatting during labor is tiring, so you might want to prepare by strengthening the muscles needed. Practice squatting frequently during these last months of pregnancy. An exercise called a wall slide also may be helpful.

How to do them

Squat. Stand with your feet about shoulder-width apart. Slowly lower into a squat position, keeping your back straight and your heels flat on the floor. If your heels start to come up, widen your stance. Hold the squat for 10 to 30 seconds, resting your hands on your knees. Slowly stand back up, pushing up from your knees with your arms. Repeat five times.

Wall slide. Stand with your back against a wall, your feet about shoulder-width apart. Slide down the wall until you're in a sitting position, but don't slide down so far that your knees jut out over your toes. Rest your hands on your thighs for better balance, and keep your knees and feet pointing forward. Hold the position for a few seconds and then slide back up. Repeat three to five times, gradually working up to 10 repetitions.

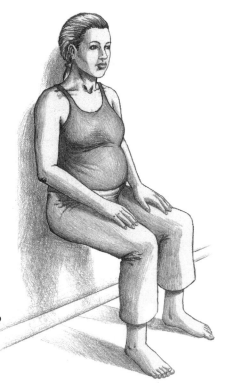

Pelvic tilt

Why do it?
This exercise strengthens the muscles in your abdomen, helps relieve backache during pregnancy and labor, and may help make for an easier delivery. Pelvic tilts can also improve the flexibility of your back and help prevent back pain.

How to do it
Get down on your hands and knees with your head in line with your back. Tilt your hips forward and pull in your abdomen, rounding your back slightly. Hold the position for several seconds, then relax your abdomen and back, keeping your back relatively flat. Don't let your back sag. Repeat three to five times, working up to 10 repetitions.

You can also do pelvic tilts while standing up. Stand up straight with your back against a wall and push the small of your back against the wall. Or simply stand up straight and rock your pelvis back and forth.

Perineal massage

Why do it?
Massaging the area between your vaginal opening and anus (perineum) in the last weeks before labor may help to stretch these tissues in preparation for childbirth. This may help minimize stinging when your baby's head

emerges from your vaginal opening. It may even help you avoid the need for an incision in your perineum that enlarges your vaginal opening (episiotomy) as the baby's head is emerging. Midwives have long recommended perineal massage. There isn't yet definitive evidence that it prevents trauma to the perineum, but some studies have shown promising results.

How to do it

Wash your hands thoroughly with soap and hot water and make sure your nails are trimmed. Then put K-Y jelly or some other mild lubricant on your thumbs and insert them inside your vagina. Press downward toward the rectum, stretching the tissues. Repeat daily for about eight to 10 minutes. Your partner can help with this process, if you wish. You may experience a little burning or other discomfort as you massage your perineum. This is normal. However, stop if you feel sharp pain.

A couple of additional points: You don't have to practice perineal massage if the idea of it makes you feel uncomfortable. And if you do it, it's no guarantee that you won't have an episiotomy. Certain birth situations, such as those involving a large baby or a baby in an abnormal position, require an episiotomy for the safety of the baby. You'll just have to wait and see what your experience of labor and childbirth brings.

Your emotions during weeks 33 to 36

Preparing for labor

You're probably thinking a lot this month about when labor will start and how your childbirth experience will go. A growing sense of tension during this time is understandable, as are worries and fears about whether your baby will be healthy.

You may also be spending some time contemplating the coming pain of childbirth. How bad will it be, really? How long will it last? How will I cope? These questions may be particularly persistent if this is your first baby.

It's natural to feel a bit anxious about labor and childbirth. After all, there isn't any way of knowing in advance just how your labor will go. But realize that women go through labor and give birth every day. It's a natural process.

You can do things now that can help you prepare for labor.

- Educate yourself. Knowing what's going to happen to your body when you give birth will likely make you less tense and fearful as it actually happens. With less fear and tension, your pain may be less, too. Childbirth classes are an excellent place to meet other moms-to-be and learn about the changes your body goes through in labor and childbirth.

- Talk with women who have had positive birth experiences. Learn what techniques worked for them during the labor and childbirth process.
- Tell yourself that you'll just do the best you can, given your circumstances and strengths. There's no right or wrong way to have a baby.
- Familiarize yourself with the various pain-relief options that will be available to you during labor. Try not to develop fixed ideas about what you'll use and what you won't. Until you're actually in the moment, you won't know what your needs will be. For more information on pain relief during labor, see "Decision Guide: Understanding pain relief choices in childbirth" on page 325.

Appointments with your health care provider

You'll probably see your health care provider twice this month, an increase from the once-a-month visits you've had up to this point. As during previous visits, your health care provider will likely check your weight and blood pressure, as well as the activity and movements of your baby. Your health care provider will likely also measure your uterus and ask you about any signs and symptoms you may be experiencing. Your uterus will probably measure between 33 and 34 centimeters in the first half of this month — roughly equal to the number of weeks of your pregnancy. After that, your fundal height won't track quite so closely with the number of weeks of your pregnancy.

Your health care provider will likely screen you for group B streptococcus (GBS), which typically lives harmlessly in the body. A culture taken from just inside the vaginal and rectal area is tested for the bacterium. Although GBS poses no risk to you, women who harbor it may pass the bacterium to their babies during labor and delivery. If GBS is found, antibiotics will likely be given to you once you go into labor.

During your visits this month, your health care provider may also check the baby's position. By the 33rd week of your pregnancy, your baby probably will have moved into the position he or she will be in for delivery, whether it's headfirst, rump first or feet first. If you've had several children, though, there's a greater possibility that your baby may change position in the final weeks.

To determine how your baby is positioned inside your uterus, your health care provider can check to see which part of your baby's body is farthest down in your pelvis, ready to be born first. This is called the presenting part. In most cases, it's the baby's head.

To determine your baby's presentation, at most visits your health care provider likely will attempt to feel the baby's position through the outside of the abdomen. As your due date nears, your health care provider may perform a vaginal exam if there's uncertainty about the baby's position. With a vaginal exam, your health care provider reaches inside the vagina to feel which part of the baby is above the opening to the cervix. If your health care provider is still uncertain about the baby's position, an ultrasound may be used to determine the presenting part.

If your baby is positioned headfirst, you're good to go. If your baby is positioned rump first or feet first, there may be problems ahead. This is what's called breech presentation, and it's a major cause of Caesarean births.

If your baby is in a breech position and isn't already too far down in your pelvis, your health care provider may recommend trying to turn the baby into the proper position in a few weeks. This procedure is called an external version, and it works about like you'd think it would. Your health care provider applies pressure to your abdomen to try to move your baby into the proper headfirst position. Medication is often used to relax the uterus and relieve pain. External version is generally tried two to four weeks before the due date.

When to call a health care professional during weeks 33 to 36

Your pregnancy is nearly over — your baby will be here before you know it. However, it's still important to know about problems that could arise and when to contact your health care provider. When in doubt, call.

This month you may be interested in:
- "Decision Guide: Understanding pain relief choices in childbirth," page 325
- "Complications: Preterm labor," page 533
- "Complications: Group B streptococcus," page 563

When to call

Here's a guide to possibly troublesome signs and symptoms and when you should notify your health care provider in the ninth month.

Signs or symptoms	When to tell your health care provider
Vaginal bleeding, spotting or discharge	
Vaginal bleeding greater than spotting	Same day
Pain	
Uterine contractions, more than six each hour for two or more hours	Immediately
Occasional pulling, twinging or pinching sensation on one or both sides of your abdomen	Next visit
Occasional mild headaches	Next visit
A moderate, bothersome headache that doesn't go away after treatment with acetaminophen (Tylenol, others)	Within 24 hours
A severe or persistent headache, especially with dizziness, faintness or visual disturbances	Immediately
Moderate or severe abdominal or pelvic pain	Same day
Pain with fever or bleeding	Immediately
Vomiting	
Occasional	Next visit
Once every day	Next visit
More than three times a day or with inability to eat or drink between vomiting episodes	Within 24 hours
With pain or fever	Immediately
Other	
Chills or fever (102 F or higher)	Immediately
Steady or heavy discharge of watery fluid from your vagina	Immediately
Sudden swelling of your face, hands and feet	Immediately
Sudden weight gain	Same day
Visual disturbances (dimness, blurring)	Immediately
Severe shortness of breath	Immediately
Severe itching	Next visit
More frequent urination with burning, fever, abdominal pain or back pain	Same day

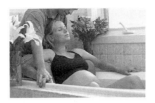

CHAPTER   10

month 10: weeks 37 to 40

I think nature's way of making moms-to-be look forward to labor is to make the final month so uncomfortable. I'm ready. After all, I've managed nine months of pregnancy. I can handle whatever comes next.

— *One mom's experience*

Your baby's growth during weeks 37 to 40

Week 37

By the end of this week, your baby will be considered full-term. He or she isn't quite done growing yet, but the rate of weight gain has slowed to about a half-ounce a day. As fat is being laid down, your baby's body is slowly becoming rounder.

Sex seems to play some role in determining size at birth. If you have a boy, he'll likely weigh a bit more than a baby girl born to you at a similar length of gestation.

Week 38

For several weeks now, your baby's development has been more about improving the function of organs than about their construction. Your baby's brain and nervous system are working better every day, but this developmental process continues through childhood and even into the later teen years. This is why exposure to drugs or alcohol may damage a baby profoundly without changing his or her appearance. This month, your baby's brain has prepared to manage the complicated jobs of breathing, digesting, keeping the right heart rate and eating.

At 38 weeks into your pregnancy, your baby weighs about 6 pounds, 13 ounces and is about 14 inches long, crown to rump.

Week 39

By this week, your baby has lost most of the vernix and lanugo that used to cover the skin, although you may see traces of them at birth.

Your baby now has enough fat laid down under the skin to hold his or her body temperature as long as there's a little help from you. This gives the baby the familiar healthy, chubby look seen at birth.

Even though the body has been catching up, the baby's head is still its largest part, and that's why it's best when babies are born headfirst.

In addition, this week your placenta is continuing to supply your baby with antibodies — protein substances that help protect against bacteria and viruses. During the first six months of your baby's life, these antibodies will help your baby's immune system stave off infections. Some of these same antibodies will be provided after birth through breast milk.

By the 39th week of pregnancy, your baby weighs about 7 to 7 1/2 pounds, but by now individual differences in babies are becoming dramatic. It's normal for a 39-week-old baby to weigh from 6 to 9 pounds.

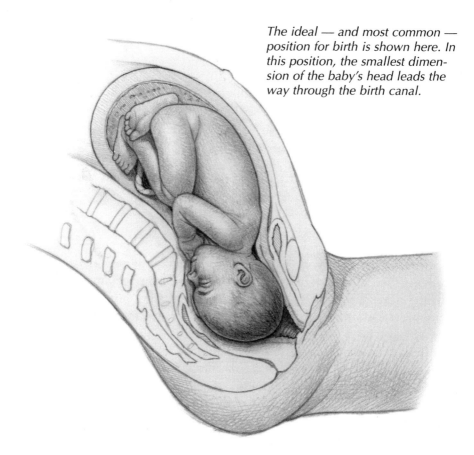

The ideal — and most common — position for birth is shown here. In this position, the smallest dimension of the baby's head leads the way through the birth canal.

Week 40

Your due date will arrive this week, but chances are good that it'll come and go without incident. Doctors and scientists estimate that only 5 percent of women deliver on their due dates. It's just as normal to have your baby a week late as it is to have him or her a week early. Try to be patient, although with all the work you've done, that's not easy!

Once labor starts, your baby will experience many changes in order to prepare for birth, including a surge in hormones. This may help maintain blood pressure and blood sugar levels after birth. It may also have something to do with communicating to your uterus that the time has come.

With labor, your baby is prepared for the blood flow to the placenta to be decreased a bit with each contraction. Your baby can coast through these interruptions so long as they aren't too frequent and don't last too long. The changes your baby will experience at birth are truly amazing. All that has gone before is prologue to this wonderful, glorious event.

At 40 weeks, the average baby weighs about 7 to 8 pounds and measures about 18 to 20½ inches long with legs fully extended. Your own baby may have a weight and size of less or more and still be normal and healthy.

Your body during weeks 37 to 40

Before you were pregnant, your uterus weighed only about 2 ounces and could hold less than a half-ounce. At term, it will have multiplied in weight by a factor of 20, to about 2½ pounds and will have stretched to hold your baby, your placenta and about a quart of amniotic fluid. At the end of this month, after 40 weeks of growth and change, you'll go through labor and delivery, giving birth to a new human being — your one-of-a-kind baby.

Here's an overview of what's happening and where:

Your respiratory system
You may still be having some shortness of breath. If your baby drops lower into your pelvis before labor begins, which is more common among first-time moms, you may feel less pressure on your diaphragm. As a result, you may be able to breathe more deeply and easily during your final weeks of pregnancy.

Your digestive system
Your digestive system remains slowed this month, influenced by hormones. As a result, you may still be experiencing heartburn and constipation. If your baby drops this month, this situation may improve. With less pressure on your stomach, digestion may be easier.

Your breasts

Stimulated by estrogen and progesterone, your breasts will reach their full size this month. As delivery time approaches, your nipples may start leaking colostrum — the yellowish milk your breasts first produce.

As your breasts have grown over the course of your pregnancy, your nipples may have become inverted, dimpling back into your breasts. If you have inverted nipples and are planning to breast-feed, don't worry. You can use some special techniques to prepare your nipples for breast-feeding. Ask your health care provider or lactation consultant for more information.

Your uterus

This month, your uterus will finish its expansion. When you reach term, it will extend from your pubic area to the bottom of your rib cage. If your baby hasn't already dropped lower into your pelvis, that may happen this month. If this is your first baby, you may experience lightening weeks before you ever go into labor. If you've been through childbirth before, lightening and the onset of labor will probably happen closer together.

Your urinary tract

This month, you'll probably again feel the need to urinate more frequently, as your baby moves deeper into your pelvis and presses on your bladder. You may find it hard to get a good night's sleep because you have to get up so often to urinate. You're probably also continuing to leak urine, especially when you laugh, cough or sneeze. Hang in there. Your pregnancy is almost over.

Your bones, muscles and joints

The aptly named hormone relaxin, which is produced by your placenta, is continuing to relax and loosen the ligaments holding your three pelvic bones together. This will allow your pelvis to open wider during childbirth — hopefully wide enough to accommodate your baby's head as it passes through. For now, you're probably continuing to feel the effects of relaxin in clumsiness and loose-feeling limbs.

If your baby drops a couple of weeks before labor begins, which is more common among first-time moms, you may also feel some pressure or aches and pains in your pelvic joints.

Your vagina

At some point in the next several weeks, your cervix will begin to open (dilate). It may start a couple of weeks before labor begins, or just a few hours. Ultimately, your cervical opening will stretch from zero to 10 centimeters in diameter so that you can push your baby out. As your cervix begins dilating, you may feel an occasional sharp, stabbing pain inside your vagina. You may also feel pressure, aches or sharp twinges in your perineal area — the area between your vaginal opening and anus — as your baby's head presses on your pelvic floor.

When your cervix begins to thin and relax, you may lose the mucous plug that's been blocking your cervical opening during your pregnancy to keep bacteria from getting into your uterus. There isn't a strong relationship between the loss of the mucous plug and the beginning of labor. It can happen up to two weeks before labor begins — or it can happen right before. When it happens, you'll likely notice that you have thick vaginal discharge or stringy mucus that's clear, pink or blood tinged. Don't worry if you don't notice this change. Some women don't even realize it when they've lost their mucous plug.

For about 10 percent of pregnant women, the amniotic sac breaks or leaks before labor begins, and the fluid that has cushioned the baby comes out as a trickle or a gush. If this happens to you, follow your health care provider's instructions. He or she will probably want to evaluate you and your baby as soon as your membranes rupture (water breaks). In the meantime, don't do anything that could introduce bacteria into your vagina. That means no tampons or sexual intercourse.

If the fluid coming from your vagina is anything other than clear and colorless, let your health care provider know. Vaginal fluid that's greenish or foul smelling, for example, could be a sign of uterine infection or that your baby has passed a bit of stool into the fluid.

Your skin

You may be continuing to experience the following pregnancy-induced skin changes this month:

- Varicose veins, particularly on your legs and ankles
- Vascular spiders, especially on your face, neck, upper chest or arms
- Dryness and itching on your abdomen or all over your body
- Stretch marks on the skin covering your breasts, abdomen, upper arms, buttocks or thighs

Many of these changes will fade or disappear after your baby is born, although evidence of stretch marks will remain.

Weight gain

Your baby is gaining weight more slowly this month. As a result, you may notice that your own weight gain has slowed or even stopped. It is even quite common to lose a pound or so at the very end of the pregnancy. By the time you reach term on your due date, you'll probably have gained a total of roughly 25 to 35 pounds. Here's a breakdown of how that weight may be distributed:

Your baby	6½ to 9 pounds
Placenta	1½ pounds
Amniotic fluid	2 pounds
Breast enlargement	1 to 3 pounds
Uterus enlargement	2 pounds
Fat stores and muscle development	6 to 8 pounds
Increased blood volume	3 to 4 pounds
Increased fluid volume	2 to 3 pounds
Total	**24 to 32½ pounds**

Self-care resources

The changes in your body during the last month of pregnancy can produce some unpleasant signs and symptoms. For more information on dealing with common complaints such as back pain, constipation, itchiness and leaking urine, see Part 3, "Pregnancy Reference Guide" on page 413.

Your emotions during weeks 37 to 40

Waiting for it to be over

By this point, you're probably tired of being pregnant. You may be having trouble sleeping because you can't find a comfortable position. Once you do drift off, your bladder may be waking you up every couple of hours. Time may seem to be standing still.

To deal with the boredom and discomfort, try to keep busy. Work on a hobby project, read the latest bestseller, and spend time with friends and family. Keeping your mind active will help the days move more quickly until the big day finally arrives and you're in labor. Plus, who knows when you'll have so much time to yourself again?

Mastering relaxation

It's a fact: If you're frightened and anxious during labor, you'll have a harder time. Stress sets in motion a whole range of reactions in your body that can ultimately interfere with labor. Childbirth educators call it the fear-tension-pain cycle.

Relaxation is the release of tension from your mind and body through conscious effort. It's a learned skill and one you have to practice regularly in order for it to be effective.

Several different relaxation techniques are helpful during labor. Progressive muscle relaxation, touch relaxation, massage and guided imagery are just some of the options. You've probably learned about these techniques in your childbirth course, but here's a quick refresher:

- **Progressive muscle relaxation.** Beginning with your head or feet, relax one muscle group at a time, moving toward the other end of your body.
- **Touch relaxation.** Starting at your temples, your partner applies firm but gentle pressure for several seconds, then moves to the base of your skull, shoulders, back, arms, hands, legs and feet. As your partner touches each part of your body, relax the muscle group in that area.
- **Massage.** Your partner massages your back and shoulders, making sweeping motions down your arms and legs and small circular motions on your brow and temples. These movements will help relax your muscles and cause your brain to release endorphins, which will enhance your sense of well-being. Experiment with different techniques until you find what feels best to you.
- **Guided imagery.** Imagine yourself in an environment that gives you a feeling of relaxation and well-being — that special, peaceful place you go to in your imagination. Concentrate on the details, such as the smells, colors or sensations on your skin. To enhance the imagery, play a nature tape or soft music.
- **Meditation.** Focus on a single point — an object in the room, a mental image or a word you repeat to yourself. When you feel yourself getting distracted, concentrate again on your focal point.
- **Breathing techniques.** Inhale through your nose, imagining cool, pure air rushing into your lungs. Exhale slowly through your mouth, imagining yourself blowing all your tension away. Practice breathing both more slowly and more quickly than normal. You can use both techniques, and others, during labor.

Practice these techniques often this month. The more you practice them ahead of time, the better they'll work when you really need them. When you practice, make sure the environment is peaceful and that you're comfortable. Use pillows if you want, or turn on some soft music.

Appointments with your health care provider

You'll probably see your health care provider once a week this month, until your baby arrives. As during previous visits, your health care provider will likely check your weight and blood pressure, as well as the activity and movements of your baby. Your health care provider may also measure your uterus and ask you about any signs and symptoms you may be experiencing.

You may have a pelvic exam this month. This exam will allow your health care provider to determine whether your baby is positioned headfirst, feet first or rump first inside your uterus. Most babies are positioned head-first. As your due date draws closer, your health care provider may refer to the station of the presenting part. *Presenting part* is the medical term for the part of your baby's body that's farthest down in your pelvis. *Station* refers to how far down in your pelvis the presenting part is.

During your pelvic exams this month, your health care provider may also check your cervix to see how much it has begun to soften, as well as how much it has opened (dilated) and thinned (effaced). If this process has started, your health care provider will probably refer to it in numbers and percentages. For example, he or she may tell you that you're 3 centimeters (cm) dilated and 30 percent effaced. When you're ready to push your baby out, your cervix will be 10 cm dilated and 100 percent effaced.

Don't put too much stock in these numbers. This type of exam doesn't tell much, with the possible exception of how well labor induction might work. You may go for weeks dilated at 3 cm, or you may go into labor without any dilation or effacement at all beforehand. In fact, unless you're being considered for induced labor, your health care provider may prefer to forgo the cervical exam entirely.

When to call a health care professional during weeks 37 to 40

Is it time to go to the hospital?

The decision about when to go to the hospital can be a tricky one. You may have read that you should wait until your contractions are three to five minutes apart for at least one hour. A friend may have told you that you should go to the hospital when you can no longer walk or talk through your contractions. Still another person may have told you to wait until the pain moves from low down in the front of your abdomen to higher up, above your navel. Your partner may want you to ignore all this advice and just go. Now!

There is no real right answer to the question of whether it's time to go to the hospital. In fact, instructions about when to go to the hospital vary from health care provider to health care provider. To help make sense of what can be a confusing issue, make it easy on yourself. Follow your health care provider's instructions — to the letter. They've been individualized for you and your pregnancy — nobody else's.

One additional point: If your labor seems to be progressing very quickly, with frequent contractions, go to the hospital sooner rather than later. Also know that if you have a history of fast labor or you know your mom and sisters did, your chances of having a fast labor are increased.

Complications during weeks 37 to 40

Here's a guide to important signs and symptoms in the last month of pregnancy that require immediate medical attention:

Vaginal bleeding

If you have bright red bleeding at any time this month, call your health care provider right away. It could be a sign of placental abruption, a serious problem in which your placenta separates from the wall of your uterus. This condition is a medical emergency. Don't confuse this kind of bleeding with the slight bleeding you may have after a recent pelvic exam. This type of light bleeding is normal and isn't cause for concern.

Constant, severe abdominal pain

If you have constant, severe abdominal pain, call your health care provider immediately. Although uncommon, this can be another sign of placental abruption. If you also have a fever and vaginal discharge, you may have an infection.

Decreased movement

It's normal for the vigor of your baby's activities to decrease somewhat during the last few days before birth. It's almost as if your baby is resting, storing energy for the big day. But generally, the number of movements shouldn't drop a great deal. Decreased frequency of movement may be a signal that something is wrong. To check your baby's movements, lie on your left side and count how often you feel the baby move. If you notice fewer than 10 movements in two hours or if you're otherwise worried about your baby's decreased movement, call your health care provider.

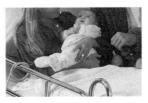

labor and childbirth

The last weeks of pregnancy may feel like a time of waiting ... and waiting. It may seem as if time is almost standing still as you anticipate the start of labor. Keep in mind, though, that your due date is nothing more than an estimate of when you may deliver. You may deliver before or after that date. In fact, labor may begin as much as three weeks before or two weeks after your due date and still be considered normal.

Making those final preparations

Make the most of the time remaining before your baby arrives. What can you do to be as ready as possible? Here's a to-do checklist.

Take childbirth classes, if you haven't already

Childbirth classes help you and your partner fully prepare for labor and childbirth. They vary in name and are available at most hospitals and birthing centers, so ask about them as part of your prenatal care. Typically, classes are offered as one- to two-hour sessions over the course of several months or as full-day sessions that take place over one or two weekends.

Childbirth classes are often taught by nurses, who cover more than just breathing techniques used for relaxation during labor, or so-called natural childbirth. They typically address all aspects of labor and delivery, as well as newborn care. You'll likely learn about signs of labor, pain relief options during labor, birthing positions, postnatal care and care of a newborn, including information on breast-feeding.

Typically, at these classes you'll also learn about what will happen to your body during labor and birth so that you feel positive rather than fearful. Especially if you're a first-time parent, you may find that childbirth classes help calm your fears and answer any of your lingering questions. In addition, you may meet other expectant couples who have questions and concerns similar to yours, which can be comforting. If you plan to have a labor coach, such as your partner or another loved one, support you throughout labor and delivery, have him or her attend childbirth classes with you.

Pregnancy books, such as this one, provide a good way to learn a lot about labor and delivery. But they're not a complete replacement for thorough childbirth classes.

Review choices for your labor and childbirth

In addition to attending childbirth classes in your final months of pregnancy, you and your partner may want to discuss with your health care provider

DON'T BE AFRAID TO ASK

When making a birth plan with your health care provider, don't be embarrassed by any question. For example, you may be wondering:

What if I have to go to the bathroom during labor?

In the past, it was normal for a woman to have an enema when she went into labor, the theory being that emptying the bowel reduced the risk of infection for the mother and baby and stimulated stronger contractions. This is no longer common practice. Your bowel usually will empty without intervention during labor. Occasionally, a small amount of stool is expelled during birth. This is perfectly normal and nothing to worry about.

Some women will be able to get up and urinate every few hours. Your health care provider will probably encourage you to do so because a full bladder may slow down the baby's descent. However, it may be difficult to sense a full bladder when you're having contractions, especially if you've had an epidural. Or you may not want to move, out of fear that doing so will worsen the contractions. Your health care team may provide you with a bedpan or intermittently empty your bladder with a catheter.

Will my pubic hair be shaved?

Not likely. Shaving a pregnant woman's pubic hair also used to be standard practice, to prepare a clean site for delivery. Now it's known that hair doesn't contribute to infection, so shaving is rarely, if ever, done.

Will I have to bare myself in front of a lot of strangers?

During labor, the health care team caring for you will perform periodic vaginal exams to check how you're progressing. During actual delivery, you're joined by your health care provider, labor coach and, typically, at least one nurse. A pediatrician also may be present to examine the baby right after birth. Who else you have in the labor room or birthing room is largely up to you. Medical professionals who help deliver babies see births almost every day, so they're used to the messy but awesome experience of birth. Some university hospital staffs

any questions you have about labor and childbirth. You can review any procedures, such as a Caesarean birth, that may become necessary.

Talk openly with your health care provider about how you want to deliver your baby. You can get ready by making some of these decisions now.

Discuss with your health care provider your preferences for pain relief. Even if you prefer to deliver without pain relief, you may want to learn about the main types of anesthetics used in childbirth. Regional anesthesia — which numbs the body from the waist down — is used most often today. An epidural is a form of regional anesthesia. It supplies a constant level of anesthetic through a flexible tube placed in your lower back. (See "Decision Guide: Understanding your pain relief choices" on page 325.)

may ask if medical students can observe labors and deliveries, including, perhaps, your own. Remember that medical students, who also are professionals, may be able to lend a hand or extra support during your child's birth, so consider their presence an advantage.

What if I make loud noises during labor?

Labor is a physical act that requires your participation. Just as when you exert yourself at home while doing chores or exercising, you may make straining or grunting noises during the workout of labor. Don't worry about making noise during labor and delivery. It's perfectly normal, and medical professionals who help deliver babies won't be shocked in the least.

Does labor hurt the baby?

Although babies don't have a far distance to travel from the uterus to the outside world, the route can be challenging. During the hardest phases of labor and delivery, your baby is squeezed and pushed down the narrow vaginal canal. Your baby must also corkscrew through the bony passageway of the mother's pelvis. During intense labor, the baby's heartbeat slows down intermittently in response to the stress of the journey. But this is expected and not serious.

Your partner may wonder:

What if something happens to my partner during labor and delivery?

Most men don't admit they have a fear that their partner might die during delivery. But that fear can be a big one, voiced or unvoiced. Maternal death is extremely rare these days. If you have anxieties about your partner's well-being during labor and delivery, talk about them ahead of time with her or her health care provider. It can be a relief to hear from a medical expert the reassurances that labor and delivery has never been safer for women in the United States, thanks to the quality of medical care available.

Labor is work, and it isn't the time to learn and make decisions about the procedures that your health care provider has recommended. So review with your health care provider beforehand his or her preferences and usual practices. For example, what are his or her views on pain relief? When would medication be used to accelerate labor? Is he or she comfortable with birthing positions other than the traditional one of lying on the back? Under what circumstances would a cut to enlarge the vaginal opening (episiotomy) be performed?

In addition, find out what steps you should take once you're in labor. When should you notify your health care provider? Should you go directly to the hospital or call the health care provider's office first? Are there any other steps your health care provider wants you to take?

From discussions during your prenatal visits, you and your health care provider can form a written or oral birth plan — a guide to how you wish to deliver your baby. But remember: Any birth plan may need to change depending on the course your labor and delivery takes, so be realistic. And being realistic means being flexible. Think of your birth plan as a guide — not a mandate.

Most women giving birth for the first time don't have an accurate perception of what it will be like, and they may think that they're going to be more in control than they actually will be. In addition, not every labor goes according to plan, because no labor is like any other. Sometimes, problems occur that no one expected. That's when the health care team needs to respond promptly. If that happens, remember that you chose your health care provider because you trusted him or her. Control what you can — but be ready to let go of what you can't control.

Preregister at the hospital

Ask about preregistering at the hospital or birthing center where you plan to deliver. Filling out the necessary paperwork and sorting out insurance matters ahead of time can save you extra work when the big day finally arrives, and you're in labor. Often, tours are included as part of childbirth classes. Seeing where you plan to give birth can help you visualize the event.

Pack your bag for the hospital

Because your due date isn't a given, it's a good idea to have your bag packed and ready for the hospital ahead of time. Here are some items you may want to have on hand.

For labor and childbirth:
- A watch with a second hand, for timing contractions
- Socks or slippers — labor rooms are often kept cool

- Glasses — you may have to remove your contact lenses
- Lip balm — your lips may become dry during relaxation-breathing techniques
- Hard candy to suck on
- A tennis ball or rolling pin for massaging the back, which can be useful if lower backache becomes a problem
- A compact disc or MP3 player
- Reading material
- Snacks for your labor coach
- A camera, with extra batteries and plenty of film or, if you have a digital camera, an extra memory card
- A video camera, with battery fully charged
- A list of phone numbers to call when the baby arrives
- A telephone credit card — use of cellular phones may not be permitted in the hospital

For after you give birth:
- Pajamas or a nightgown that opens in front to allow for easy breast-feeding
- A robe
- A nursing bra or, if you plan to bottle-feed, a supportive bra
- Underwear
- Toiletries, cosmetics and a hair dryer
- Presents "from the baby" to your other children
- A small amount of money for snacks or for items you forgot to bring

For going home:
- Loose clothing — probably a midpregnancy maternity outfit
- A baby outfit, including a hat
- A baby blanket

If you don't want to put everything into your bag yet — your cosmetics, for example — make a list so that you can gather items easily when you prepare to leave. Normally, you don't have to rush — you might even have time to shower — but it's best to be organized.

In addition, have a car seat on hand for baby's ride home.

Try to relax

Most women greet the end of their pregnancies with a mixture of anticipation and, often, nervousness. But try not to worry. Women's bodies are made to accommodate labor and delivery. Labor, as the name implies, is work, that's true. But you can help make the experience go as smoothly as possible by learning about the birth process and by practicing relaxation techniques.

Many women experience a spurt of energy in the last weeks of pregnancy, a behavior often referred to as nesting. You may find yourself cleaning like mad and anxious to start any projects that you've put to the side. Even though the thought of coming home to a clean house may be tempting, try not to wear yourself out. You'll need the energy for the work ahead.

In the last weeks of pregnancy, finish up final tasks, but more importantly, try to focus on savoring the time before your baby arrives. Treat yourself to a nice dinner or fun outing. Indulge in a favorite hobby. Read a good book. Cuddle with your partner. Visit with friends and family. Staying busy but relaxed will help time move along until the day arrives and you're in labor.

How your body prepares for labor

You're making exciting final preparations for your baby's arrival. Your body, on its own, is preparing for labor and delivery, as well.

As labor approaches, your body undergoes certain changes that signal that your baby likely will be born soon. These changes include lightening, false labor (Braxton-Hicks contractions) and bloody show.

Lightening

As you approach your due date, you may feel that the baby has dropped, settling deeper into your pelvis in preparation for labor and delivery. This natural step in carrying a child is called lightening.

Lightening may be noticeable to you. The profile of your abdomen may change — your belly may seem lower and tilt more forward. You may find that it's easier to breathe, as the baby moves down and relieves pressure on your diaphragm. Eating a full meal may become more comfortable with more room in your upper abdomen. In exchange, though, you'll likely feel increased pressure on your bladder from the weight and position of the baby. You may feel twinges of pain as the baby bumps up against your pelvic floor. Your center of gravity may feel lower, throwing you off balance slightly.

Some women, such as those who are already carrying their babies low, may not notice any changes.

If this is your first pregnancy, lightening will probably occur anywhere from two to four weeks before labor starts. With subsequent pregnancies, the babies may drop into position just hours before the onset of labor or even during labor itself. Lightening is rarely an indication of impending labor.

Your baby's position and station

As the end of your pregnancy nears, your health care provider may talk to you, in medical terms, about the position and station of your baby.

Position refers to your baby's placement in the uterus, for example, facing left or right, headfirst or feet-first. Throughout your pregnancy, your baby floats in your uterus and changes position somewhat freely. But, usually between the 32nd and 36th week of pregnancy, the baby rotates to — ideally — a headfirst position, settling into place for labor and delivery. The headfirst position is called the vertex presentation. However, babies may descend feet-first (breech presentation) or lie sideways (transverse lie) within the uterus. As your due date nears, your health care provider may check your baby's position by feeling your outer abdomen and, at times, by examining you internally or using an ultrasound.

In vaginal deliveries, your baby must pass through the bony cavity of the pelvis as it journeys downward from the uterus into the vagina (birth canal). *Station* refers to how far your baby's head has moved into the pelvic cavity and is measured in centimeters. Each station is 1 centimeter. A baby high up in the pelvic cavity is said to be at a -5 station. A baby at 0 station is midway through the pelvis.

Once actual labor begins, the baby's head continues through the pelvis to +1, +2 and +3 stations. At the +5 station, the baby's head crowns, emerging from the vagina and completing its passage through the pelvic cavity.

For most women experiencing their first labor, the baby will already be at 0 station at the onset of labor. At 0 station, the baby are said to be engaged in the pelvis, as the largest part of the baby's head has now entered the pelvic inlet. In women who are having their third or fourth babies, this may not happen until labor has progressed for several hours.

Braxton-Hicks contractions

Throughout your second and third trimesters of pregnancy, you may experience occasional, painless contractions — a sensation that your uterus is tightening and relaxing. They're especially noticeable when you place your hand on your abdomen. These are called Braxton-Hicks contractions, and they're your body's way of warming up for labor. Your uterus is exercising its muscle mass to build strength for the big job ahead: labor and the birth of your child.

As you approach your due date, these contractions typically become stronger and may even become painful at times. Sometimes, Braxton-Hicks contractions, which are also called false labor pains, are mistaken for true labor. However, Braxton-Hicks contractions are irregular and often cease if you rest. True labor pains come at regular intervals, increasing in strength and intensity, regardless of your activity.

Bloody show

During pregnancy, the opening to your uterus (cervix) is blocked by a thick plug of mucus. This plug forms a barrier between your cervix and vagina so that bacteria can't enter your uterus and cause an infection. A few weeks, days or hours before labor begins, this plug is sometimes discharged, and you may have what health care providers call bloody show. You may notice a small amount of blood-tinged, brownish mucus leaking from your vagina. Some women don't notice the loss of this plug. Bloody show may be a sign that things could happen soon, although labor may still be a week or more away.

WILL EATING SPICY FOODS START LABOR?

Most pregnant women have heard of at least one folk remedy for starting labor. You may have heard that one of the following will help get labor going as your due date nears:
- Frequent walking
- Having sex
- Exercising
- Using a laxative
- Stimulating your nipples
- Eating spicy foods
- Driving on a bumpy road
- Fasting
- Being frightened
- Consuming castor oil
- Drinking herbal tea

Is there any truth to any of these old wives' tales? A few such folk remedies have some basis in science. Nipple stimulation can cause uterine contractions, similar to what happens when a baby breast-feeds right after birth. It's biologically plausible that sex might trigger contractions because semen contains substances similar to those used in labor-inducing medications. These facts don't mean that your health care provider will advise that you try either of these methods. In fact, he or she may advise against sex in your ninth month of pregnancy to avoid intrauterine infections, and nipple stimulation could stimulate contractions that are long and hard enough to harm the baby.

Most folk remedies aren't based in science and simply don't work. Some are even ill-advised. For example, fasting really isn't good for you or the baby. Is there anything you can do to get labor going? Not really. Just be patient and let Mother Nature takes its course.

Signs that you're in labor

As your due date approaches, after about the 36th week of your pregnancy, your health care provider may want to examine you more often, typically weekly. The principal medical reason for this is to watch for preeclampsia, the serious form of high blood pressure in pregnancy. He or she likely will also check for the early signs of labor (pre-labor signs) in addition to monitoring your health and that of your unborn child. Your health care provider likely also will review signs of labor with you and your partner.

It's probably one of the most common questions medical professionals hear from expectant mothers: "How will I know when I'm in labor?" You may have heard from other mothers that "you will just know." You may not find that information very comforting.

First-time parents commonly worry that the baby will be born on the way to the hospital. But, in reality, this situation seldom occurs. Labor can start suddenly and progress quickly. More often, though, it doesn't. Usually, more subtle signs announce the start of labor.

Thinning and softening of the cervix

One sign that labor is starting is that your cervix begins to thin (efface) and soften (ripen) in preparation for delivery. As labor progresses, the cervix eventually will go from an inch or more in thickness to paper thinness. You won't be aware of this thinning process unless your cervix is checked during a pelvic exam. Effacement is measured in percentages or in terms of cervical length, and if your health care provider says, "You're about 50 percent effaced," it means that your cervix is half its original thickness.

When your cervix is 100 percent effaced, it's completely thinned out. This thinning out is what allows your cervix to stretch, enabling the baby to move downward through the opening of the cervix into the vagina (birth canal) for delivery.

WHAT TRIGGERS LABOR?

For some 270 days, your unborn child has been developing within your uterus. The time is now nearing for your baby to make his or her entrance into the outside world.

But what triggers the miracle of birth is still somewhat of a medical mystery. Somehow, your body knows — accurately most of the time — when your baby has matured enough to live outside the uterus.

Our current understanding of how labor begins involves the chemical signals produced by your body (prostaglandins), which thin, soften and dilate your cervix. At term, something triggers your body to produce prostaglandins in large amounts, which cause the uterine contractions you may have felt throughout your pregnancy to become stronger. These contractions, in turn, cause even more production of prostaglandins, and the cycle accelerates into labor. By definition, labor is a series of uterine contractions that open your cervix for birth. It seems that a complex cross talk between the baby's glandular system, the placenta and the mother's uterus triggers the production of these prostaglandins. Arriving at a complete understanding of this interaction remains one of the challenges of science.

Dilation of the cervix

In your final days of pregnancy, your health care provider might also tell you that your cervix is beginning to open (dilate), another sign that labor is getting closer. With a first pregnancy, effacement usually begins before dilation. With subsequent pregnancies, the opposite is generally true.

Dilation is measured in centimeters, with the cervix opening from 0 to 10 centimeters (4 inches) during the course of labor. Your health care provider estimates how far dilated you are by feeling the opening of your cervix during a pelvic exam. Thinning, softening and dilation of the cervix may precede other signs of labor, such as contractions.

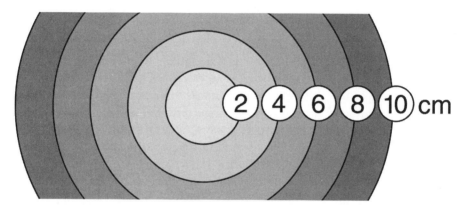

WHAT DOES LABOR FEEL LIKE?

What do contractions (labor pains) *feel* like? Except for perhaps menstrual cramps, the sensation may be unlike any other you've experienced. That's because you're not accustomed to feeling your uterine muscles contracting.

In true labor, the contraction usually begins high in the uterus and radiates down the abdomen and into the lower back. The pain may be felt in the lower abdomen, lower back, hips or upper thighs. The sensation has been described as an aching feeling, pressure, fullness, cramping and backache.

Women respond to the pain of labor in different ways. For some, contractions may seem like strong menstrual cramps. For others, the pain may be stronger and difficult to bear. How will you handle the pain? How bad will it be? How will you cope?

The pain of childbirth may end up being easier or harder than you imagined. The best way to prepare for either outcome is to take childbirth classes so that you have realistic expectations of labor and delivery.

Don't let fear add to your pain. Remember that contractions have a positive purpose, which is to help you deliver your baby. The pain won't last forever; it has a definite time limit. And pain relief options are available, one or more of which many women choose as part of their birth plans.

Breaking of water

At some point during labor, the bag of water (amniotic sac) housing your baby begins to leak or break, and the fluid that has cushioned your baby flows out of your vagina in a trickle or gush. Like other pregnant women, you may fear that your labor will start with your water breaking (membranes rupturing) while you're out in public.

In reality, few women experience a dramatic breaking of water, and if they do, it usually happens at home, often in bed. Most often, a woman's water breaks while she's in active labor and at the hospital or under the care of her health care provider. In fact, your health care provider may break your water for you during labor, if it hasn't broken on its own.

Digestive disturbances

Many women experience diarrhea or nausea at the start of labor.

Contractions

At the beginning of labor, the uterus begins to contract (squeeze). These contractions are what move your baby down the birth canal. Contractions (labor pains) often begin with cramping or discomfort in your lower back and abdomen that doesn't stop when you change position. Over time, these contractions become stronger and more regular.

Contractions alone may or may not be an indication that you're in labor. Many women experience false labor (Braxton-Hicks contractions) and believe that they're in real labor. To distinguish between false and true labor, consider:

The frequency of your contractions
Using a watch or clock, measure the frequency of your contractions by timing them from the beginning of one to the beginning of the next. True labor will develop into a regular pattern, with your contractions growing closer together. In false labor, contractions remain irregular.

The length of your contractions
Measure the duration of each contraction by timing when it begins and when it stops. True contractions last about 30 seconds at the onset and get progressively longer — up to 75 seconds — and stronger. False labor contractions vary in length and intensity.

So, when will your labor start? It's really anyone's call. Your health care provider can make an educated guess, but the fact is, your cervix can begin to thin, soften and open (efface and dilate) gradually over a period of weeks or even a month or more in some women. In others, these changes can occur in a matter of hours.

Is it time to go to the hospital?

Once you've started having regular contractions, the next question is: When is it time to leave for the hospital or birthing center, or to call your health care provider?

Your health care provider probably will give you instructions on when to leave for the hospital or birthing center. For example, you may be told to call your health care provider when it becomes hard to walk or talk through contractions. Many women are told to go to the hospital or birthing center after an hour of contractions that come five minutes apart. You may need to leave sooner if your labor seems to be progressing rapidly.

As your due date approaches, keep the gas tank full and make a practice run or two to the hospital or birthing center. It's a good idea, especially, to become familiar with where to park your car when the time arrives and how to get to the obstetrical floor. Make arrangements for your other children, including an emergency plan for a friend or neighbor to help out in case you have to leave in the middle of the night or someone who's coming from out of town to help you hasn't yet arrived.

Or is it a false alarm?

On television and in the movies, a pregnant woman wakes in the night, places a hand knowingly on her abdomen and calmly rouses her husband with the words: "Honey, it's time." In real life, you may doubt your ability to judge the start of labor, especially if this is your first baby.

You might leave for the hospital or birthing center with regular contractions that are five minutes apart, and after you arrive, they simply stop. It's possible that your health care provider may send you home if your contractions aren't to the stage called active labor and your cervix isn't dilating. If this happens, try not to feel embarrassed or frustrated. Instead, regard it as a good practice run.

Telling real labor from false labor can be tricky. Sometimes, the only way to be certain is to have a vaginal exam to assess whether your cervix is opening (dilating). When in doubt or if you have questions about whether this is the real thing, call your health care provider.

Most health care providers want you to come to the hospital if your water breaks. If there are concerns about your health, your health care provider may instruct you to go to the hospital or birthing center sooner. It's always a good idea to discuss this plan with him or her.

The stages of labor and childbirth

Labor is not a static, one-time event. It's a sequence of events, or a process, that takes place over the span of an hour to as long as 24 hours or more.

How long will your labor last? That depends on many factors. As a rule, labor is usually longer with first babies. That's because the openings of the uterus (cervix) and vagina (birth canal) of first-time mothers are less flexible, and therefore it takes longer for labor and birth. For women giving birth for the first time, labor usually lasts between 12 and 24 hours, with an average of 14 hours. For women who have given birth before, labor usually lasts between four and eight hours, with an average of six hours.

How long labor lasts and how it progresses differs from woman to woman and from birth to birth. Even though every labor is unique, the sequence of events that takes place remains roughly the same.

Labor is formally divided into three natural stages. Stage 1 occurs when the uterus, on its own, opens the cervix to allow descent of the baby. Stage 2 is pushing and delivery — the birth of your baby. Stage 3 is delivery of the placenta (afterbirth). The first stage is the longest of these stages and is, itself, divided into three phases — early labor, active labor and transition.

Stage 1: Early labor, active labor and transition

Early labor

During labor, the cervix opens (dilates) so that your baby can move downward into the vagina in preparation for pushing and delivery. Over time, the cervix will go from being completely closed to being completely open (complete) at 10 centimeters (cm), which is 4 inches in width. This opening is large enough for the baby's head to pass through.

The uterus, which houses the baby, is a muscular, hollow organ. Think of it as a large, upside-down elastic bottle. The opening of the uterus (cervix) is the neck of the bottle. When labor begins, the cervix is closed. But contractions cause the cervix to open by creating pressure downward through the uterus. This force is directed through the uterus in two ways. During a contraction, your baby is subjected to pressure that forces him or her against the cervix. The contractions also cause the cervix to thin and pull up around the baby's head. Repeated contractions eventually stretch the cervix to a full 10 cm.

What's happening

Early labor is the phase when your cervix dilates from 0 cm to a little over 3 cm. This period is usually the longest and, fortunately, the least intense phase of labor. Early labor begins with the start of contractions, which vary tremendously from woman to woman. Some women may not even recognize that they're in labor if their contractions are mild and irregular. Other women dilate the full 10 cm in just a few hours with clear contractions.

In general, contractions during early labor last 30 to 60 seconds. They may be irregular or regular, ranging between five and 20 minutes apart. They're usually mild to moderately strong.

Along with contractions, you may experience backache, upset stomach and, possibly, diarrhea. Some women report a sensation of warmth in the abdomen

FACTORS THAT AFFECT LABOR

Many factors can affect how your labor will progress. They include:

Size of your baby's head

Because the bones of the skull aren't yet fused together, your baby's head molds itself to the shape and size of your pelvis as it moves through the vagina (birth canal). If the head moves through at an awkward angle, it can affect the location and intensity of your discomfort and the length of your labor.

Position of your baby

Birth is easiest if your baby comes headfirst through the birth canal, with its chin tucked down on the chest so that the smallest diameter leads the way. But babies aren't always so accommodating — sometimes their heads aren't in the best position, and sometimes they're breech, with their buttocks or feet coming first. They may even be sideways in the uterus or come shoulder-first.

Shape and roominess of your pelvis

Your pelvis, which consists of three bones forming a hollow cavity, must be roomy enough for your baby's head to pass through. Fortunately, babies are generally well-matched to the size of their mothers. Women who have smaller frames, for example, tend to have smaller babies. Nature helps in another way, too. Near term, the placenta releases a hormone called relaxin. This hormone relaxes the ligaments of the pelvis, widening it and contributing to that feeling that you're waddling in your later months of pregnancy. This widening, along with the molding of the baby's head, usually allows the head enough room to move through the pelvis.

Ability of your cervix to thin and open

Rarely, the cervix may be unable to thin (efface) and open (dilate). In most labors, the cervix opens as expected, but the speed of that dilation may vary considerably.

Your ability to push

Because you use your abdominal muscles to help push the baby out, the better shape you're in physically, the more you can assist. If you've had a long labor and you're tired, your pushing may be less effective.

as labor begins. You may also experience bloody show at this time — a blood-tinged, mucous discharge from your vagina — as the cervix begins to open.

Early labor (latent labor) can last for hours to days, so you may need to be patient. Your cervix needs to soften before it can dilate. Labor doesn't always begin when your contractions start. You may have irregular, painful contractions for hours or even several days before your cervix dilates, especially if this is your first baby.

Your physical state

If you go into labor healthy and well-rested, you'll have more strength to work through your contractions. But if you're ill or tired or the early phase of your labor is particularly long, you may already be exhausted when it comes time to push. Your energy level can affect your ability both to cope with pain and to concentrate during labor.

Your outlook on labor

If you have a positive outlook, know generally what to expect, trust your health care team and have thought through your choices, you're ready to take an active part in your labor and delivery. Women who are frightened or anxious about labor and birth tend to have a harder time. That's because stress can lead to a range of physiologic reactions in the body that can ultimately interfere with labor.

Support from staff and your labor coach

Your health care provider, the nurses, your labor coach or other loved ones in the labor room with you — they all work together to support you and help you stay relaxed during labor. Through their presence and coaching, they can enhance the coping skills necessary for labor and delivery. Especially important is your relationship with the health care team caring for you. Medical professionals who explain why things are done and what your options are, in an atmosphere of caring support, give you peace of mind and promote a more positive birth experience.

Medication

Certain medications for pain relief can both help and hinder labor. Some health care providers believe that if medications relieve pain early on, they can leave you rested and better equipped for the work ahead, and if they help you relax, you can concentrate on getting the baby out. But if the medications slow down labor or interfere with your ability to push, they can undo some of their usefulness. Remember, only you can decide when you need help for labor discomfort.

How you may be feeling
During those early hours to days of labor, you'll likely labor at home. Many women do. They use that time to rest or nap, while they still can, to conserve energy for the work ahead. Some women continue a normal schedule, barely aware that the process has begun.

With the onset of your first real contractions, you may be giddy with excitement and full of relief that after all the long months of waiting, your baby is soon to be born. At the same time, though, you may be scared about the unknown. Try to remain relaxed. Remember: You've done a lot to prepare yourself for this moment. You're ready!

What you can do
Until your contractions pick up in frequency and intensity, you may feel like doing household chores, watching television or a movie, playing games or making phone calls. Choose activities that you find most comfortable and that help distract you from your contractions. You may want to relax in a chair or get up and move around. Walking is a great activity because it may help your labor along.

During early labor, you may also find it helpful to:
• Take a shower or bath.
• Listen to relaxing music.
• Ask your partner for a massage.

TIPS ON DEALING WITH BACK LABOR

Some women experience back labor — intense and relentless back pain, especially during active labor and transition. Often, back labor occurs when the baby is in an awkward position as it enters the birth canal. The baby's head is pressing against the mother's tailbone (sacrum). But that doesn't have to be the case. During labor and delivery, some women simply feel more tension in their backs than others do.

To relieve back labor:
• Have your labor coach apply counterpressure to your lower back. Have him or her massage the area or use hands or knuckles to apply direct pressure.
• Apply counterpressure by placing a tennis ball or rolling pin — if you brought either with you — under your tailbone.
• Have your labor coach apply heat or cold, whichever feels better to you, to your lower back.
• Change to a more comfortable position.
• If possible, take a shower and direct the warm water spray on your lower back.
• Ask for an epidural or spinal anesthetic, if desired, to try to help relieve the pain.

- Try slow, deep breathing.
- Change positions often.
- Drink water, juice or other clear liquids.
- Eat a light, healthy snack.
- Cool yourself with a wet washcloth.
- Use lip balm on dry lips.
- Use the bathroom often.

For lower backache, try ice packs or heat, or switch between hot and cold. Use a tennis ball, rolling pin or doorknob to apply pressure to the lower back. But don't take aspirin or any other pain reliever except acetaminophen (Tylenol, others) for your discomfort.

Without an examination, there's no way to know when you've moved into the more active phase of labor, but many signs suggest that you're ready to go to the hospital or birthing center. The timing and intensity of your contractions can help you and your health care provider pinpoint which phase of labor you're in. Follow your health care provider's instructions about when to leave for the hospital or birthing center.

At the hospital or birthing center
Once you check into the hospital or birthing center, you're typically taken to your room, often a labor room, where admission procedures are completed. After you've changed into a hospital gown or your own nightgown, you'll probably be examined to see how dilated your cervix is. You'll likely be connected to a fetal monitor to time your contractions and check your baby's heart rate. Your vital signs — your pulse, blood pressure and temperature — are taken on admission and at intervals throughout your labor and delivery.

You may have an intravenous (IV) needle placed into a vein, usually on the back of your hand or arm. This needle is attached to a plastic tube leading to a bag of fluid that drips into your body. The bag hangs on a movable stand, which you can wheel with you when you take a walk or go into the bathroom.

The fluid you receive through the IV helps to keep you hydrated during labor. Medications such as oxytocin also can be administered through your IV, if they're needed. Many health care providers routinely request an IV early on in labor. Some wait until there's a clear need for one before requesting it for you. In some situations, no IV is required. In normal labor, without anesthesia, it's more of an insurance policy against trouble than a necessity.

If your contractions aren't forceful enough to open the cervix, you may be offered a medication to make your uterus contract. Contractions can sometimes start regularly, but then stop halfway through your labor. If this happens and the progress of your labor halts for a few hours, your health care provider may suggest breaking your water (rupturing your membranes) — if it hasn't already broken — or artificially stimulating your labor with oxytocin.

Active labor

Active labor is the second phase of the first stage of labor. It's the period of time when your cervix dilates from a little more than 3 or 4 cm to nearly 7 cm.

What's happening

Active labor is when the real work begins for the mother-to-be. Your contractions will become stronger and progressively longer. They may last 45 seconds to a minute or longer. They may be three to four minutes apart, or perhaps even two to three minutes apart. There's definitely less rest for you between contractions.

The good news is that your contractions are accomplishing more in less time. Your baby is on the move down through the stations of your pelvis as your cervix continues to open. During active labor, the average woman in

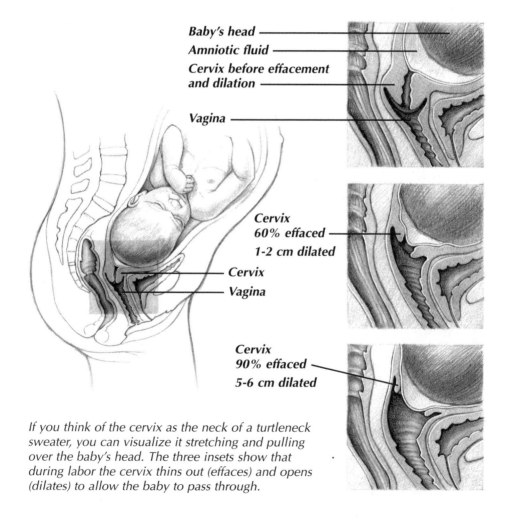

Baby's head
Amniotic fluid
Cervix before effacement and dilation
Vagina

Cervix
60% effaced
1-2 cm dilated

Cervix
Vagina

Cervix
90% effaced
5-6 cm dilated

If you think of the cervix as the neck of a turtleneck sweater, you can visualize it stretching and pulling over the baby's head. The three insets show that during labor the cervix thins out (effaces) and opens (dilates) to allow the baby to pass through.

What's that for?

If you've never been hospitalized, you may find medical surroundings slightly intimidating. But if you understand what's going on around you while you're laboring and delivering, you can better relax. Here is a list of equipment and supplies often found in a typical delivery room and what each item is used for during the birthing process.

Birthing bed

A birthing bed (delivery bed) is usually a twin bed that's high off the ground. Delivery beds are designed to be practical. The bed can be raised or lowered, and the end of the bed can be removed to facilitate delivery. The bed may have a bar that you can hold onto while you push. Most delivery beds have stirrups that can be pulled out. Sometimes the stirrups are helpful during delivery, or you may need them if you require stitches after the birth.

Fetal monitor

This piece of equipment records your contractions and your baby's heart rate. In external fetal monitoring, two wide belts are placed around your abdomen. The one high on your uterus measures and records the strength and frequency of your contractions. The other belt, usually secured across your lower abdomen, records the baby's heart rate. The two belts are connected to a monitor that displays and prints out both tracings at the same time so that their interactions can be observed.

Why is fetal monitoring used? The baby's reaction to your contractions can be monitored by observing the baby's heart rate. The baby's heart can respond to contractions with both increased and decreased rates, but a drop in the baby's heart rate just after a contraction may suggest that your baby isn't getting enough oxygen.

During labor, if your baby's heartbeat is normal and your labor is progressing well, you can periodically be disconnected from the monitor so that you can change position or take a walk.

Blood pressure monitor (sphygmomanometer)

This device measures your blood pressure throughout your labor and delivery. A cuff goes around your arm just above the elbow and is attached to a measuring instrument.

Bassinet

After birth, your baby is laid on a bassinet while being examined by the nurse or health care provider.

Other items

Some rooms also have extra comforts, such as a rocking chair or a birthing chair, stool or ball. You can request extra pillows, blankets and towels. Some rooms have a tub or shower for your use during labor.

her first labor dilates about 1 cm an hour after she has reached 4 cm. If you've had a baby before, you usually progress faster. Active labor lasts, on average, between three and eight hours, generally shorter in duration than early labor, but much more intense.

You'll probably be in the hospital or birthing center by the time you're in active labor. Throughout your labor, you'll have occasional pelvic exams to see how your cervix is changing. Your health care provider can check to see how you and your baby are responding to your contractions. Your vital signs will probably be checked. A fetal monitor may be used to check your baby's heart rate. Sometimes, if you haven't yet received an intravenous (IV) line, one is started to give you medication and fluids. If your amniotic sac hasn't broken already, it may break as your cervix dilates further. Or your health care provider may break the water (rupture the membranes) for you.

How you may be feeling
During active labor, your contractions become more painful and you may feel increasing pressure in your back. You may be unable to talk through your contractions now.

Between contractions you may still be able to talk, watch television or listen to music, at least during the early part of active labor. You may feel upbeat, excited and encouraged that things are starting to happen.

But that initial excitement usually gives way to seriousness as your labor progresses and the pain intensifies. Your smile may fade, as you become inwardly focused. You may feel tired and restless. Some women report feeling sensitive and irritable. You may reach a point that you no longer want to talk much.

As the tone in the room changes, you may begin to realize the importance of your childbirth classes and that you may actually need to use the breathing and relaxation techniques to get through your contractions. You may wonder, "Am I really going to be able to do this?" Your confidence may begin to waver, and you may feel as if labor is never going to end.

You might turn inward to find the strength to deal with what your body is going through. You may even need to have the room quiet and the lights dimmed so that you're completely free to concentrate on the job at hand.

During active labor, you may wish to lean more on your labor coach, seeking encouragement as your contractions peak and wane. Or you may resist being touched or coached, in an attempt to stay focused and in control.

What you can do
To combat your growing discomfort, use your breathing and relaxation techniques. If you have never practiced or learned natural childbirth techniques,

your health care team can demonstrate some simple breathing exercises to help you through your contractions. But don't feel you have to use breathing techniques if you're uncomfortable with them or they simply don't relax you.

Many women request pain medication during active labor. If you're having an epidural, it's usually given during this phase. Don't be afraid to discuss pain relief with your health care provider if you feel you need some relief.

Some women find that as the pain intensifies, rocking in a rocking chair, rolling on a birthing ball or taking a warm shower helps them relax between contractions. Changing your position also helps your baby descend. Walking especially helps labor progress because of the motion and the influence of gravity. If walking feels comfortable, continue with it, stopping to breathe through contractions. Vary your activities because no single approach is likely to work throughout labor.

Try to concentrate on relaxing between your contractions. Doing so will help you stay energized through each stage of labor and delivery. Use that time to give yourself a mental pep talk. Your contractions may be hard, but you're doing a great job getting through each one as they come. Your labor won't last forever, and the only way through labor and delivery, really, is to go through it with as much determination and concentration as possible.

During active labor, try to urinate every hour or so. You may not feel the urge to urinate because of the pressure from the descending baby, so ask your labor coach to remind you, if necessary, to empty your bladder. At times, your health care team may use a catheter to empty your bladder, especially if an epidural is used for pain relief.

You may feel slightly nauseated during active labor. Your health care provider may permit you to drink clear liquids or to eat a light snack, such as gelatin or applesauce. But most times, you're discouraged from eating or drinking as labor progresses. To keep your mouth and throat from becoming dry, suck on ice chips or hard candy. Apply lip balm to your lips to keep them moist.

Transition

The last phase of the first stage of labor is called transition. It's the shortest but most difficult phase. During transition, your cervix opens the remaining centimeters, dilating from 7 to 10 cm.

During transition, your contractions increase in strength and frequency, with little break between them. There may be time for only a hurried breath before the next one hits. Your contractions reach peak intensity almost immediately, and they now last 60 to 90 seconds. In fact, it may feel as if your contractions never completely disappear.

What's happening

Transition is a demanding time. You'll likely feel a lot of pressure in your lower back and rectum. In addition, you may feel nauseated and vomit. One minute you may feel hot and sweaty, the next, cold and chilled. Your legs may begin to shake or cramp, which is fairly common.

If you haven't had any pain relief medication, your discomfort will probably be greatest during transition. Pain medications are rarely given so close to your baby's birth, but options are still available. At this point, IV pain medication may not be as advisable because it could affect your baby's breathing once he or she is born. There may still be time for an epidural. Trust your health care provider to help you make decisions about pain medication.

POSITIONS FOR LABOR AND CHILDBIRTH

There's no best position for labor. Once you're in labor, experiment to find what's most comfortable for you. Listen to your body to discover what feels good. One tip: Give each new position a chance. The first few contractions may be stronger until you get used to a new position.

Lying flat on your back isn't recommended for labor or childbirth. It can cause the weight of your uterus to compress major blood vessels and decrease blood flow to your uterus.

Some of the positions for labor and delivery that you may want to try include:

The semireclining position

In the semireclining position, you lean back as if you're in a reclining chair. The head of the bed is elevated, and your head and shoulders rest against pillows. During each contraction you grab your legs behind the knees or handles near the stirrups and pull back toward your body. Or you may pull your body forward into a more upright position.

Standing or walking

If it's helpful — especially during early labor — stand up or take a walk. In particular, a labor that hasn't been progressing may gain some momentum if the mother stands or walks. During contractions, lean on your labor partner or a stationary object. Of course, it may not be possible for you to stand or walk if you've had an epidural and your legs are numbed or you're connected to a monitor and can't easily leave your bed. Most women use walking earlier in the course of labor, often before an epidural has been initiated.

Kneeling

If you're having a lot of back pain, kneeling on a pillow on the floor and leaning forward against your bed or a chair may feel good. This position relieves backache by directing the baby's weight away from your spine. Many birthing beds have two sections, one which can be lowered and the other which can be raised. The beds are designed so that you can kneel on the lower portion while resting your arms and upper body on the raised portion.

How you may be feeling

Transition may go quickly. You may suddenly be past it and ready to push. Or you may feel as if the pain is never going to end, and you're unsure whether you can hold on one more minute. Many women, especially those practicing natural childbirth, feel exhausted and somewhat overwhelmed during transition.

Don't worry if you lose control of your emotions. But to help you stay focused, try to remember the real reason you're there: to deliver and meet your new baby. And you're almost there! Your body was designed to give birth, and you're capable of making it through any tough times of labor. So let your uterus do its work and try not to fight or fear the pain.

Squatting

Squatting opens your pelvis a little wider, giving your baby more room to rotate as he or she moves through the birth canal. Squatting also allows you to bear down more effectively. If it feels right to you, squat on your bed or ask someone to support your weight as you lean on the bed or a chair and squat during contractions.

Sitting

During labor, you may want to sit up and have your labor partner sit behind you, supporting your weight. Or you may find it comfortable to straddle a chair, leaning against a pillow on the chair's back while your partner massages your back. Some centers have birthing stools, chairs or balls that allow you to sit during pushing and delivery. Find out what's available at your birthing center by talking with your childbirth class instructors or health care provider.

On your hands and knees

Don't be embarrassed to get down on your hands and knees during labor and delivery. Many women find this position comfortable. A hands-and-knees position allows your baby to fall forward during delivery, taking the pressure off your spine, which may help rotate the baby into a favorable position for birthing. Your health care provider may suggest this position to help maximize delivery of oxygen to your baby.

Lying on your side

Many women find it easiest to labor lying on their sides. Your partner can hold your upper leg, while you lie on your side and prop your head up with pillows. Lying on your side maximizes blood flow to your uterus and baby. This position also helps support the weight of your baby, which can ease back discomfort.

It's a good idea to discuss with your health care provider your preferences about positions for labor and childbirth, although you won't know what the best position is for you until you have a chance to experience it.

What you can do

During transition, concentrate on getting through each contraction. If it helps, focus on getting through just the first half of each contraction. After a contraction peaks, the second half gets easier. If your contractions are being monitored, your partner can watch their progress, letting you know when they've peaked so that you know when the hardest part is over.

During transition, you may not want things like radio or television distracting you. You may want to try some of the following techniques for making it through this challenging phase:

- Changing positions
- Placing a cool, damp cloth on your forehead
- Getting a massage between contractions
- Doing breathing, relaxation and focusing techniques learned in classes

Don't think about the contraction you just had or the contractions to come. Just take each one as it comes.

As difficult as transition can be, remember that it means you're almost finished. The average length of time for transition is about 15 minutes to three hours. Soon it will be time to push your baby out!

If you feel the urge to push, try to hold back until you've been told you're fully dilated. This will help prevent your cervix from tearing or swelling, which can delay delivery. It can be hard to resist this sensation when your body is telling you to bear down. To fight the urge to push, instead pant or blow, unless you've been instructed otherwise.

Stage 2: The birth of your baby

Pushing has a purpose, and you're actively involved in making it happen — the birth of your baby. Soon the top of your baby's head appears (crowns) at the opening of your vagina. Unfortunately, even though your partner and the health care team can see the baby when you push, it may take another 30 to 40 minutes of your effort to deliver the baby, especially if an incision (episiotomy) is to be avoided.

Occasionally, the baby needs to be delivered promptly and from this position. In such cases, an episiotomy can be made that will allow for more rapid delivery. Anesthesia will be provided for you if this procedure is necessary. In most cases, you'll be able to push the baby out without this intervention.

After you push the baby's head out, you'll probably be instructed to stop pushing for a moment while your health care provider clears the baby's airway and makes sure that the baby's umbilical cord is free.

You may find it difficult to stop pushing when told to, but try. It may help to pant instead of pushing. Slowing down gives your vaginal area time to stretch rather than tear. To stay motivated, you may be able to put your

How the baby comes out

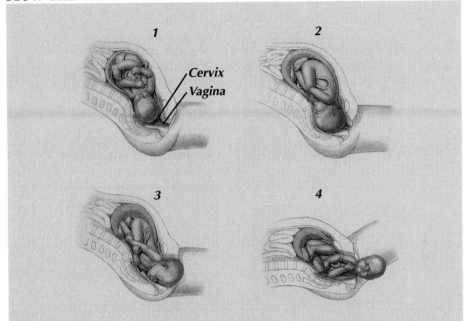

The human pelvis has a complex shape, making your baby negotiate several maneuvers during labor and delivery. Your pelvis is widest from side to side at the top (inlet) and from front to back at the bottom (outlet). The baby's head is widest from front to back, and the shoulders are widest from side to side. As a result, your baby must twist and turn on the way through the birth canal.

Because almost every mother's pelvis is widest side to side at the entrance, most babies enter the pelvis looking left or right (visual 1). The exit from the pelvis is widest from front to back, so babies almost always turn faceup or facedown (visual 2). These maneuvers occur as a result of forces of labor and the resistance provided by the birth canal.

In addition to making these turning maneuvers, the baby is simultaneously descending farther down the vagina. Finally, the top of your baby's head appears (crowns), stretching your vaginal opening (visual 3). When the vulva has stretched enough, the baby's head will emerge — usually by extending the head, lifting its chin off the chest and thus emerging from under your pubic bone. The baby usually emerges facedown but will turn to one side very quickly as the shoulders turn to take the same route (visual 4).

Next, the shoulders are born one at a time, and with a great slippery rush, the rest of the body is delivered — and now you can hold your new baby.

hand down and feel the baby's head or see it in a mirror. You're very close now! Then, when you're encouraged to, push again. With just a few more pushes, your baby is born!

WHAT YOU CAN DO AS THE LABOR COACH

You may be the father-to-be, a partner, parent, sibling, or friend. Whatever your other roles, your job as labor coach is to support the mother-to-be both physically and emotionally during labor and delivery. Here are some ways that you can help your partner through each phase of childbirth:

During early labor

Time her contractions
Measure the time from the beginning of one contraction to the next. Keep a record. When contractions are coming five minutes apart, it's usually time to call the health care provider.

Keep her calm
Once contractions begin, you both may feel some initial butterflies. After all, it's the big moment you've been anticipating for the past nine months. But during labor and delivery, your goal is to keep the expectant mother relaxed. That means staying as calm as possible yourself. Take some deep breaths together. Between contractions, practice those relaxation techniques you learned in childbirth class. For example, suggest that she let her muscles go limp or that she concentrate on relaxing her jaw and hands. Gently massage her back, feet or shoulders. Reassure her with your words and actions that you're both ready to have this baby.

Help distract her
Suggest activities — such as watching television or taking a walk — that will help keep both your minds off labor. Humor can be a great distraction, too. Enjoy some laughs, when appropriate.

Ask her what she needs
If you're unsure what to do for your partner, ask her what would make her more comfortable. If she isn't sure what she needs, do your best to suggest something that you think might make her feel better. But don't take it personally if she doesn't take you up on your suggestions or focuses inward during contractions.

Give encouragement
Offer her encouragement and praise through each contraction. Remind her that with each contraction, and with each passing hour of labor, she's getting closer to meeting the baby. What you don't want to do is criticize her or pretend that the pain doesn't exist. She needs your empathy and support, even if she's not complaining.

Take care of yourself, too
To keep up your strength, have some refreshments periodically. But respect that your partner may not want you to eat in front of her or to leave her for an extended period to eat. If you feel faint at any time during labor and delivery, sit down, and then tell someone on the health care team.

During active labor

Quiet the room
If it's possible, keep the labor room or birthing room as calm as possible by keeping the doors closed and the lights dimmed. Some women find it relaxing to listen to soft music during labor.

Help her through contractions
Learn to recognize the start of your partner's contractions. If she's on a fetal monitor, ask the health care team how to read it. Or place your hand on your partner's abdomen and feel for the telltale tightening of the uterus. You can then alert your partner when a contraction is beginning. You can also offer encouragement as each contraction peaks and wanes. If it helps her, breathe with her through difficult contractions. Try to make her more comfortable by massaging her abdomen or lower back or by using counterpressure or any other techniques you've learned.

Some women prefer not to be touched during labor, so take your cues from your partner. If she's uncomfortable, suggest a change of position or a walk — if possible — to help labor progress. Offer her water or ice chips, if she's permitted them. Mop her brow with a cool, damp cloth, if she likes that.

Be an advocate
As much as possible, serve as her go-between with the health care team. Don't be afraid to ask questions about how her labor is progressing or to ask for explanations about any procedures or the need for medications. If your partner requests pain medication, discuss pain relief options with her health care providers, openly or in private. Remember: Labor isn't a test of pain endurance. A woman doesn't fail at labor if she chooses pain relief medication.

Continue to give encouragement
By the time a woman is in active labor, she's likely feeling quite tired and uncomfortable, and perhaps edgy. As in early labor, be supportive and encouraging by saying things such as: "You did a good job to get through that contraction," or "You're doing great! I'm really proud of you."

Don't take things personally
Things may be said in labor that aren't meant. Don't take it personally if your partner seems irritated with your thoughtful attempts to comfort her or if she doesn't respond to your questions. Your presence alone is comforting and sometimes is all that's needed.

During transition

Continue to help her through contractions
Transition, as the baby progresses down the birth canal, is usually the hardest time for the mother. Now is the time to give her even more encouragement and praise. Remind her to take it one contraction at a time. If it helps her, talk her

through each contraction again or breathe with her. Some women find that they don't want to have someone coaching them as contractions intensify. Give space, if needed. In fact, holding her hand, making eye contact or simply saying, "I love you," may convey more than many words.

Put her needs first
Throughout labor and delivery, stay conscious of her needs. Offer her water or ice chips, if allowed. Massage her body. Suggest position changes periodically. Keep her informed of how labor is progressing and how well she's doing. It's more important for you to take care of her than to record everything on film or call friends and family.

During pushing and delivery
Help guide her pushing and breathing
Using cues from the health care team or from what you learned in childbirth classes, help guide her breathing while she pushes. Support her back or hold one of her legs while she's pushing. Whatever seems to help her — that's the thing to do!

Stay close by
A lot may happen quickly when it comes time for her to push. Or she may have to keep pushing on and off for several hours. Once she gets ready to push, don't feel that you're in the way as the health care team takes charge. Your presence is important, particularly as labor nears completion.

Point out her progress
As the baby's head crowns, if allowed, hold up a mirror so that she can see for herself how she's progressing. Or tell her how close the baby is to being born!

Cut the cord, if desired
If offered the opportunity to cut the cord, don't panic. You'll get clear directions from the health care team on just what to do. Don't feel pressured to do this, if you're uncomfortable with the idea.

After labor and delivery
Celebrate!
Once the baby has arrived, enjoy bonding with the new baby. But don't forget to give your partner some well-earned words of praise, and congratulate yourself, too, for a job well done!

Immediately after birth

At birth, your baby is still connected to the placenta by the umbilical cord. Often the parents can assist with the clamping and cutting of the cord. If you'd like to assist, make your wishes known, and you'll be shown what to do.

There's usually no particular urgency to cut the umbilical cord. Two clamps are placed on the cord, and then a scissors is used to snip painlessly between the clamps. If the umbilical cord has looped snugly around the baby's neck, the cord may be clamped and cut before the shoulders are delivered.

Immediately after birth, your baby may be placed in your arms or on your abdomen. Or occasionally, the baby may be passed to a nurse or pediatrician for evaluation and attention.

Shortly after birth, your baby is weighed and examined. He or she is dried off and wrapped in blankets to keep warm. The Apgar scores (see page 212) are recorded at one- and five-minute intervals. An identification band is placed on your baby so that there's no mix-up in the nursery. This is just the first of many safeguards to ensure no mistake in identification is made.

In most cases, you'll be able to hold and breast-feed your baby right after birth. But if your baby shows any signs that help is needed, such as trouble breathing, he or she may need to be evaluated more thoroughly in the nursery.

Stage 3: Delivery of the placenta

After your baby is born, a lot is happening. You and your partner are celebrating the excitement of the birth and, perhaps, sharing some private moments. You're likely both decompressing, relieved that labor and childbirth is finally over. Meanwhile, a health care provider in the background is examining your baby as he or she takes the first breaths and you hear those wonderful first cries.

The third — and final — stage of labor and childbirth is delivery of the placenta. The placenta is an organ inside the uterus attached to the baby by the umbilical cord. It's the organ that has nourished your baby throughout your pregnancy.

For most couples, the placenta — also called the afterbirth — is of little significance. For the medical personnel attending the birth, delivering the placenta and ensuring that the mother doesn't bleed excessively are important.

What's happening

After your baby is born, you continue to have contractions. These are mild, and they're necessary for several reasons — one of which is to help you deliver the placenta.

Usually about five to 10 minutes after the birth, the placenta separates from the wall of the uterus. Your final contractions push the placenta out from the uterus and down into the vagina. You may be asked to push one more time to deliver the placenta, which usually comes out with a small gush of blood. Sometimes, it may take up to 30 minutes for the placenta to detach from the wall of the uterus and be expelled.

Your health care provider may massage your lower abdomen after you have delivered your baby. This is to encourage your uterus to contract, to help expel the placenta.

After delivery of your placenta, you may be given a medication such as oxytocin by injection or by intravenous (IV) drip to encourage uterine contractions. Uterine contractions after birth are important. They help close off blood vessels and minimize bleeding. They also help your uterus shrink back to the size it was before it expanded to house your baby.

How you may be feeling
You shouldn't feel much pain while your uterus contracts to push out the placenta. The hardest part may be simply being patient as you wait for the delivery of the placenta. The deep massages of your abdomen by your health care provider may hurt.

What you can do
You can help expel the placenta by pushing when directed. As you push, your health care provider may pull gently on the leftover umbilical cord attached to the placenta.

You can also try to accelerate the process by breast-feeding your baby. Stimulation of the breasts signals your body to release the hormone oxytocin, which causes uterine contractions.

In most instances, delivery of the placenta is a routine part of childbirth. But complications can arise if your placenta doesn't spontaneously detach from the uterine wall (retained placenta). In the case of a retained placenta, the health care provider must reach inside the uterus and remove the placenta by hand.

Once the placenta is out, your health care provider examines it to make sure it's normal and intact. If it's not intact, he or she must remove any remaining fragments inside the uterus. Rarely, surgery is needed to remove placental fragments. Remnants that aren't removed could cause bleeding and infection.

After delivery, your health care provider disposes of the placenta. Most women never see the placenta. If you're interested, ask to see it. It's usually round and flat, red, about 6 to 8 inches in diameter and about 20 ounces in weight.

In multiple pregnancies, there may be more than one placenta to deliver. Or there may be one placenta with more than one cord coming from it.

Meeting your new baby

For most parents, all the preparation, pain and effort that went into bringing this newborn into the world are quickly forgotten as they hold their own child. This is one of the most significant moments in your life. You are a new parent. A new human being has taken his or her place among all of us in the human family. It is an absolute miracle. Savor this moment, cherish it and embrace the joy that nothing else in life can quite match.

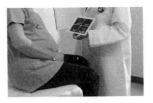

CHAPTER   12

Caesarean birth

Caesarean birth is the birth of a baby by means of an incision in the uterus. It's done when your health care provider decides it's safer — either for you or for your baby — than a vaginal birth. Most first-time Caesareans occur unexpectedly. For that reason, it's a good idea to educate yourself about Caesarean birth as you come to the end of your pregnancy. That way, you'll be more prepared for the possibility, should it arise.

Why a Caesarean birth might be necessary

Many different factors can lead to the decision to perform a Caesarean birth.

Your labor is failing to progress normally

The failure of labor to progress normally is one of the most common reasons that doctors deliver babies by Caesarean. In fact, about a third of all Caesareans are done because labor is progressing too slowly or stops altogether. The causes of slow or stalled labor are varied. Your uterus may not be contracting vigorously enough to dilate your cervix completely. Or your baby's head may simply be too big to fit through your pelvis. This is what's known as cephalopelvic disproportion (CPD). It, too, can stop your cervix from dilating completely.

Your baby has an abnormal heart rate pattern during labor

Certain patterns of fetal heart rate are very reassuring in labor. Other patterns may indicate a problem with the baby's oxygen supply. When these heart rate patterns cause concern, your health care provider may recommend a Caesarean birth. This scenario accounts for 10 percent to 15 percent of all Caesarean births. These abnormal fetal heart rate patterns can arise when the baby isn't getting enough oxygen, because the umbilical cord is compressed or because the placenta isn't functioning optimally. For more information on problems with your placenta or umbilical cord, see the sections "There's a problem with your placenta" and "There's a problem with the umbilical cord" on page 190.

Unfortunately, abnormal fetal heart rate patterns may occur without indicating any real risk to your baby. At other times, these findings may indicate a serious problem. One of the most difficult decisions in obstetrics is determining when the risk is genuine. To help make that decision, your health care provider may attempt to test the baby's blood by obtaining a sample through the scalp. Or your health care provider may try certain maneuvers, such as massaging the baby's head, to give rise to reassuring heart rate changes.

Deciding when a Caesarean is necessary depends on a lot of variables, such as how long labor is likely to continue before delivery and what other problems, such as an overdue baby, make the abnormal heart rate patterns more likely to be significant. Although there are times a baby is clearly in trouble, many other times it's a difficult assessment.

Your baby is in an abnormal position

Babies whose feet or buttocks enter the birth canal before the head are in what's known as the breech position. Most of these babies are born by Caesarean section, primarily because of the severity of the possible complications of vaginal birth. For example, in vaginal breech births, it's more common to have the umbilical cord slip through the cervix before the baby (prolapsed umbilical cord). This can cut off the baby's oxygen supply. Plus, the baby's head could become trapped in the birth canal, even if the rest of the body emerges easily.

If your baby is lying horizontally across your uterus, the position is called a transverse lie. This position, too, calls for Caesarean birth.

If your baby is in the breech position, your health care provider may be able to move the baby into a more favorable position by pushing on the baby through your abdomen, before labor starts. This procedure is called an external version. If this doesn't work, Caesarean birth will probably be considered.

You have a serious health problem

If you have diabetes, heart disease, lung disease or high blood pressure, you may need a Caesarean birth. Often, these conditions lead to the decision to deliver a baby earlier in pregnancy by starting (inducing) labor. Early inductions of labor often lead to failure of the cervix to dilate or abnormal fetal heart rate patterns, which increase the chances of Caesarean birth.

In many of these cases, vaginal delivery would be preferable for mother's care. For example, good evidence suggests that women with coronary artery disease should deliver vaginally, especially if they also have pulmonary vascular disease. For these women, Caesarean birth seems to worsen their outcome. Women with severe complications of pregnancy-induced high blood pressure (preeclampsia) may also do better if a vaginal delivery can be accomplished. If you have a serious health problem, discuss your options with your health care provider well before the end of your pregnancy.

Another unusual cause for a Caesarean birth is to protect a baby from acquiring herpes simplex infections. If a mother has primary (first episode) herpes in the genital tract, it can be passed to a birthing baby, giving rise to serious disease. A Caesarean birth is often used to prevent that complication.

Your baby's head is in the wrong position

When your baby enters your pelvis, he or she should be head-down and facedown. His or her chin should be tucked down to the chest so that the back of the head, which has the smallest diameter, is leading the way. If your baby's chin is up or head is turned so that the smallest dimensions aren't leading the way, a larger diameter of the head has to fit through your pelvis. The fit can be quite tight. In these cases, the top of your baby's head, forehead or face may be the body part farthest down in the pelvis, ready to be born first. Even though your cervix might be fully dilated, your baby simply may be unable to fit through your pelvis, and Caesarean birth may be necessary.

Some babies also move into the birth canal head-down but faceup, in what's known as an *occiput posterior* position. Most babies will turn during labor and be born facedown. Your health care provider might have you get on your hands and knees with your buttocks in the air, a position that causes the uterus to drop forward and seems to help babies turn. Sometimes the health care provider may try to turn the baby's head during a contraction by way of a vaginal exam. Occasionally, turning the baby with forceps and helping the baby be born that way is the safest route to delivery. If that doesn't work, a Caesarean birth may be the safest option.

Many women, especially those of African ancestry, have perfectly normal labors with their baby in the faceup position. It may not be a problem for you and your baby.

You're carrying twins, triplets or other multiples

About half of all women who have twins have Caesarean births. Twins can often be born vaginally, depending on their position, estimated weight and gestational age. Triplets and other multiples are a different story. Studies show that more than 90 percent of triplet births are by Caesarean birth.

When more than one baby is present inside your uterus, it's not unusual for one to be in an abnormal position. In this case, Caesarean birth is often safer than vaginal birth, especially for the twin born second. In fact, some research suggests that second twins born vaginally are at greater risk of death due to complications during labor and childbirth than are the twins delivered first.

Each multiple pregnancy is unique. If you're carrying twins, triplets or other multiples, discuss your birth options with your health care provider and decide together what's best for you. Remember to stay flexible. Even if both babies are head down during your examinations, that may not be the case after the first baby is born.

There's a problem with your placenta

Two problems with the placenta may warrant Caesarean birth: placental abruption and placenta previa.

Placental abruption occurs when your placenta detaches from the inner wall of your uterus before labor begins. It can cause life-threatening problems for you and your baby. If your health care provider suspects that you have a placental abruption, he or she can recommend steps to manage it based on your condition and the condition of your baby.

If electronic fetal monitoring shows that your baby is not in immediate trouble, you may be hospitalized and monitored closely. If your baby is in jeopardy, immediate delivery will likely be required. Caesarean birth may be necessary, although in some situations vaginal birth may be possible.

The decision-making process is quite different with placenta previa. With this condition, your placenta lies low in your uterus and partially or completely covers the opening of your cervix.

Women with a placenta previa in late pregnancy will likely need a Caesarean birth. The placenta can't be born first, as the baby would no longer have access to oxygen. In addition, it's very unlikely that the mother would be able to tolerate the blood loss that resulted. So for both mother and baby, Caesarean birth is safest.

There's a problem with the umbilical cord

Once your water has broken, it's possible that a loop of umbilical cord will slip out through your cervix, before your baby is born. This is called umbilical cord prolapse, and it poses grave danger to your baby. As your baby presses against your cervix, the pressure on the protruding cord can block your baby's oxygen supply.

If the cord slips out after your cervix is completely dilated, and if birth is imminent, you might still be able to deliver vaginally. Otherwise, Caesarean birth is the only option. Fortunately, this problem is very rare when babies are head down.

Similarly, if the cord is wrapped around your baby's neck or is positioned between your baby's head and your pelvic bones, or if you have decreased amniotic fluid, each uterine contraction will squeeze the cord, slowing blood flow and the delivery of oxygen to your baby. In these cases, Caesarean birth may be the best option, especially if cord compression is prolonged or severe. This is a common cause of abnormal heart rate patterns, but it usually isn't possible to know for sure where the umbilical cord is until after birth.

Your baby is very large

Some babies are just too large to deliver safely vaginally. Your baby's size may be of particular concern if you have an abnormally small pelvis, which may prevent the baby's head from passing through. This is rare unless you have had a pelvic fracture or another deformation of the pelvis.

If you've developed gestational diabetes during your pregnancy, your baby may have gained too much weight before birth — a condition called macrosomia. If your baby is overly big — generally defined as 9 pounds, 14 ounces or more — Caesarean birth is more likely.

For the most part, electing to do a Caesarean birth because of the anticipated size of the baby isn't warranted. Ultrasound and clinical examination (just feeling the baby through the abdomen) are about equally accurate at guessing a baby's weight once the baby exceeds about 8½ pounds. There's enough error in this estimation that if Caesarean births were recommended for all babies estimated to be over nine pounds, a good number of babies who actually weighed only 8 pounds would never have the chance to be born vaginally.

Your baby has a health problem

If your baby has been diagnosed in the womb with a developmental problem, your health care provider may recommend that you have a Caesarean birth. Examples include spina bifida (a spine defect resulting in failure of the vertebrae to fuse) or hydrocephalus (increased size of the fluid-filled cavities of the brain). For babies with the most common severe form of spina bifida called myelomeningocele, some evidence shows that Caesarean births lead to a better neurological outcomes than vaginal births do.

Unfortunately, few definitive studies are available to help health care providers and parents-to-be decide between Caesarean and vaginal birth for babies with birth defects and other health problems.

Work with your health care provider to gather the facts that apply to your situation. Discuss your birth options with your health care provider, and decide together what's best for you and your baby. In these situations, a Caesarean birth might not be necessary to prevent damage to a baby, but being born in a controlled situation with a team of surgeons on hand may benefit the baby greatly. Often, the only way to orchestrate this kind of timing is through Caesarean birth.

You've had a previous Caesarean birth

If you've had a Caesarean birth before, you may need to have one again. But this isn't always the case. See "Considering vaginal birth after Caesarean birth" on page 345.

CAN YOU PREVENT A CAESAREAN?

Can you prevent having a Caesarean birth? Probably not. If your baby is in a breech position, you can ask your health care provider whether it would be possible for him or her to turn the baby into the proper position for a vaginal birth, a procedure called an external version. But the decision to perform a Caesarean will depend on your doctor's assessment of your health and the health of your baby. If either of you is in danger, a Caesarean birth may be necessary. Remember, your aim is to be a healthy mom for a healthy baby, no matter what it takes. Be sure you have a trusting relationship with your health care provider and her or his team. When something goes wrong in labor, it's best to have confidence in those who are advising you.

Risks of Caesarean birth

A Caesarean birth is major surgery. Although it's considered a very safe procedure, it carries certain risks, including the risk of death. Although a woman's risk of death after a Caesarean birth is very low — estimated at about two in 10,000 — it's about twice as great as the risk is if she was to deliver vaginally. One important point to remember: Caesarean deliveries are often performed to resolve life-threatening complications. It's to be expected that more complications would arise in those women.

Risks for you

Other risks are higher with Caesarean birth than with vaginal delivery. These include:

- **Increased bleeding.** On average, blood loss during Caesarean birth is about twice that as during vaginal birth. However, blood transfusions are rarely needed during Caesarean birth, typically only about 3 percent of the time.

- **Reactions to anesthesia.** The medications used during surgery, including those used for anesthesia, can sometimes cause unexpected responses, including breathing problems. In rare cases, general anesthesia can lead to pneumonia when a woman aspirates stomach contents into the lungs. However, general anesthesia is used in less than 20 percent of Caesarean births, and precautions are specifically taken to avoid these complications.
- **Inadvertent injury to your bladder or bowel.** These surgical injuries are rare, but they're recognized complications of Caesarean birth.
- **Endometritis.** This condition causes an inflammation and infection of the membrane lining your uterus. It's the most frequent complication associated with Caesarean birth. It occurs when bacteria that normally inhabit your vagina make their way into your uterus. Endometritis is up to 20 times more likely to occur after a Caesarean birth than after a vaginal childbirth.
- **Urinary tract infection.** Urinary tract infections, such as bladder infections and kidney infections, rank second to endometritis as a cause of complications after a Caesarean birth.
- **Decreased bowel function.** Most women have few if any gastrointestinal problems after a Caesarean birth. In some cases, though, the drugs used for anesthesia and pain relief may lead the bowel to slow down for a few days after surgery, resulting in temporary distention of the abdomen, bloating and discomfort.
- **Blood clots in your legs, lungs or pelvic organs.** The risk of developing a blood clot inside a vein is about three to five times greater after a Caesarean childbirth than after a vaginal delivery. If untreated, a blood clot in the leg can travel to your heart and lungs. There it can obstruct blood flow, causing chest pain, shortness of breath and even death. Clotting can also occur in the pelvic veins. This, too, is more common after Caesarean birth.
- **Wound infection.** Wound infection rates following Caesarean birth vary. An elective, repeat Caesarean birth generally has a wound infection rate of about 2 percent. Caesareans that follow labor, particularly if your membranes have ruptured (your water has broken), have a wound infection rate of 5 percent to 10 percent. Your chances of developing wound infection after a Caesarean birth are higher if you abuse alcohol, have type 2 diabetes (formerly called adult-onset or noninsulin-dependent diabetes) or are obese, which is defined as having a body mass index of 30 or higher.
- **Wound rupture.** When a wound is infected or healing poorly, it's more likely to split open along the surgical suture lines. This occurs in only about 5 percent of wound infections.

- **Placenta accreta and hysterectomy.** Placenta accreta is the term used to describe a placenta attached too deeply and too firmly to the wall of the uterus. If you've had a previous Caesarean birth, your risk of developing placenta accreta in a subsequent pregnancy is increased. Placenta accreta is closely associated with placenta previa — abnormal position of the placenta inside the uterus. About 25 percent of women having a Caesarean birth for placenta previa, and who've also had a previous Caesarean, need a post-Caesarean hysterectomy for placenta accreta. In fact, placenta accreta is currently the most common reason for post-Caesarean hysterectomy.
- **Rehospitalization.** A recent study found that compared with women who deliver vaginally, women who deliver by Caesarean birth are twice as likely to be hospitalized again in the two months after giving birth.

Risks for your baby

Caesarean birth also poses potential risks for your baby. These include:
- **Premature birth.** In a Caesarean birth by choice, it's important that dates are very accurately assessed or a sample of the amniotic fluid is tested for lung maturity. Delivering a baby prematurely may lead to difficulty breathing and low birth weight.
- **Breathing problems.** Babies born by Caesarean are more likely to develop a minor breathing problem called transient tachypnea, a condition marked by abnormally fast breathing during the first few days after birth.
- **Fetal injury.** Although rare, accidental nicks to the baby can occur during surgery.

Managing anxiety about Caesarean birth

Getting the unexpected news that you need a Caesarean can be stressful, both for you and your partner. In an instant, your expectations about giving birth and caring for your new baby abruptly change. To make things worse, this news often comes when you're tired and discouraged from ineffective labor. In addition, there's often not much time for your health care provider to explain the procedure and answer your questions. This is especially true in the case of an emergency Caesarean birth.

It's normal to have some worries about how you and your baby will fare during a Caesarean birth. But don't let these worries get the better of you. Almost all mothers and babies recover well after Caesarean birth, with few problems. If you're feeling disappointed that you need a Caesarean, try to let it go. Although you would probably have preferred a vaginal birth, remind yourself that your health and the health of your baby are much more important than the method of delivery.

If you're scheduled for a repeat Caesarean birth, you may also be anxious. You may have disturbing memories of your last Caesarean. You may be concerned about how you'll care for your new baby and your other child or children while recovering from major surgery. On the other hand, you may feel relieved that you won't have to go through labor. Being able to schedule your baby's arrival may give you a sense of calm. Each woman is different.

If you're feeling anxious about a scheduled repeat Caesarean birth, discuss your fears with your health care provider, childbirth educator or partner. Sharing your feelings will probably make you feel less worried. Tell yourself that you made it through once before — and you can do it again. If anything, recovering from a Caesarean will probably be easier this time around. You know more than you once did, and your coping skills are probably better now, too.

What you can expect during a Caesarean birth

Preoperative preparation

Whether your Caesarean childbirth is planned or unexpected, you'll undergo a series of steps to prepare for the surgery. The standard steps are listed below. In an emergency, some of these steps might be cut short or left out entirely.

Discussing your anesthesia options

An anesthesiologist can come to your hospital room to assess your condition and circumstances and to recommend which type of anesthesia (spinal, epidural or general) is best. The recommendation depends on many factors. Which type of anesthesia is safest for your baby? Which is safest for you? Which options are feasible right now?

Spinal, epidural and general anesthesia are all used for Caesarean births. Spinal and epidural anesthesia numb your body from the chest down, allowing you to remain awake for the procedure. You feel little or no pain, and little or no medication reaches your baby.

The differences between spinal and epidural anesthesia are fairly small. With a spinal block, pain-relieving medication is injected into the fluid surrounding your spinal nerves. With an epidural, this medication is injected just outside the fluid-filled space surrounding your spinal cord. An epidural takes about 20 minutes to administer and lasts almost indefinitely. A spinal block can be performed more quickly but usually only lasts about two hours. In an emergency situation, there's often not enough time for an epidural. Spinal block and epidural are each used in about 40 percent of Caesarean births.

General anesthesia, during which you're completely unconscious, is typically used in emergency Caesarean births, when your baby needs to be delivered as quickly as possible. Some of the medication does reach your baby, but this doesn't cause any problems that an attendant pediatrician can't readily deal with. Most babies show no effect of general anesthesia, since the mother's brain absorbs the medication promptly and to a large extent. If necessary, your baby can be given medications to counteract any effects of the anesthesia.

Undergoing other preparations

Once you, your doctor and the anesthesiologist have decided which type of anesthesia you'll have, preparations begin in earnest. These typically include:

- **Getting an IV.** Your nurse can insert an intravenous (IV) needle into your hand or arm. This will allow you to receive fluids and medications during and after surgery.
- **Providing blood samples.** Your nurse will likely collect these samples and send them to the hospital lab for analysis. These lab tests will allow your doctor to have a more complete picture of your baseline condition — that is, your presurgery condition.
- **Taking an antacid.** You may be given an antacid to neutralize your stomach acids. This simple step greatly diminishes the possibility of damage to your lungs if stomach contents were to enter during anesthesia.
- **Placement of monitors.** Your anesthesiologist or nurse will probably wrap a blood pressure cuff around your arm so that your blood pressure can be monitored during surgery. You can also be hooked up to a cardiac monitor through electrodes stuck to your chest to monitor your heart rate and rhythm during surgery. A saturation monitor can be clamped onto your finger to monitor the oxygen level in your blood.
- **Receiving a urinary catheter.** A thin tube called a catheter can be inserted into your bladder to drain urine so that your bladder will stay empty during surgery.

In the operating room

Getting ready

Most Caesarean births are performed in operating rooms specially set aside for that purpose. The atmosphere in the operating room may be a lot different from what you've experienced in the birthing room. Because surgery is a team effort, many more people will be there. In fact, if you or your baby have a complex medical problem, as many as 12 people may be in the room.

If you don't already have an IV, you'll get one now. You might receive extra oxygen through a face mask.

If you're going to have an epidural or spinal block and your anesthesiologist hasn't administered it yet, you'll sit up with your back rounded or lie curled up on your side. The anesthesiologist can scrub your back with antiseptic solution and inject a medication to numb the site. Then he or she can administer the blocking medication by inserting a needle between two vertebrae and through the tough tissue next to your spinal column.

You may receive just one dose of medication through the needle, which will then be removed. Or your anesthesiologist may thread a narrow catheter through the needle, slide the needle out and tape the catheter to your back to keep it in place. This will allow you to receive repeat doses of anesthetic as needed.

If you need to have general anesthesia, all preparations for surgery, including washing your entire abdomen with antiseptic solution, will be done before you receive an anesthetic agent. Your anesthesiologist can administer the general anesthetic drugs by injecting the drugs into your IV. These drugs will circulate in your bloodstream to all areas of your body, including your brain, causing you to lose consciousness.

Once you're anesthetized, awake or not, you'll be placed lying on your back with your legs positioned securely in place. A wedge may be placed under the right side of your back so that you're turned to the left. This shifts the uterine weight left, which can help ensure good uterine blood flow.

Your arms likely will be outstretched and secured on padded platforms. A nurse may shave the hair on your abdomen and the upper portion of your pubic hair, if it will interfere with surgery or removing bandages after surgery. Alternatively, a portion of your pubic hair may be clipped.

A nurse will likely scrub your abdomen with an antiseptic solution and drape it with sterile cloths. A drape (anesthesia screen) can be placed below your chin to help keep the surgical field clean.

Abdominal incision

Once you're in position, your abdomen is clean and you're numb or asleep, your surgeon will make the first incision. This will be the abdominal incision, made in your abdominal wall. The incision on your abdomen will probably be about 6 inches long, going through your skin, fat and muscle to reach the lining of your abdominal cavity, called the peritoneum. Bleeding blood vessels can be sealed with heat (cauterized) or tied off.

The location of your abdominal incision will depend on several factors, such as whether your Caesarean birth is an emergency and whether you have any previous abdominal scars. Your baby's size or the position of placenta also will be considered.

A bikini incision, curved across your lower abdomen along the line of an imaginary bikini bottom, is the generally preferred abdominal incision. It heals well and causes the least pain after surgery. It's also preferred for cosmetic reasons and gives your surgeon a good view of the lower pregnant uterus.

However, sometimes a low vertical incision, made from just below your navel to just above your pubic bone, is the best option. This incision allows faster access to the lower portion of your uterus, allowing your surgeon to remove your baby more quickly. Occasionally, time is of the essence. Seconds matter. Low vertical incisions also have less blood loss and allow for the incision to be extended around the belly button, should that be necessary.

Uterine incision

Once your abdominal incision is complete, your surgeon can safely move the bladder off of the lower part of the uterus and make a second incision in the wall of your uterus. Your uterine incision may or may not be the same type as you have on your abdomen. The uterine incision is usually smaller than the abdominal incision.

As with the abdominal incision, the location of the uterine incision will depend on several factors, such as whether your Caesarean is an emergency, how big your baby is and how your baby or placenta is positioned inside the uterus.

The low transverse incision, made sideways across the lower portion of the uterus, is the most common, used in more than 90 percent of all Caesarean births. It provides greater ease of entry, bleeds less than incisions higher on the uterus and poses less risk of bladder injury. It also forms a strong scar, presenting little danger of rupture during future labors. This makes vaginal birth after Caesarean (VBAC) a real option for future pregnancies.

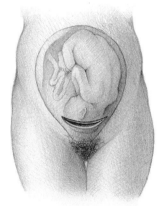 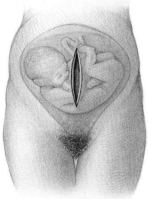 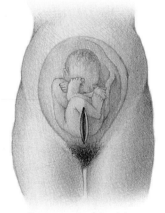

Low transverse incision *Classical incision* *Low vertical incision*

In some cases, a vertical uterine incision is more appropriate. A low vertical incision, made vertically in your lower uterus where the tissue is thinner, may be used if your baby is positioned feet-first, rump-first or sideways in your uterus (breech or transverse lie). It may also be used if your surgeon thinks your incision may need to be extended to a high vertical incision — what doctors sometimes call a classical incision.

In the past, Caesarean births were almost always done with a classical incision, made in the upper portion of the uterus. Today, classical incisions are used in less than 10 percent of all Caesarean births, mainly because of the increased risk of bleeding and rupture of the uterus in later pregnancies. In fact, women with classical Caesarean incisions who become pregnant again are at increased risk of uterine rupture even before labor starts. The main advantage of the classical incision is the speed by which your surgeon can enter your uterus and remove your baby. This can be vitally important if your baby is acutely ill. A classical incision may occasionally be done to avoid bladder injury if a woman has decided this is her last pregnancy.

Birth
With your uterus exposed, your surgeon can open your amniotic sac so that your baby can make his or her grand appearance. If you're awake, you will probably feel some tugging, pulling or pressure as your baby is pulled out. This is because your surgeon is trying to keep the incision in your uterus as small as possible. You should not feel any pain.

After your baby is born, your surgeon can clamp the umbilical cord and hand your baby to another member of your health care team. This person can make sure your baby's nose and mouth are free of fluids and that your baby is breathing well. In just a matter of minutes, you'll have your first look at your baby. If your partner is in the room, he may have the option of cutting the umbilical cord. At this point, you may also receive a dose of antibiotics through your IV to help prevent uterine infection.

Removal of the placenta and closing of the incision
After your baby is delivered, your surgeon can detach and remove your placenta from your uterus. He or she can then begin to close your incisions, layer by layer. Because you may feel drowsy, the time will probably pass quickly.

The stitches on your internal organs and tissues can dissolve on their own and won't need to be removed. With the incision on your skin, your surgeon may use stitches to close it or may use a type of staples — small metal clips that bend in the middle to pull the edges of the incision together. Throughout this repair, you may feel some movement but no pain. If your incision is closed with staples, your doctor or nurse can remove them with a tiny pair of pliers before you go home.

Seeing your baby

Although a Caesarean typically takes 45 minutes to an hour, your baby will likely be born in the first five to 10 minutes of the procedure. If you're feeling up to it and are awake, you may be able to hold your baby as your surgeon closes the incisions in your uterus and abdomen. At the very least, you'll probably be able to see your baby snuggled into your partner's arms. Before giving your baby to you or your partner, your health care team can suction your baby's nose and mouth and do the first Apgar check, which is a quick assessment of a baby's appearance, pulse, reflexes, activity and respiration taken at one minute after birth.

In the recovery room

Immediately after surgery, you'll be taken to a recovery room. There, your vital signs can be monitored frequently, about every 15 minutes, until the anesthesia has worn off and your condition is stable. This generally takes an hour or two, but it can take longer if you've had general anesthesia. During your time in the recovery room, you and your partner may have a few minutes alone with your baby so that you can start to get acquainted.

If you've chosen to breast-feed your baby, you may be able to do it for the first time in the recovery room, if you're feeling up to it. When it comes to breast-feeding, the sooner you start, the better. Pillows placed behind you can help you get into a comfortable position. In fact, if you've had an epidural, breast-feeding may be more comfortable for several hours after surgery, while the anesthesia is still working. However, if you've had general anesthesia, you may be groggy and uncomfortable for a few hours after surgery. You may want to wait until you've received medication for pain before beginning breast-feeding.

Recovery from Caesarean birth

After a couple of hours in the recovery room, you'll be moved to a room in the maternity unit of the hospital. Over the next 24 hours, your doctor and nurses can continue to monitor your breathing rate, heart rate, temperature and blood pressure. They'll also monitor the condition of your abdominal dressing, the amount of urine you're producing and the amount of post-pregnancy bleeding (lochia) you're experiencing. Your nurses will also periodically check your uterus, making sure that it's remaining contracted.

During the course of your hospital stay, your health care team will continue to carefully monitor your condition. Your nurses can periodically take your vital signs and assess the condition of your incision, uterus and lochia. Your

Your partner's involvement in Caesarean birth

If your Caesarean birth isn't an emergency requiring general anesthesia, your partner may be able to come into the operating room with you. Many hospitals allow this. Your partner may be thrilled by the idea. Or he may be squeamish or downright scared. It can be difficult to be so close to surgery when it involves someone you know and love.

If you and your partner choose for him to be present for your Caesarean birth, he'll have to wear surgical scrubs, a covering for his hair, shoe covers and a face mask. If he decides he wants to watch the procedure, he may have that option. But if he doesn't, he can sit near your head and hold your hand, where the anesthesia screen will block his view. Having your partner close by will probably make you feel more relaxed. This has its advantages. There is, however, a potential disadvantage: Fathers frequently have fainted in the delivery room, giving rise to a second patient who can't be given too much immediate attention.

Most hospitals encourage your photos of your baby, and the surgical team may take some shots of you, your partner, and the baby before the surgery is even over. Be aware, though, that most hospitals don't allow direct filming of the operation. Before your partner starts snapping photos or rolling tape, make sure he asks permission.

nurses also want to know that your bowels and urinary tract are returning to normal and that your legs and feet are getting enough blood circulation. If you have questions about anything that's happening, ask a member of your health care team.

Relieving pain

You may not like the idea of taking pain-relieving drugs after surgery, especially if you plan to breast-feed. But it's important to be medicated for pain when the anesthesia wears off so that you can stay comfortable. Also, to be successful with breast-feeding, it's important to be comfortable. Comfort is especially crucial during the first several days of your recovery, when your incision is beginning to heal.

In the period immediately after your Caesarean birth, you'll likely receive pain-relieving medications called narcotics. This class of drugs includes morphine and its derivatives. These can be given through your IV or injected into a muscle, if your IV has been removed. During the first 24 hours after surgery, narcotics can also be given through an epidural catheter left in place.

Many hospitals connect a small pump to your IV so that you can self-administer small doses of narcotic when you feel you need it, simply by pressing a button. This is called patient-controlled analgesia. Because the drug goes directly into your IV, pain relief is fast. The pump has a lockout device, which limits the amount of narcotic you can receive. This prevents you from overmedicating yourself.

After a day or so, your health care provider will probably recommend that you switch to a combination of narcotic and non-narcotic pain relievers and ultimately to non-narcotic pain relievers only. Non-narcotic pain relievers include nonsteroidal anti-inflammatory drugs (NSAIDs), such as ibuprofen. You can also try relaxation techniques, soft music, dim lights and simple breathing exercises to relieve pain. You can be confident that your health care provider won't recommend any medications that are inadvisable for you or your baby.

In addition to the incision pain, you may also have afterbirth pains — uterine contractions that help control bleeding. These can start anytime after surgery and can last four to five days. They may be especially noticeable when you're breast-feeding. That's because breast-feeding causes your body to produce oxytocin, which stimulates uterine contractions. To help relieve afterbirth pains, try relaxation techniques or coordinate breast-feeding with taking your pain medication.

If you're still experiencing pain when it's time for you to be discharged, your health care provider may prescribe a small supply of narcotic medication for you to take at home.

Keeping your lungs clear

To prevent fluid from building up in your lungs after surgery, you may be encouraged to change positions in bed frequently and to cough and take slow, deep breaths. Coughing and turning may pull on your incision. But if you splint it by holding a pillow across your stomach and applying slight pressure, it shouldn't be as painful.

Eating and drinking

You'll probably be allowed to have only ice chips or sips of water for the first 12 to 24 hours after your surgery. You'll receive fluids intravenously in order to prevent dehydration. Once your digestive system starts to come back on line, you'll be able to drink more fluids and probably eat some easily digested food. You'll know you're ready to start eating if you begin to pass gas. It's a sign that your digestive system is waking up and starting to again function the way it should. You typically can begin eating solid foods the day after the surgery.

Walking

You'll probably be encouraged to take a brief walk about six to eight hours after your surgery, if it's not too late in the day. Walking may be the last thing you feel like doing. Your incision probably hurts every time you move. However, walking is good for your body and an important part of your recovery. It helps clear your lungs, improves your circulation, promotes healing and helps get your urinary and digestive systems back to normal. If you're having gas pains, walking can help relieve them. Walking also helps prevent blood clots, which were a common complication back in the days when women were kept in bed for weeks after surgery. Once you can get out of bed and walk to the bathroom, you may have your urinary catheter removed.

For your first venture out, be sure to have a supporting arm nearby. You'll probably be anxious the first time you try it. But once you're under way, you'll see that slow walking isn't as difficult or painful as you feared it might be.

After your first little stroll, you'll probably be encouraged to take brief walks a couple of times a day until it's time for you to go home.

Dealing with lochia

With the birth of your baby, your hormone levels have shifted. These shifts cause a vaginal discharge called lochia — a brownish to clear discharge that lasts for several weeks. Some women who've had Caesarean births are surprised at the amount of vaginal discharge they have after surgery. Even though the placenta is removed at the operation, the uterus still needs to heal and this discharge is part of the process. During your hospital stay, you'll use sanitary pads to absorb your lochia.

Incision care

The bandage on your incision will likely be removed the day after surgery, when your incision has had enough time to seal shut. During your hospital stay, your doctors and nurses will probably check the incision frequently.

As your incision begins to heal, it may itch. Don't scratch it. Applying lotion is a better, safer alternative.

If your incision was closed with surgical staples, they'll be removed before you go home. Once you're home, shower or bathe as usual. Afterward, dry the incision thoroughly with a towel or a hair dryer at a low setting.

Breast-feeding

Some techniques may be helpful when you start breast-feeding after a Caesarean birth. You may want to try the football hold, in which you hold your baby much the way a running back tucks a football under his arm. This breast-feeding position is just as effective as any other, but it keeps your baby from putting pressure on your still-sore abdomen.

To do the football hold, hold your baby at your side on your arm, with your elbow bent and your open hand firmly supporting your baby's head, near the level of your breast. Your baby's torso should be resting on your forearm. Put a pillow at your side to support your arm. In the first weeks after you're home from the hospital, a chair with broad, low arms typically works best.

With your free hand, get your breast into the proper position, gently squeezing it so that the nipple is aligned horizontally. Move your baby to your breast until your baby's mouth opens. Then pull your baby in close to latch on snugly. Repeat on the other side.

You may also want to try nursing your baby while lying down, especially in the first few days after surgery. To do this, lie on your side and place your baby on his or her side facing you. Make sure your baby's mouth is close to the nipple of your lower breast. Use the hand of your lower arm to help keep your baby's head in the proper position at your breast.

With your upper arm and hand, reach across your body and grasp your breast, touching your nipple to your baby's lips. Once your baby has latched on firmly, you can use your lower arm to support your own head and your upper hand and arm to help support your baby.

Being discharged

The typical hospital stay after a Caesarean birth is three days. Some women are discharged as early as two days after surgery

Before leaving the hospital, be sure that your questions are answered. Know what your health care provider recommends for relieving pain and what restrictions he or she is placing on your activity. Be aware of the signs and symptoms of possible post-Caesarean complications.

In addition, schedule an appointment with your health care provider for a postpartum exam. Most mothers will return for their next visit at six weeks, just as after vaginal delivery.

Recovery after Caesarean birth is a longer process than recovery after vaginal birth. It will probably take four to six weeks before you feel like you're back to normal. You'll have to take things slowly and ask for help when you need it.

Post-Caesarean restrictions

During your first week at home after a Caesarean birth, restrict your activities to taking care of yourself and your newborn. Avoid heavy lifting or other activities that could put a strain on your healing wound. Ask your health care provider for recommendations about everyday activities, such as walking up and down stairs or lifting anything heavier than your baby.

Many women find it hard to adhere to their restrictions as they start to feel better. After a Caesarean, you might feel very tired when you first try to exert yourself. Give yourself a chance to heal. After all, you did have an operation.

Until you can make quick movements with your legs or torso without pain, don't drive. Although some women recover from a Caesarean birth more quickly than others, the typical no-driving period is two weeks.

Once your health care provider gives you the OK, you can begin exercising. But take it easy. Swimming and walking are good choices. By the third or fourth week after leaving the hospital, you'll likely feel like resuming your normal activities at home.

Possible post-Caesarean complications

In general, report these signs and symptoms to your health care provider if they occur once you're home from the hospital:
- Fever of 100.4 F or greater
- Painful urination
- Vaginal discharge (lochia) heavier than a normal period
- Pulling apart at your incision
- Redness or oozing at the incision site
- Severe abdominal pain

For more on these and other postpartum complications, see page 579.

THE EMOTIONAL EFFECTS OF A CAESAREAN BIRTH

Once you're discharged from the hospital, you may begin to experience negative feelings about having had a Caesarean birth, even if you were accepting of the surgery at first. You may be angry that childbirth didn't happen the way you had hoped it would. You may grieve that you weren't able to give birth vaginally. You may feel like a failure as a woman, doubting your femininity and self-worth. To make things worse, you may feel guilty about having these feelings! Comments from friends and family like, "You took the easy way out," or "Are you going to have your next baby naturally?" may be making you feel even worse.

Suppress any feelings of inadequacy. Almost one out of four women give birth by Caesarean today, and the most important product of your pregnancy is a healthy baby. If you find yourself struggling with uncomfortable feelings, discuss them with your health care provider. Postpartum depression is a common disorder and a serious one. In addition, talk it over with friends, family and your caregiving team. It can help to know what happened and to understand fully the circumstances of your baby's birth. There are many resources to help work through postpartum concerns, so make your concerns known.

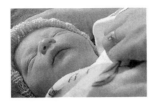

CHAPTER   13

your newborn

When the nurse put my baby boy in my arms for the first time, the chaos of the delivery room disappeared. I was surprised at how natural it felt to hold this new little life. I looked over everything — his hands, his feet, his eyes ... and his incredible mass of curly black hair! It was such a relief to see for myself the beautiful child I had delivered.

— One mother's experience

The wait is over. In the last nine months, you've spent endless hours in preparation and anticipation of the day you'd look into your baby's face. And now that day is here.

Your labor and delivery — whether a marathon session or shockingly short — is behind you. Now is the time to hold, caress and enjoy that precious little person you've been waiting to meet.

Even though you're probably eager to go home and start your new life, take advantage of your time in the hospital or birthing center. Many mothers are surprised by how much privacy time they want after birth. Although your family and friends will want to hear about your labor and birth and how you and the baby are doing, you might feel that you'll need to limit calls and visits. It's OK to turn off the phone, and the nurses can help restrict visitors to ensure your privacy. Good friends — especially if they're parents themselves — will understand if you need time to focus on yourself and your baby.

Your body has been through a significant workout, and new babies are demanding. So sit back and let the hospital staff help take care of you and your baby. It's not a luxury you'll be afforded for long.

You'll likely have many questions, and — fortunately — answers are just down the hall. You can feel comfortable calling on your hospital staff anytime, day or night. Part of their job is to help you make the transition to parenthood, whether this is your first baby or your fifth. Take advantage of their expertise.

In addition, many hospitals provide literature and videos about the care of newborns, ranging from feeding your baby to car seat safety. Your nurse can suggest which materials might be most helpful to you. If you have the opportunity, take some time to review this information. Once you get home, spare moments may be few and far between.

Many hospitals allow your baby to room in with you. This is a wonderful opportunity to get to know and spend time with your newborn. Realize, though, that it's perfectly acceptable to request some quiet time away from your baby. Once you go home, you won't have much time to rest — or, as some moms will attest, possibly even brush your teeth. If you're tired or just need a break, trust that your nurses will take excellent care of your baby in the nursery.

Before you let anyone take your newborn from your room, however, be sure they have identified themselves and are wearing a hospital name tag. If you're uncomfortable with or unsure about someone who wants to handle your baby, alert the nurses' station immediately. Although infant abduction is extremely rare, hospitals have procedures to identify and protect your baby. This means that you or a family member shouldn't move your baby away from the mother-and-baby area of your hospital without notifying one of the nurses. When your baby is dismissed from the hospital, don't leave until the nurse signs you out.

In this chapter, you'll learn about your newborn's first days of life — what he or she may look like, and what exams and immunizations your baby may undergo. The chapter also includes common problems some newborns have.

Your baby's appearance

Considering what they've just been through during labor and childbirth, it's no wonder that newborn babies don't look like the sweet little angels seen on television. Instead, your newborn will first appear somewhat messy looking. If your baby is like most, his or her head will be a bit misshapen and larger than you expected. The eyelids may be puffy, and his or her arms and legs may be drawn up as they were in the uterus. He or she may be somewhat bloody, wet and slippery from amniotic fluid.

In addition, most babies will be born with what appears like skin lotion. Called vernix, it'll be most noticeable under your baby's arms, behind the ears and in the groin. Premature babies, especially, are coated with it. Most of this vernix will be washed off during your baby's first bath.

Molded head

At first, your baby's head may appear flat, elongated or crooked. This peculiar elongation is one of the common features of the newly born baby.

A baby's skull consists of several sections of bone flexibly joined so that the head shape can change to correspond to the shape of your pelvis as your baby moves through the birth canal. A long labor usually results in an elongated or tall skull shape at birth. The head of a breech baby may have a shorter, broader appearance. If a vacuum extractor was used to assist in the birth, your baby's head may look particularly elongated.

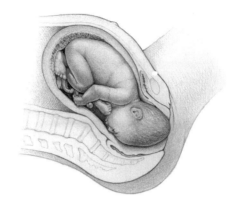

Fontanelles

When you feel the top of your baby's head, you'll notice two soft areas. These soft spots, called fontanelles, are where your baby's skull bones haven't grown together yet.

The fontanelle toward the front of the scalp is a diamond-shaped spot roughly the size of a quarter. Though it's usually flat, it may bulge when your baby cries or strains. By nine to 18 months, this fontanelle will be filled in with hard bone.

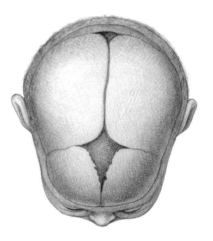

The smaller, less noticeable fontanelle at the back of the head is the size of a dime and closes around six weeks after birth.

Skin blemishes and bruises

Most babies are born with some blotchiness, bruising and skin blemishes.

A rounded swelling of the scalp (caput succedaneum) is usually seen on the top and back of the baby's head when a baby is born the usual way — headfirst. Caput succedaneum is simply puffiness of the skin that disappears within a day or so.

Pressure from your pelvis during labor can cause a bruise (cephalohematoma) on your baby's head. A cephalohematoma will be noticeable for several weeks, and you might feel a bump that persists for several months. You may also see scrapes or bruises on your baby's face and head if forceps were used during delivery. In most cases, these blemishes will go away within two weeks.

Other skin conditions common in newborns include:

- **Milia.** Most babies have milia, which look like tiny white pimples on the nose and chin. Although they appear to be raised, they are nearly flat and smooth to the touch. Milia disappear in time, and they don't require treatment.
- **Salmon patches.** These red patches may be found over the nape of the neck, between the eyebrows or on the eyelids. Also called stork bites or angel kisses, they usually disappear over the first few months. The medical term that's commonly used to describe a salmon patch is *nevus flammeus.*
- **Erythema toxicum.** It sounds scary, but *erythema toxicum* is simply the medical term for a skin condition that typically is present at birth or appears within the first few days afterward. It's characterized by small white or yellowish bumps surrounded by pink or reddish skin. This condition causes no discomfort, and it's not infectious. Erythema toxicum disappears in a few days.
- **Newborn acne.** Newborn (infantile) acne, which is also called miliaria, has nothing to do with acne in the mother. And this condition doesn't necessarily mean that a baby will have acne later in life. The red bumps and blotches similar to acne are seen on the face, neck, upper chest and back. This condition is most noticeable at a month or two and typically disappears without treatment within another month or two.
- **Mongolian spots.** Also known as the blue-gray macule of infancy, these large, flat areas containing extra pigment appear gray or blue on the lower back or buttocks. They're especially common in black, American Indian and Asian infants and in babies with dark complexions. Sometimes mistaken for bruises, Mongolian spots don't change color or fade like a bruise would. They generally go away in later childhood.
- **Pustular melanosis.** These small spots look like small white sesame seeds that quickly dry and peel off. They sometimes look similar to skin infections (pustules), but pustular melanosis isn't an infection, isn't red and disappears without treatment. These spots are most commonly seen in the folds of the neck and on the shoulders and upper chest. They're more common in dark-complected babies.
- **Strawberry hemangiomas.** Caused by overgrowth of blood vessels in the top layers of skin, strawberry (capillary) hemangiomas are red, raised spots that may resemble a strawberry. Usually not present at birth, a hemangioma begins as a small, pale spot that becomes red in the center. A strawberry hemangioma enlarges during the baby's first few months and eventually disappears without treatment.

Hair and lanugo

Your baby may be born bald, with a full head of thick hair — or almost anything in between! Don't fall in love with your baby's locks too quickly. The hair color your baby is born with isn't necessarily what he or she will have six months down the road. Blond newborns, for example, may become lighter or darker blond as they get older, and sometimes a reddish tinge isn't apparent at birth.

You may be surprised to see that your newborn's head isn't the only place he or she has hair. Downy, fine hair called lanugo covers a baby's body before birth and may temporarily appear on your newborn's back, shoulders, forehead and temples. Most of this hair is shed in the uterus before the baby is delivered, making lanugo especially common in premature babies. It disappears in the weeks following birth.

Early eye characteristics

It's perfectly normal for your newborn's eyes to be puffy. In fact, some infants have such puffy eyes that they aren't able to open their eyes wide right away. But don't worry, within a day or two, your baby will be able to look into your eyes.

You may also notice that your new baby sometimes looks cross-eyed. This, too, is normal and will be outgrown within several months.

Sometimes babies are born with red spots on the whites of their eyes. These spots are caused by the breakage of tiny blood vessels during birth. The spots are harmless and won't interfere with your baby's sight. They'll probably disappear in about 10 days.

Like hair, a newborn's eyes give no guarantee of future color. Although most newborns have dark bluish brown, blue-black, grayish blue or slate-colored eyes, permanent eye color may take six months or even longer to establish itself.

First bowel movements

Your baby's first soiled diaper — which will probably occur within 48 hours — may surprise you. During these first few days, your newborn's stools will be thick and sticky — a tar-like greenish black substance called meconium.

After the meconium is passed, the color, frequency and consistency of your baby's stools will vary depending on how your baby is fed. In babies who breast-feed, stools will be more frequent, generally soft, watery and golden yellow. In bottle-fed babies, stools will be less frequent, more formed and tan-colored, and have a stronger odor.

Initial health care for the newborn

From the moment your newborn emerges from the birth canal, he or she is the focus of much activity.

Once your baby has been delivered, your health care provider or a nurse likely will quickly clean his or her face. To make sure your baby can breathe properly, the nose and mouth are cleared of fluid as soon as the head appears — and again immediately after birth.

While the baby's airway is being cleared, the heart rate and circulation can be checked with a stethoscope or by feeling the pulse in the umbilical cord. The baby's color can be noted to make sure circulation is normal.

Your baby's umbilical cord is clamped with a plastic clamp, and you or your partner may be given the option to cut it. Then, the moment arrives: You can hold your baby for the first time.

In the next few days, the medical team likely will conduct newborn examinations, administer screening tests and give immunizations. Here's what to expect.

Examinations

Apgar scores
Apgar scores — a quick evaluation of a newborn baby's health — are noted at one minute and five minutes after birth. Developed in 1952 by anesthesiologist Virginia Apgar, this test rates newborns on five criteria: color, heart rate, reflexes, muscle tone and respiration.

Each of these criteria is given an individual score of zero, one or two. Then all scores are totaled for a maximum possible score of 10. Higher scores indicate the healthier infants, while scores below 5 mean an infant needs help at birth.

Today, many doctors downplay the significance of Apgar scores because most babies with lower scores ultimately turn out to be perfectly healthy.

Other checks and measurements
Soon after birth, your newborn's weight, length and head circumference can be measured. Your baby's temperature can be taken, and breathing and heart rate can be measured. Then, usually within 12 hours of your baby's birth, a physical exam is conducted to detect any problems or abnormalities.

Immunizations and vaccinations

Eye disease prevention
To avert the possibility of gonorrhea being passed from mother to baby,

all states require that infants' eyes be protected from this infection immediately after birth. Gonorrheal eye infections were a leading cause of blindness until early in the 20th century, when postnatal treatment of babies' eyes became mandatory.

Soon after your baby's birth, an antibiotic ointment or solution, commonly either erythromycin or tetracycline, is placed onto his or her eyes. These preparations are gentle to the eyes and cause no pain.

Vitamin K injection
In the United States, vitamin K is routinely given to infants shortly after they're born. Vitamin K is necessary for normal blood coagulation, the body's process for stopping bleeding after a cut or bruise. Newborns have low levels of vitamin K in their first few weeks. The injection can help prevent the rare possibility — one in 4,000 births — that a newborn would become so deficient in vitamin K that serious bleeding might develop. This problem is unique to babies in their first several weeks of life. It's not related to hemophilia.

Hepatitis B vaccination
Hepatitis B is a viral infection that affects the liver. It can cause such illnesses as cirrhosis and liver failure, or it can result in the development of liver tumors. Adults contract hepatitis through sexual contact, shared needles or exposure to the blood of an infected person. Babies, however, can contract hepatitis B from their mothers during pregnancy and birth.

The hepatitis B vaccine can protect infants from any possible contact with this virus. Therefore, your baby may be given this vaccine in the hospital or birthing center shortly after birth. Alternatively, the hepatitis B vaccinations may be given along with other immunizations at two months.

Screening tests

Before your baby leaves the hospital, a small amount of his or her blood is taken and sent to the state health department. This sample, which may be taken from a vein in your baby's arm or a tiny cut made on the heel, is analyzed to detect the presence of rare but important medical conditions. Results should be available by your baby's first office exam.

Occasionally, a baby needs to have the test repeated. Don't be alarmed if this happens to your newborn. To ensure that every newborn with any of these conditions is identified, even borderline results are rechecked. Retesting is especially common for premature babies.

Although newborn screening tests differ slightly from state to state, disorders that are commonly tested for include:

• **Phenylketonuria (PKU).** Babies with PKU retain excessive amounts of phenylalanine, an amino acid found in the protein of almost all foods. Without treatment, PKU can cause mental and motor retardation, poor growth rate and seizures. With early detection and treatment, growth and development should be normal.

- **Congenital hypothyroidism.** About one in 3,000 babies have a thyroid hormone deficiency that slows growth and brain development. Left untreated, it can result in mental retardation and stunted growth. With early detection and treatment, normal development is possible.
- **Congenital adrenal hyperplasia (CAH).** This group of disorders is caused by a deficiency of certain hormones. Signs and symptoms may include lethargy, vomiting, muscle weakness and dehydration. Infants with mild forms are at risk of reproductive and growth difficulties. Severe cases can cause kidney dysfunction and even death. Lifelong hormone treatment can suppress the disease.
- **Galactosemia.** Babies born with galactosemia can't metabolize galactose, a sugar found in milk. Although newborns with this condition typically appear normal, they may develop vomiting, diarrhea, lethargy, jaundice and liver damage within a few days of their first milk feedings. Untreated, the disorder may result in mental retardation, blindness, growth failure and, in severe cases, death. Treatment includes eliminating milk and all other dairy (galactose) products from the diet.
- **Biotinidase deficiency.** This deficiency is caused by the lack of an enzyme called biotinidase. Signs and symptoms include seizures, developmental delay, eczema and hearing loss. With early diagnosis and treatment, all signs and symptoms can be prevented.
- **Maple syrup urine disease (MSUD).** This disorder affects the metabolism of amino acids. Newborns with this condition typically appear normal but will experience feeding difficulties, lethargy and failure to thrive by the first week of life. Left untreated, MSUD can result in coma or death.
- **Homocystinuria.** Caused by an enzyme deficiency, this disorder can lead to eye problems, mental retardation, skeletal abnormalities and abnormal blood clotting. With early detection and management — including a special diet and dietary supplements — growth and development should be normal.
- **Sickle cell disease.** This inherited disease prevents blood cells from circulating easily throughout the body. Affected infants will have an increased susceptibility to infection and slow growth rates. The disease can cause bouts of pain and damage to vital organs such as the lungs, kidneys and brain. With early medical treatment, the complications of sickle cell disease can be minimized.
- **Medium-chain acyl-CoA dehydrogenase (MCAD) deficiency.** This rare hereditary disease results from the lack of an enzyme required to con-

vert fat to energy. Serious life-threatening signs and symptoms and even death can occur. With early detection and monitoring, children diagnosed with MCAD can lead normal lives.

- **Cystic fibrosis (CF).** This genetic disease causes the body to produce abnormally thickened mucous secretions in the lungs and digestive system. Signs and symptoms include salty-tasting skin, persistent coughing, shortness of breath and poor weight gain. Affected newborns can develop life-threatening lung infections and intestinal obstructions. With early detection and treatment plans, infants diagnosed with CF can live longer and in a better state of health than they did in the past.
- **Hearing screening.** While your baby is in the hospital, he or she may have a hearing test. Although not done routinely at every hospital, newborn hearing screening is becoming widely available. Hearing loss affects about five out of 1,000 newborns. This screening can detect possible hearing loss in the first days of a baby's life. If a possible hearing loss is found, further tests can confirm the results.

  These two tests are used to screen a newborn's hearing. Both are quick (about 10 minutes), painless and can be done while your baby sleeps.

  - **Automated auditory brainstem response.** This test measures how the brain responds to sound. Clicks or tones are played through soft earphones into the baby's ears while electrodes taped on the baby's head measure the brain's response.
  - **Otoacoustic emissions.** This test measures responses to sound waves presented to the ear. A probe placed inside the baby's ear canal measures the response when clicks or tones are played into the baby's ear.

Circumcision

If your new baby is a boy, you may decide to have another procedure performed: circumcision. When a baby boy is circumcised, a doctor surgically removes the foreskin covering the tip of the penis. The procedure exposes the end of the penis. It can be performed before you bring your baby home. There are advantages and disadvantages to circumcising your baby. You can learn more about this important decision in the decision guide titled "Considering circumcision for your son" on page 355.

Common newborn problems

Some babies have trouble adjusting to their new world. Luckily, most of these newborn problems are minor and soon resolved. Here are some common newborn problems.

Jaundice

More than half of all newborn babies develop jaundice, a yellow tinge to the skin and eyes. Most affected babies show signs a few days after birth. Jaundice usually lasts several weeks.

A baby has jaundice when bilirubin, which is produced by the breakdown of red blood cells, builds up faster than his or her liver can break it down and pass it from the body. Jaundice usually disappears on its own. It doesn't cause any discomfort to your baby.

Your baby may develop jaundice for a few reasons:
- Bilirubin is being made more quickly than the liver can handle.
- The baby's developing liver isn't able to remove bilirubin from the blood.
- Too much of the bilirubin is reabsorbed from the intestines before the baby gets rid of it in a bowel movement.

Although mild levels of jaundice don't require treatment, more severe cases can require a newborn to stay longer in the hospital. Currently, jaundice may be treated in several ways:
- You may be asked to feed the baby more frequently, which increases the amount of bilirubin passed with bowel movements.
- The doctor may place your baby under a bilirubin light. This treatment, called phototherapy, uses a special lamp to help rid the body of excess bilirubin.
- The doctor may give your baby intravenous immune globulin (antibodies) to decrease the severity of the jaundice if the bilirubin level becomes extremely high.
- Rarely, an exchange blood transfusion is done to reduce the bilirubin level.

Infection

A newborn's immune system isn't adequately developed to fight infection. Therefore, any type of infection can be more critical for newborns than for older children or adults.

Serious bacterial infections, which occur in about two or three of 1,000 newborns, can invade any organ or the blood, urine or spinal fluid. Prompt treatment with antibiotics is necessary, but even with early diagnosis and treatment, a newborn infection can be life-threatening.

For this reason, doctors are cautious when treating a possible or suspected infection. Newborns who have difficulty breathing, are unusually sleepy, eat poorly, or have persistently high or low temperatures may have sepsis — the body's response to infection. Antibiotics often are given early, and their use is stopped only when an infection doesn't seem likely. Although the majority of the test results come back showing no evidence of infection, it's better to err on the side of safety by quickly treating a baby than to risk not treating a baby with an infection soon enough.

Viruses can cause infections in newborns, although they do so less often than bacterial infections do. Some viruses cause serious infection in the mother, and others may interfere with the growth and development of an unborn fetus. Certain viral infections such as herpes, varicella, HIV and cytomegalovirus may be treated with antiviral medication.

Difficulty learning to eat

Whether you choose to breast-feed or bottle-feed, for the first few days after your baby's birth, you may find it difficult to interest your newborn in eating. This isn't uncommon. Some babies just seem to adopt a slow-and-sleepy approach to eating. If you're concerned that your baby isn't getting enough nourishment, talk to your baby's nurse or doctor. Occasionally, pokey eaters require tube feedings to help them along for a few days. Soon they'll catch on and breast-feed or bottle-feed with enthusiasm.

Over the first week, a newborn will lose about 10 percent of his or her birth weight. Monitoring changes in a baby's weight helps gauge the amount of milk a baby is taking. Work with your baby's health care provider to monitor your baby's growth throughout his or her first year of life.

Baby's new world

As you recover from childbirth and adjust to being a parent, remember that your baby is adjusting, too. Your newborn has gone from the safe, dark and reasonably quiet womb to the bright lights and jarring sounds of a whole new world. Your quiet voice and gentle touch are the calming influences in this strange new environment.

The premature newborn

Every parent dreams of having a healthy, full-term baby. Unfortunately, that dream isn't always the reality. Although most infants are born full-term and free of medical problems, some are born too early. Prematurity is often accompanied by medical complications.

Due to medical progress, the outlook for these newborns is much more hopeful than it once was. Still, many infants experiencing problems will require special care. This section explains some of the types of problems and treatments that can arise with prematurity.

When a baby is born prematurely

Each year, about 11 percent of babies in the United States are born prematurely — that is, before they've completed 37 weeks of development. If your baby is among these ranks, you'll likely feel a range of emotions — including fear, disappointment and worry. This is natural and understandable.

The good news is that today's neonatal intensive care has dramatically improved the outlook for premature infants. In fact, more than two-thirds of babies born at 24 to 25 weeks can survive with the proper medical care. Because most premature babies can survive, much of the medical care given to mothers in preterm labor and to premature newborns focuses on minimizing possible complications of prematurity.

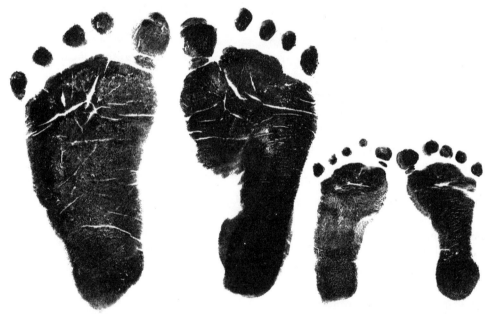

Footprints of a full-term baby girl whose birth weight was 8 pounds, 4 ounces.

Footprints of a premature baby boy whose birth weight was 1 pound, 8 ounces.

What your premature baby may look like

Your first close-up look at your premature baby will likely be in the neonatal intensive care unit (NICU). You'll probably be amazed, overwhelmed — and perhaps a little shocked — by this first look.

You may first notice the array of tubes, catheters and electrical leads taped to your tiny baby. This equipment may be overwhelming and intimidating at first. It's important to remember that it helps keep your baby healthy and the medical staff continuously informed about your baby's condition.

You'll also notice right away your baby's tiny size. He or she will probably be considerably smaller than a full-term infant. Some very premature babies are so small that a man's wedding ring can serve as a loose-fitting bracelet.

Because premature babies have less body fat than full-term babies do, they need help to stay warm. They're often placed in an enclosed and warmed plastic box (isolette) to help them maintain a normal body temperature.

A premature baby's skin will have a number of notable characteristics not found on a full-term baby. Your baby's features will appear sharper and less rounded than a full-term baby's. The skin and cartilage that form your baby's outer ears will be especially soft and pliable. The skin may be covered with more fine body hair (lanugo) than is common in full-term babies. Your baby's skin may look thin, fragile and somewhat transparent — allowing you to see the blood vessels underneath it.

These characteristics will be easy to see because most premature babies won't be dressed or wrapped in blankets. This is so the nursery staff can closely observe their breathing and general appearance.

In the neonatal intensive care unit (NICU)

Immediately after birth, your premature baby is likely to undergo many of the same procedures as a full-term baby. But, of course, special precautions are necessary after a premature birth. For example, your baby's breathing, heart rate and blood pressure may be monitored.

Soon after birth, a baby born at less than 35 weeks may be transferred to an NICU or a special care nursery, sometimes called a level 3 or level 2 nursery. If your premature baby is born in a hospital without such a facility, he or she may be transferred to a nearby NICU.

In the NICU, your baby will receive specialized care — including a feeding plan tailored to your baby's specific needs. For the first few days or weeks after delivery, premature babies are usually fed intravenously because their gastrointestinal and respiratory systems may be too immature to safely start formula feedings. When your baby is ready, the intravenous feeding will end and a new form of feeding, called tube feeding, will likely be the next step. In tube feedings, your baby receives breast milk or formula through a tube that delivers the food directly to the stomach or upper intestine.

Getting involved

Become physically involved with your baby as early as possible. Loving care is important to your baby's physical and psychological growth and development.

When you were pregnant, you probably daydreamed about holding, bathing and feeding your new baby. As the parent of a premature baby, you probably won't be able to spend these first weeks with your baby in the way you had envisioned. Still, you can be involved with your baby in important ways.

The neonatal intensive care unit team

In the neonatal intensive care unit (NICU), your baby is cared for by many specialized and qualified people. The team attending to your baby may include:

- Neonatal nurses — registered nurses with special training in caring for premature and high-risk newborns
- Neonatal respiratory therapists — staff trained to assess respiratory problems in newborns and adjust ventilators and other respiratory equipment
- Neonatologists — pediatricians who specialize in the diagnosis and treatment of problems of the newborn
- Pediatric surgeons — surgeons trained in the diagnosis and treatment of newborn conditions that may require surgery
- Pediatricians — doctors who specialize in treating children
- Pediatric resident physicians — doctors receiving specialized training in treating children

Until your baby is ready to be held, you can reach through the openings in the isolette to hold your baby's hand or gently stroke him or her. Gentle contact with your premature baby can help him or her thrive. Help your newborn get to know you by humming a lullaby or talking softly to him or her.

As your baby's condition improves, you'll be able to hold and rock your baby. Skin-to-skin contact, sometimes called kangaroo care, can be a powerful way to bond with your baby. In kangaroo care, a nurse can help place your baby on your bare chest, then loosely cover him or her with a blanket. Some studies have shown that premature babies respond positively to this skin-to-skin contact with their parents and that kangaroo care can improve babies' recovery times.

Another important way the mother can be involved in her baby's health is by providing breast milk, which contains proteins that help fight infection and promote growth. In the NICU, your baby will likely be fed every one to three hours through a tube that goes from the nose or mouth to the stomach. Nurses can show the mother how to pump breast milk, which can be refrigerated and stored for use as the baby needs it.

Complications of prematurity

Babies born prematurely are at risk of several medical problems because they haven't had the chance to fully develop in the uterus. Recent years have seen an increase in the use of maternal medications given to prepare the premature baby for birth and improvements in NICU care. Today, survival rates and outcomes are excellent for all but the youngest or most ill newborns.

Some babies' problems are apparent at birth. Others may develop weeks to months later. The earlier a baby is born, the greater his or her chances are of developing problems. Some of these conditions may include the following:

Respiratory distress syndrome

Respiratory distress syndrome (RDS) is the most common breathing problem among newborns, occurring almost exclusively in premature infants. In RDS, a baby's immature lungs lack an important liquid substance called surfactant, which gives normal, fully developed lungs the elastic qualities required for easy breathing. Mothers in premature labor at less than 35 weeks might be given injections of corticosteroid medication to increase the baby's lung maturity before birth.

RDS is usually diagnosed within the first minutes to hours after birth. The diagnosis is based on the extent of breathing difficulty and on abnormalities seen on the baby's chest X-ray.

Treatment

Babies with RDS require various degrees of help with their breathing. Supplemental oxygen is usually required until the lungs improve. The air contains 21 percent oxygen. Premature babies with RDS may require up to 100 percent oxygen.

Many babies with RDS require supplemental breaths. A ventilator, sometimes called a respirator, can give the baby carefully controlled breaths. These can range from helping with a few extra breaths per minute to entirely taking over the work of breathing.

Some babies will benefit from breathing assistance called continuous positive airway pressure (CPAP). A plastic tube that fits in the nostrils provides additional pressure in the air passages to keep the tiny air sacs in the lungs properly inflated.

Babies with severe RDS are given doses of surfactant preparation directly into the lungs. Other medications are frequently used in babies with RDS. These include medications that increase urine output and rid the body of extra water, reduce inflammation in the lungs, reduce wheezing and minimize pauses in breathing (apnea).

Babies who require assistance with their breathing or extra oxygen are monitored carefully. A device called an oximeter (saturation monitor) continuously indicates the baby's blood level of oxygen.

In addition, blood samples can check levels of oxygen and carbon dioxide and the pH (acid-base balance) of the blood. These tests indicate how well the baby is breathing and whether it's necessary to make changes in how much help is given to the baby.

Bronchopulmonary dysplasia

A premature baby's lung problems generally improve within several days to several weeks. Babies who still require help with ventilation or supplemental oxygen a month after birth are often described as having bronchopulmonary dysplasia (BPD). This condition is also called chronic lung disease.

Treatment

Babies with BPD continue to need supplemental oxygen for an extended period. If they develop a bad cold or pneumonia, they may need breathing assistance, such as that provided by a ventilator. Some of these babies may need to continue using supplemental oxygen, even after they go home from the hospital. As these babies grow, their need for supplemental oxygen lessens, and their breathing becomes easier. However, they are more likely than are other children to have episodes of wheezing or asthma.

Apnea and bradycardia

Premature babies typically have immature breathing rhythms that cause them to breathe in spurts: 10 to 15 seconds of deep breathing followed by five- to 10-second pauses. This condition is called periodic breathing.

If the intervals of pauses in breathing last longer than 10 to 15 seconds, the baby is said to be having an apneic episode, or an A and B spell. *A* stands for apnea, a pause in breathing. *B* stands for bradycardia, the medical term for a slow heartbeat. Sometimes the oxygen level also briefly drops, which is termed a *desaturation episode* (desat).

Almost all babies born under 30 weeks gestational age will experience A and B spells. This reduction in breathing, heart rate and oxygen saturation will trigger alarms from your baby's monitoring device to alert the baby's medical caregivers.

Treatment

A premature baby's reduced breathing, heart rate and oxygen saturation typically promptly return to normal on their own, which is called a self-limited A and B spell. If they don't, the nurse may gently stimulate the baby by rubbing or wiggling him or her awake. In more severe spells, the baby may need brief assistance with breathing. If your baby experiences frequent A and B spells, your baby's doctor may prescribe a medication to help regulate breathing.

Patent ductus arteriosus

Before birth, a baby's lungs aren't used and therefore require minimal blood flow. Because of this, a short blood vessel called the ductus arteriosus diverts blood away from the lungs to maximize blood flow to the placenta.

Before birth, a chemical compound called prostaglandin-E circulates in the baby's blood, keeping the ductus arteriosus open. In full-term infants after birth, levels of prostaglandin-E fall sharply, causing the ductus arteriosus to close. Then the circulation works properly.

Occasionally, especially in premature babies, prostaglandin-E circulates at about the same level after birth as it did before. This causes the ductus arteriosus to remain open, possibly resulting in respiratory or circulation difficulties.

Treatment
This condition is often treated with a medication that stops or slows the production of prostaglandin E. If this medication isn't effective, an operation might be needed.

Intracranial hemorrhage
Premature babies who are born at less than 34 weeks of gestation are at risk of bleeding in their brains. This is called intracranial hemorrhage (ICH) or intraventricular hemorrhage (IVH). The earlier a baby is born, the higher the risk of complication. Therefore, if premature birth seems inevitable, the mother may be given certain medications to help lessen the likelihood of a severe intracranial hemorrhage in the newborn.

Intracranial hemorrhages ranging from minor to significant occur in about one-third of babies born at 23 to 26 weeks of gestational age. These very premature infants have delicate, immature blood vessels that may not tolerate the changes in circulation that take place after birth. Bleeding usually occurs within the first three days. It's detected with an ultrasound exam of the baby's head.

Treatment
Babies with minor degrees of intracranial hemorrhage require only observation. Those with serious degrees of bleeding may undergo various treatments. Babies with severe intracranial hemorrhage are at risk of developmental problems such as cerebral palsy, spasticity and mental retardation.

Necrotizing enterocolitis
For reasons that aren't entirely clear, some premature babies — usually those at less than 28 weeks of gestation — develop a serious problem called necrotizing enterocolitis. In this condition, a portion of the baby's intestine develops a poor blood flow. This can lead to infection in the bowel wall. Signs include a bloated abdomen, feeding intolerance, breathing difficulty and bloody stools.

Treatment
Babies with necrotizing enterocolitis may be treated with intravenous feedings and antibiotics. In severe cases, an operation may be required to remove the affected portion of the intestine.

Retinopathy of prematurity

Retinopathy of prematurity (ROP) is abnormal growth of the blood vessels in an infant's eye. It's most common in very premature babies. Most babies born at 23 to 26 weeks of gestational age, for example, will experience at least some ROP, and babies beyond about 30 weeks of gestational age rarely have it.

ROP results from a disturbance in the development of the retina. Because during fetal life the retina develops from the back of the eye forward, the process is complete just about the time a baby is full term. When a baby is born prematurely, the retinal development isn't finished, which may allow a number of factors to disturb it.

Treatment

If your baby is at risk of ROP, an eye specialist (ophthalmologist) can examine the eyes after six weeks of age. Fortunately, most cases of ROP are mild and will resolve without additional treatment. More severe degrees of retinopathy are often successfully treated with procedures such as laser treatment or cryotherapy. Today, retinal detachment and blindness are uncommon and affect only the very smallest and most unstable premature babies.

This month, you may be interested in:
- **"Decision guide: Considering circumcision for your son," page 355**
- **"Decision guide: The breast or the bottle?" page 363**

WHEN YOUR BABY IS HOSPITALIZED

- Spend time touching and talking to your newborn.
- Learn as much as you can about your baby's medical condition, especially what parents should watch for and how parents can care for their baby's conditions.
- Don't be afraid to ask questions. Medical terminology can be confusing. Have the doctor or nurse write down any key diagnoses. Ask for printed patient information sheets or recommended Web sites for further information.
- Take an active role in your baby's care, especially as your baby becomes close to leaving the hospital.
- Ask if you can be given or mailed a copy of your baby's hospital dismissal summary.
- Inquire if public health nurses or visiting nurses can assist with your baby's care after you're home.
- Ask if your baby should be enrolled in special infant follow-up or infant development programs.
- Lean on someone. Talk the situation over with your partner or other family members. Invite family members and friends to join you at the hospital. Ask to meet with the hospital social worker.

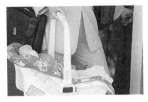

taking your baby home

Finally, the moment you've been anticipating is here — you're bringing home the newest member of your family! You've set up the crib and nursery, bought and borrowed the cute little outfits, and stocked up on diapers, wipes, blankets and other supplies. You've been thinking about all of the changes this new baby will bring to your life and probably alternated between feeling excited and scared.

Now you wonder: Am I ready? Are we ready?

Probably not — and that's perfectly normal. No matter how many pregnancy and baby-care books you've read, or how meticulous you've been in getting everything in place, nothing can fully prepare you for the first few weeks after your baby's birth. This time can be exciting — and overwhelming.

During the postpartum weeks, you're dealing with many different physical, practical and emotional issues all at once. You're getting used to your new baby and trying to understand his or her needs and habits. At the same time, your body is recovering from pregnancy and childbirth.

Given all these changes, the first few weeks after you bring your baby home are likely to be one of the most challenging times of your life. It may take months or even a year to feel back to normal. Be patient with yourself and your baby. You'll get there in your own way, in your own time.

This chapter gives you a glimpse into your newborn's world and tells you what you need to know to take care of your baby and keep him or her safe. Having a new baby in your life is a special, life-changing experience. By taking good care of your baby and yourself, you'll be able to enjoy it.

Your baby's world

In the first few weeks of a newborn's life, it may seem like all he or she does is eat, sleep, cry and keep you busy changing diapers. But your baby is also taking in the sights, sounds and smells of his or her new world, learning to use his or her muscles and expressing a number of innate reflexes.

As soon as babies are born, they begin to communicate with you. Infants can't use words to communicate their needs, moods or preferences, but they have other ways of expressing themselves, especially by crying.

You won't always know how your newborn is feeling, and sometimes it will seem as though he or she is communicating in a foreign language. But you can learn about how your baby experiences the world and relates to you and others. In turn, your baby will learn your language of touching, holding, and making sounds and facial gestures.

Crying

Crying is the first and primary form of communication that newborns use. And they do plenty of it — young babies typically cry an average of one to as many as four hours a day. It's a normal part of adjusting to life outside the womb.

Common reasons for crying include:

- **Hunger.** Most babies eat six to 10 times in a 24-hour period. For at least the first three months, babies usually wake for night feedings.
- **Discomfort.** Your baby may cry because of wet or soiled diapers, gas or indigestion, and uncomfortable temperatures or positions. When babies are uncomfortable, they may look for something to suck on. But feeding won't stop the discomfort, and a pacifier may help only briefly. When the discomfort passes, your baby will probably settle down.
- **Boredom, fear and loneliness.** Sometimes, a baby will cry because he or she is bored, frightened or lonely and wants to be held and cuddled. A baby seeking comfort may calm down with the reassurance of seeing you, hearing your voice, feeling your touch, being with you, being cuddled or being offered something to suck on.
- **Overtiredness or overstimulation.** Crying helps an overtired or overstimulated baby to shut out sights, sounds and other sensations. It also helps relieve tension. You may notice that your baby's fussy periods occur at predictable times during the day, often between early evening and midnight. It seems nothing you do at these times can console him or her, but afterward the baby may be more alert than before and then may sleep more deeply. This kind of fussy crying seems to help babies get rid of excess energy.

As your baby matures, you'll be able to distinguish the different messages in your baby's cries.

How to calm a crying baby

In general, respond promptly to your infant when he or she cries during the first few months. You won't spoil the baby by doing so. Studies show that newborns who are quickly and warmly responded to when crying learn to cry less overall and sleep more at night.

When your baby's crying seems incessant, run down a simple list to determine what might be needed:

- Is your baby hungry?
- Does your baby need a clean diaper?
- Does your baby need to be burped?
- Is your baby too warm or too cold?
- Does your baby need to be moved to a more comfortable position? Is something pinching, sticking or binding your baby?
- Does your baby just need to suck, whether on a finger or a pacifier?
- Does your baby need some tender care — walking, rocking, cuddling, stroking, a baby massage, gentle talking, singing or humming?
- Has there been too much excitement or stimulation? Does the baby just need to cry for a while?

Try to meet your baby's most pressing needs first. If hunger seems to be the problem, feed him or her. If the crying is shrieking or panicky, check to make sure nothing is poking or pinching the baby.

If your baby is warm, dry, well-fed and well-rested but still wailing, these suggestions may help:

- Try swaddling the baby more snugly in a blanket, as shown here.

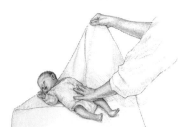

Step 1. Bring one corner of the blanket up and pull it taut. Bring the blanket across your baby's body with one arm tucked inside. Tuck the corner under your baby's bottom snugly.

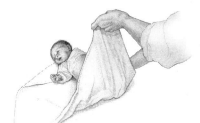

Step 2. Fold the bottom point up, leaving room for your baby's legs to move freely.

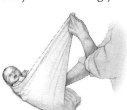

Step 3. Bring up the other corner of the blanket, pull it taut and tuck it under your baby. Leave one hand and arm free.

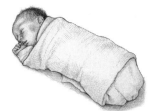

Step 4. Aah ... a cozy bundle.

- Gently talk or sing to your baby face to face.
- Use gentle motion, such as rocking the baby in your arms, walking with the baby against your shoulder or carrying him or her in a front carrier.
- Gently stroke the baby's head or rub or pat his or her chest or back.
- Hold the baby tummy-down on your lap.
- Hold the baby in an upright position on your shoulder or against your chest.
- Put the baby in a car seat and go for a drive.
- Give the baby a warm bath or put a warm — not hot — water bottle on his or her stomach.
- Play soft music.
- Go outside — take your baby for a walk in a stroller or carriage.
- Offer your baby your finger or a pacifier to suck on as you rock or rhythmically walk him or her.
- Reduce the noise, movement and lights in the area where your baby is. Or try introducing white noise, such as the continuous, monotonous sound of a vacuum cleaner or a recording of ocean waves. Often it can relax and lull babies by blocking out other sounds.

If your baby is dry, full, comfortable, and wrapped snugly, but is still crying, he or she may need a 10- to 15-minute period alone. Stay within earshot, and check on the baby every few minutes from a distance. Although many parents find it difficult to let their baby cry, it may give the infant an opportunity to unwind and let off steam.

Remember that you won't always be able to calm your baby, especially when the fussing is simply a way to release tension. Babies do cry. It's a normal part of being a baby. Rest assured that the crying won't last forever — the amount of time your baby spends crying usually peaks at about six weeks after birth and then gradually decreases.

It's also a normal part of parenting to find excessive crying frustrating. Make arrangements with family, friends or a baby sitter for needed breaks. Even an hour's break can renew your coping strength.

If your baby's crying is making you feel out of control, put your baby in a safe place, such as a crib. Then immediately contact your health care provider, your hospital emergency room, a local crisis intervention service or a mental health help line.

Normal crying or colic?

Every baby is fussy at times, but some babies cry much more than others. If your baby is healthy but has frequent fussy episodes, especially during the evening, or has prolonged, inconsolable crying for three or more hours a day, chances are the baby has colic. It's not a physical disorder or disease — *colic* is just the term for recurring bouts of crying that are difficult to relieve.

A colicky baby's crying is not simply due to hunger, a wet diaper or any other apparent cause, and the baby can't be calmed down. Experts aren't sure what causes the condition. Colic typically peaks at about six weeks after birth and usually goes away by three months.

Remember, though, that a baby's fussiness may not be colic but rather a sign of illness. Colicky babies will still have a healthy appetite, like to be cuddled and handled, and have normal stools.

Coping with colic

For parents of a baby with colic, it may seem that the baby will never outgrow this phase. It's common to feel frustrated, angry, tense, irritable, worried and fatigued.

No single treatment consistently provides relief to infants with colic. Experiment with various methods to calm the baby, such as those listed on pages 227-228. Try not to get discouraged if many of your efforts seem futile; your baby will outgrow colic eventually.

The more relaxed you can stay, the easier it'll be to console your child. Listening to a newborn wailing can be agonizing, but your own anxiety, frustration or panic will only add to the infant's distress.

Take a break and allow others to watch your baby so that you can relax. Sometimes a new face can calm the baby when you've used up all your tricks.

Call your baby's health care provider about crying if:
- Your baby seems to cry for an unusual length of time
- The cries sound odd to you
- The crying is associated with decreased activity, poor feeding, or unusual breathing or movements
- The crying is accompanied by other signs of illness, such as vomiting, fever and diarrhea
- A parent or someone else is having trouble dealing with a crying baby

You can also call an emergency help line such as that offered by Childhelp USA: (800) 4-A-CHILD, or (800) 422-4453. For more information, see the Childhelp Web site at *www.childhelpusa.org/report_hotline.htm.*

No matter how impatient or angry you get, never shake a baby. Never let anyone else shake a baby. Shaking an infant can cause blindness, brain damage or even death.

Eating and sleeping

Two important items on a newborn's agenda are eating and sleeping. Because most of a baby's energy goes into growing, many nonsleeping hours are spent eating. During the first several weeks, most babies will be hungry six to 10 times during a 24-hour period. Their stomachs don't hold enough breast milk or formula to satisfy them for long. That means you could be feeding your baby every two or three hours, including during the night. But there's tremendous variation among infants in how often and how much they eat.

Your baby probably won't have a feeding routine at first. Although you can roughly estimate the amount of time between feedings, the baby's schedule will be erratic. During growth spurts, feedings will be more frequent for a day or two.

You'll soon learn to read the signals that your baby is hungry, such as crying, opening the mouth, sucking, putting a fist in the mouth, fidgeting and turning toward your breast. Babies will also let you know when they've had enough by pushing the nipple or bottle out of their mouth or turning their head away.

As with eating, it takes awhile for newborns to get on any kind of schedule for sleeping. During the first month, they usually sleep and wake around the clock, with relatively equal parts of sleep between feedings.

In addition, newborns don't know the difference between night and day. It takes time for them to develop circadian rhythms — the sleep-wake cycles and other patterns that revolve on a 24-hour cycle. As a baby's nervous system gradually matures, so do his or her phases of sleep and wakefulness.

Sleep patterns and cycles

Although newborns don't usually sleep for more than about 4 1/2 hours at a stretch, altogether they sleep 12 or more hours a day. They'll stay awake long enough to feed or for up to about two hours before falling asleep again. By the time your baby is 2 weeks old, you'll probably notice that the periods of sleeping and being awake are lengthening. By 3 months, many babies shift more of their sleep to nighttime. But each baby is unique, and some babies may not sleep through the night until they're 1 year or older.

You can help adjust your baby's body clock toward sleeping at night by following these tips:

- Avoid stimulation during nighttime feedings and diaper changes. Keep the lights low, use a soft voice and resist the urge to play or talk with your baby so that you reinforce the message that nighttime is for sleeping.
- Start to establish some kind of bedtime routine. This might be reading or singing or having a quiet time for an hour before putting your baby to bed.

Feeding a sleepy baby

Many pediatricians recommend that parents shouldn't let newborns sleep too long without feeding. But you'll no doubt have times when your baby rouses to eat, only to doze again when you begin feeding.

Developing good sleep habits

Drooping eyelids, rubbing the eyes and fussiness are the usual signs that a baby is tired. Many babies cry when they're put down for sleep, but if left alone for a few minutes, most will eventually quiet themselves.

If your baby is not wet, hungry or ill, try to be patient with the crying and encourage self-settling. If you leave the room for a while, your baby will probably stop crying after a short time. If not, try comforting him or her and allow the baby to settle again.

In the first few months, it's common for a pattern to evolve in which a baby is fed and falls asleep in a parent's arms. Many parents enjoy the closeness and snuggling of this time. But eventually this may be the only way the baby is able to fall asleep. When the baby wakes up in the middle of the night, he or she can't fall asleep again without being fed and held.

To avoid these associations, put your baby in bed while he or she is drowsy but still awake. If babies fall asleep in bed without assistance when they're first laid down, it's more likely that they'll fall asleep easily after waking in the middle of the night.

Babies who stir during the night aren't necessarily distressed. Infants typically cry and move about when they enter different sleep cycles. Parents sometimes mistake these signs for waking up and begin an unnecessary feeding. Instead, wait a few minutes to see if your baby falls back to sleep.

Try these tips to feed a sleepy baby:
- Watch for and take advantage of your baby's alert stages. Feed during these times.
- A sleeping baby may squirm and root around or gently fuss when hungry. If your baby naps for more than three hours, watch closely for these subtle signs. If your baby is partially awake, sit him or her up and gently encourage eating.
- Partially undress your baby. Because the baby's skin is sensitive to temperature changes, the coolness may wake up the baby long enough to eat.
- Rock your baby into a sitting position. The baby's eyes often open when he or she is positioned upright.
- Give your baby a massage by walking your fingers up his or her spine.
- Stroke a circle around your baby's lips with a fingertip a few times.

Call your baby's health care provider about sleeping and eating if:
- Your baby is unusually difficult to rouse from sleep, sleeps through feedings or seems uninterested in eating.

Urinating and bowel movements

New parents often wonder what's normal when it comes to their baby's urination and bowel movements. By the time a baby is three or four days old, he or she should have at least six wet diapers a day. As your baby gets older, he or she may have wet diapers with every feeding. However, if the baby is ill or feverish or if the weather is very hot, the usual output of urine may drop by half and still be normal.

If urine output decreases when a baby is sick, especially if the baby is vomiting or feeding poorly, it could indicate dehydration. In older children, the presence of tears would suggest adequate hydration, but in young infants, tears don't serve as a reliable guide. So if you're worried about dehydration in the baby, have the baby examined by his or her health care provider.

In a healthy infant, urine is light to dark yellow in color. Sometimes, highly concentrated urine dries on the diaper to a pinkish color, which may be mistaken for blood. Actual blood in the urine or a bloody spot on the diaper is cause for concern, however.

As for stools, the range of normal is quite broad and varies from one baby to another. Babies may have a bowel movement as frequently as after every feeding, as infrequently as once a week, or in no consistent pattern. By 3 to 6 weeks of age, some breast-fed babies may have only one bowel movement a week because breast milk leaves little solid waste to be eliminated from the digestive system. If a baby is being fed formula, he or she will likely have at least one bowel movement a day.

If you're breast-feeding, your baby's stools will resemble light mustard with seed-like particles. They'll be soft and even slightly runny. The stools of a formula-fed infant are usually tan or yellow and firmer than those of a breast-fed baby, but no firmer than peanut butter. Occasional variations in color and consistency are normal. Different colors may indicate how fast the stools moved through the digestive tract or what the baby ate. The stool may be green, yellow, orange or brown.

Mild diarrhea is common in newborns. The stools may be watery, frequent and mixed with mucus. Constipation is not usually a problem for infants. Babies may strain, grunt and turn red during a bowel movement, but this doesn't mean they're constipated. A baby is constipated when bowel movements are infrequent, hard and perhaps even ball-shaped.

Check with your baby's health care provider about urination and stools if:
- You notice any signs of distress when your infant is urinating
- Your baby is wetting fewer than four diapers a day
- The baby's urine is unusually dark or strong smelling
- You see blood in the urine or a bloody spot on the diaper
- Your baby seems to have ongoing difficulty with bowel movements
- Your baby has hard or only ball-shaped stools
- Your baby is formula-fed and has fewer than one bowel movement a day

- You notice a drastic change in the baby's stool patterns
- You see blood, mucus or water are in the stool
- Diarrhea is severe or persistent and the diaper area looks red and sore

Your baby's reflexes

Newborns are just learning to enjoy the freedom of movement outside the cramped quarters of the uterus. In their first few days, they may seem a bit reluctant to experiment with their new mobility, preferring to be wrapped and held snugly. Over time, however, they will begin to explore a range of movements.

Babies are born with a number of reflexes (automatic, involuntary movements). Some of these movements — such as turning the head to avoid suffocating — seem to be protective responses. Some may be preparing babies for voluntary movements. Most reflexes diminish after a few weeks or months and then disappear completely as they're replaced with new, learned skills.

In the meantime, watch for some of these reflexes:

- **Rooting.** This reflex prompts babies to turn in the direction of the food source, whether it's a breast or bottle. If you gently stroke a newborn's cheek, he or she will turn in that direction, with his or her mouth open, ready to suck.
- **Sucking.** When a breast, bottle nipple or pacifier is placed in a baby's mouth, he or she will automatically suck. This reflex not only helps the newborn eat but also can calm him or her.
- **Hand to mouth.** Babies will try to find their mouths with their hands. This reflex may be why many babies bring their hands to the breast or bottle.
- **Stepping.** When you hold infants under their arms and let the soles of their feet touch the ground, they may place one foot in front of the other as if they're walking. This stepping reflex is most apparent after about the fourth day and disappears at about two months. Most babies won't actually learn to walk until almost a year later.
- **Startle (Moro reflex).** When startled by a noise or sudden movement, babies may throw both arms outward and cry. You may notice this if you put your baby in the bassinet or crib too quickly.
- **Fencing (tonic neck reflex).** If you turn your baby's head to one side while he or she is lying on his or her back, you may see this classic baby pose, in which one arm is crooked and raised behind the head and the other is straightened and extended away from the body in the direction the head is turned. Sometimes the baby's fist grabs a clump of hair and won't let go.

- **Smiling.** In the first few weeks of life, most of a newborn's smiles are involuntary, but it won't be long before the baby begins smiling in response to a person or situation.

If you're observant, you may notice some of these reflexes, but don't worry if you don't notice them. Your baby's health care provider may check for them during physical examinations.

If you want, you can encourage your baby's movement by gently cycling the arms and legs as he or she lies on his or her back. Or you might let the baby kick at your hands or a squeaky toy.

Your baby's senses

It's a new world for your baby, and all of his or her senses are coming alive to explore and make sense of it. You'll notice when an object, light, sound, smell or touch engages your baby. Watch for him or her to settle down or become quiet when something new is introduced.

Sight

Your newborn is nearsighted and sees best at 12 to 18 inches. That's the perfect distance for seeing the most important things to babies — their parents' faces as they hold or feed them. Your baby will love to fixate on your face, and it will be the favorite entertainment for a while. Give your newborn plenty of face-to-face time to get to know you.

In addition to being interested in human faces, newborns are also engaged by brightness, movement and simple, high-contrast objects. Many toy stores sell black-and-white and brightly colored toys, mobiles and nursery decorations.

Because newborns can't fully control their eye movement, they may appear to be cross-eyed at times, or their eyes may briefly diverge and look walleyed. This is normal. Your baby's eye muscles will strengthen and mature during the next few months.

When your baby is quiet and alert, provide simple objects for him or her to look at. Try slowly moving an object to the right or left in front of him or her. Most babies will briefly follow moving objects with their eyes, and sometimes with their heads. But don't overload the baby — one item at a time is plenty. If your baby is tired or overstimulated, he or she won't want to play this game.

Check with your baby's health care provider regarding vision if:
- Your child's eyes increasingly tend to cross or diverge
- Your child's eyes appear cloudy or filmy
- Your child's eyes seem to wander randomly and rarely focus
- You have other concerns about your newborn's ability to see

Hearing

Once the baby is born, new sounds will capture his or her attention. In response to noises, babies may pause in sucking, widen their eyes or stop fussing. They may startle at a loud noise such as a dog barking, and they may be soothed by the hum of the vacuum cleaner or the whirring of the clothes dryer. But babies can easily adapt and tune out noises, so they may react to a particular sound only once or twice.

Newborns can tell the difference between human voices and other sounds. Babies are most curious about their parents' voices. Your baby will learn quickly to associate your voice with food, warmth and touch. He or she will listen carefully when you talk to him or her, and even infants enjoy music and being read to. Talk to your baby whenever you can. Even though he or she won't understand what you're saying, the sound of your voice is reassuring and calming.

Improvements in hearing tests have made newborn hearing screening possible. Many hospitals now routinely test every newborn's hearing. If this testing isn't offered where you give birth, you might want to ask your baby's medical health care provider to refer you to an audiologist for newborn hearing screening. This is particularly important if someone in the family has hearing problems.

Touch

Infants are sensitive to touch and can detect differences in texture, pressure and moisture. They respond quickly to changes in temperature. They may startle when cold air wafts across their skin and become quiet again when they're wrapped warmly. Your touch provides comfort and reassurance to your baby and can rouse a sleepy baby for feeding.

Smell and taste

Infants have a good sense of smell. Even when very young, they can recognize their mother by scent. They may show interest in a new smell by a change in movement or activity. But they easily become familiar with a new smell and no longer react to it.

The sense of taste is closely related to the sense of smell. Although newborns aren't exposed to many tastes beyond breast milk or formula, research shows that from birth babies prefer sweet tastes over bitter or sour tastes.

Baby-care basics

Throughout your pregnancy, most of your preparation and instruction probably focused on childbirth. It was a time of anticipation and dreaming about seeing your baby for the first time. Once the excitement of birth is over and you're traveling home from the hospital, the reality may sink in that you and your partner are on your own now with a tiny person whose life depends on you. It's normal to wonder how you'll take care of your baby and to feel nervous or anxious about it.

No doubt you'll become a whiz at changing diapers, maneuvering the car seat and bathing the baby. The following sections give you the basics you need to get started with baby care and home safety.

Car seat know-how

One of the most important pieces of baby equipment is a car seat, which you'll use right away, starting with your baby's first ride home from the hospital. Car seats are required by law in every state, and correct and consistent use of them is one of the best ways parents can protect their children. It's never safe to hold an infant or child on your lap in a moving vehicle.

An infant must never ride in a rear-facing car seat in the front seat of a vehicle that has passenger air bags. The safest place for all children to ride is in the back seat.

The two types of car seats for infants are infant-only seats and convertible seats, which accommodate both babies and toddlers. Whichever type you use, be sure to install it rear-facing, which is the only safe position for infants in cars. When your child reaches 1 year of age and weighs at least 20 pounds or more, depending on the car seat model, you can switch to a bigger car seat or turn around the convertible seat so that the child faces the front. Until that time, a baby's neck muscles aren't very strong. In a collision, a forward-facing baby is at greater risk of head and neck injuries because the head may be thrown forward.

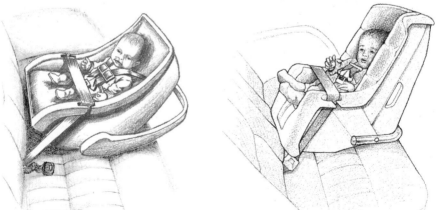

Infant-only car safety seats (left) fit newborns best, but convertible safety seats (right) can be used longer.

When you buy a new car safety seat, register it using the registration card that comes with it. That way, the manufacturer can let you know if your child's seat has been recalled.

You can find out if an older car seat has been recalled by calling the manufacturer or the Department of Transportation's Auto Safety Hotline, (888) DASH-2-DOT, or (888) 327-4236. This information is also available online at *www.nhtsa.dot.gov/cars/problems/recalls/index.cfm*.

Infant-only seats

These are used for babies who weigh up to 20 pounds or more, depending on the safety seat. They're the best seats for newborns and may be the best fit for premature infants. Many models come with a detachable base, which allows you to carry your baby in and out of the car in the car seat without having to reinstall the base. The base attaches to the car, and the car seat easily snaps into the base.

Infant-only car seats come with either a three-point or a five-point harness. The harness is made of straps that secure your baby into the seat. A three-point harness fastens snugly between the baby's legs, and a five-point harness comes from either side of the hips to snap into the crotch piece. An advantage of five-point harnesses is that they provide more stability than do three-point harnesses. They allow even the smallest baby to fit snugly inside a car seat.

Convertible seats

These are bigger and heavier than infant-only seats and can be used longer and for heavier children, up to 40 pounds. Although you'll save some money using a convertible seat, an infant-only seat may be easier to use and may fit a newborn better.

Convertible seats have one of three types of harnesses:
- A five-point harness made of five straps — two at the shoulders, two at the hips and one at the crotch
- An overhead shield that swings down around the child
- A T-shield — a T-shaped or triangular shield attached to shoulder straps

If you're using a convertible seat for a small infant, it's best to use one with a five-point harness. A small baby's face can hit a shield in a crash.

Choosing a car seat

How do you know which car seat to buy? No one seat is safest or best. The best car seat is one that fits your child's size and weight and can be installed correctly in your car. Choose a seat with a label that says it meets or exceeds Federal Motor Vehicle Safety Standard 213 (FMVSS 213).

CAR SEAT SAFETY TIPS

Here are some tips for installing and using child car seats:
- Never substitute any type of regular infant seat for a child car safety seat. Regular infant seats simply allow babies to sit up — they're not designed to protect a baby in a crash. Some car safety seats can double as infant seats, however.
- Child safety seats should always be placed in the back seat of a vehicle.
- Safety seats should face the rear of your vehicle until your child is at least 1 year old and weighs at least 20 pounds. It's recommended that you keep your child safety seat facing the rear as long as the weight limit allows it.
- Safety seats should never be installed in a seat with an air bag.
- Read your vehicle owner's manual and the car seat instruction manual to ensure that you're installing the seat correctly.
- Become familiar with your vehicle's rear seat belt system or anchor system. Newer vehicles and car seats use an anchor system called LATCH (Lower Anchors and Tethers for Children), which makes installation easier because you don't have to use seat belts to secure the car seat. But unless both your vehicle and your car seat have this anchor system, you'll still have to use seat belts to secure the car seat.
- When the safety seat is properly installed, you shouldn't be able to move it more than 1 inch from side to side or front to back.

Look at several different models. When you find a seat you like, try it out. Try adjusting the harnesses and buckles. Be sure you understand how to use it. If possible, try installing the car seat in your vehicle before you buy the seat. Choose a seat that can be held tightly against the vehicle seat back. A car seat that's upholstered in fabric may be more comfortable for your baby.

If you decide to borrow a car seat or buy a used one, make sure it's safe. Don't use a car seat that:

- Was in a crash
- Is more than six years old
- Has no labels
- Doesn't come with instructions
- Has cracks or rust
- Is missing parts
- Has been recalled

Holding and carrying your baby

At first you may feel a little awkward or nervous about holding and carrying your baby. But over time you'll feel more and more comfortable. And you'll soon learn what positions the baby likes — all babies have their

- Tilt the rear-facing car safety seat back so it's reclined at the angle specified in the manufacturer's instructions, usually 45 degrees.
- Check to see that the harness is tight enough. You shouldn't be able to fit more than one finger width between the torso harness and the baby.
- Make sure the harness straps lie flat and aren't twisted. Straps should be at or below the baby's shoulders. If a plastic harness clip is provided, place it at armpit level to hold the shoulder straps in place.
- Always keep the carrying handle on an infant-only car seat in the down position when the seat is in the vehicle.
- To keep a newborn from slouching, roll up a couple of small blankets or cloth diapers and tuck them in along the sides of the baby's body and head. If the baby still slumps, put a rolled-up diaper between the legs. Never put padding or head rolls behind or under the baby.
- Dress your baby in clothes that keep the legs free. If you want to cover the baby, place a blanket over your baby after he or she is secured in the car seat with the harness buckled and adjusted.
- Make sure you use the seat correctly every time you're in the vehicle.

own preferences. Newborns generally love being held close, soothed by the warmth of your body. They also feel secure and calm when they're cradled in the crook of an elbow, with their head, legs and arms firmly supported.

During the first few months of life, babies differ in their ability to control their neck muscles and head. Until you're sure your baby can hold up his or her head quite well, lift the baby gently and slowly so that his or her body is supported and the head doesn't flop back. When putting your baby down, gently support the head and neck with one hand and the bottom with the other.

With experience you'll discover the best position for calming and comforting a fussy baby. You might try holding him or her along the length of your arm, facedown, with the baby's head at the bend of your elbow and his or her crotch at your hand. Or you can hold the baby facedown across your lap, with his or her tummy lying against your thigh. Another comforting position is to lie on your back and put your baby facedown on your chest while gently rubbing his or her back.

Your baby will probably also develop a preference for how he or she wants to be carried. Some infants enjoy facing outward, looking at the world, and others prefer the security of snuggling close to your body. Your baby may like being carried with arms and legs tucked in, or he or she may prefer a more relaxed position with just the body and head supported.

Baby carriers

Infant carriers allow you to keep your baby nestled close to your body while your hands are free for other activities. A variety of carriers are available, including front carriers, slings and back carriers. They're especially useful for the first several months. By the time your baby weighs 15 to 20 pounds, he or she may be too heavy to carry this way. When the baby begins to sit up, at about 6 months, you can use a baby backpack.

A front carrier consists of two shoulder straps supporting a deep fabric seat. A sling is a wide swath of fabric worn across your torso and supported by a single shoulder strap. Breast-feeding is easier if you're wearing a sling instead of a front carrier. But some people find slings to be bulky and cumbersome.

Remember that it's never safe to ride a bicycle or drive or ride in a car while holding your baby in a carrier.

When choosing a baby carrier, consider these tips:

- Choose a carrier that holds and supports your baby securely. Look for padded head support.
- Make sure the carrier is comfortable for both you and your baby. Look for wide padded shoulder straps, a padded waist or hip belt, adjustable straps and leg holes that aren't too tight and are banded with elastic or padded fabric. Make sure a sling isn't so large that your baby gets lost in it. Both you and your baby should try on the carrier before buying it.
- Check for ease of use. Make sure you can easily slip the carrier on and off.
- Select a carrier with a fabric that's durable and easy to clean. Cotton is a good choice because it's warm, soft, breathable and washable.
- Look for a carrier with pockets or zippered compartments, which are handy for storing frequently used items.
- Choose a carrier that allows the baby to face both inward and outward.

Crib and sleeping safety

Because your newborn will spend at least half of the time sleeping, where and how you put the baby to sleep is no small matter. For the first weeks, many parents place their newborn's crib or bassinet in their own bedroom. Some families welcome the child into the "family bed," while others provide a separate room and crib for the baby. Your choice will depend on personal preference and needs.

Some breast-feeding mothers prefer to nurse while lying in their own bed. After feeding, they may place the infant in a nearby bassinet, cradle or crib, or the baby may remain in the parents' bed and nurse on demand throughout the night. Keep in mind that many adult beds may pose a serious risk of the baby falling to the floor or becoming trapped between the mattress and bed frame. Waterbeds are not safe for babies.

Crib and bassinet precautions

Falls are the most common injury associated with cribs. But it's easy to prevent falls if you follow a few safety rules. All safety guidelines for cribs also apply to bassinets. If you use a bassinet for the first few weeks, keep in mind that your baby will quickly outgrow it. A baby who's too large will make the bassinet unstable. Start using a crib by the end of the first month or when the baby weighs 10 pounds. Your child should be able to use a crib from birth until nearly age 3.

You may want to buy a portable crib or playpen for traveling, but it shouldn't take the place of a full-size, permanent crib. Portable cribs aren't subject to the same federal safety requirements as permanent cribs.

All new cribs are required to meet stringent safety requirements. Whether you opt for a new or used crib, be sure to follow these safety guidelines:

- Side slats should be less than 2 3/8 inches apart.
- End panels should be solid, without decorative cutouts.
- Drop sides should be operated with a locking, hand-operated latch, secure from accidental release.
- Corner posts should fit flush with end panels.
- The mattress should be snug fitting — you shouldn't be able to get more than two fingers between the mattress and the crib side.
- The top edge of the raised crib sides should be at least 20 inches above the mattress surface. The lowered crib side should be at least 4 inches above the mattress.
- Periodically check the crib to make sure it has no rough edges or sharp points on metal parts and no splinters or cracks in the wood. If you notice tooth marks on the railing, cover the wood with a plastic strip. Such strips are available at most children's furniture stores.
- Place bumper pads around the entire crib. Keep them in place until your baby is big enough to stand up. These prevent the baby from hurting his or her head. Be sure to tie all the strings on the pads, and make sure the strings are less than 6 inches long to prevent strangulation.
- Never use any type of thin plastic as a mattress cover. If you cover the mattress with heavy plastic, be sure the cover fits tightly. Zippered covers are best.
- Some older cribs — those made before 1974 — were painted with lead-based paint, which can cause lead poisoning in children. The simplest way to avoid that problem is to use a crib made later than 1974.
- Be sure that the hardware fits properly and that all joints are tight.
- Never place the crib near a hanging window blind or drapery cords. Avoid placing a crib next to a window.
- When choosing bedding for your baby's crib, don't use pillows or large quilts and comforters. Instead, use crib sheets and baby blankets.

Similarly, don't put stuffed animals in an infant's crib. Excessive bedding and stuffed animals might cause risk of suffocation or lead to overheating a baby.

- If you hang a mobile over your baby's crib, make sure it's securely attached to the side rails. Hang it high enough so that the baby can't reach it to pull it down, and remove it when the baby is able to get up on hands and knees.
- If you use a playpen or portable crib with mesh sides, make sure the mesh has a tight weave and keep all sides raised at all times.

'Back to sleep'

Always place your baby on his or her back to sleep, even for naps. This is the safest sleep position for reducing the risk of sudden infant death syndrome (SIDS). SIDS, sometimes called crib death, is the sudden and unexplained death of a baby under 1 year of age. Typically with SIDS, a peacefully sleeping baby simply never wakes up. In most cases, no cause is ever found.

Research shows that babies who are put to sleep on their stomach are much more likely to die of SIDS than are babies placed on their back. Infants who sleep on their side are also at increased risk, probably because babies in this position can roll onto their stomach. Since 1992, when the American Academy of Pediatrics began recommending the back-sleeping position for infants, the incidence of SIDS has declined nearly 50 percent in the United States.

The only exceptions to the back-sleeping rule are babies who have health problems that require them to sleep on their stomach. If your baby was born with a birth defect, spits up often after eating or has a breathing, lung or heart problem, talk to your baby's health care provider about the best sleeping position for your baby.

Make sure everyone who takes care of your baby knows to place the infant on his or her back for sleeping. That may include grandparents, child-care providers, baby sitters, friends and others.

Some babies don't like sleeping on their back at first, but most get used to it quickly. Many parents worry that their baby will choke if he or she spits up or vomits while sleeping on his or her back, but doctors have found no increase in choking or similar problems.

Other tips that may help reduce the risk of SIDS include:
- Breast-feed your baby. Although it's not entirely clear why, breast-feeding may protect babies against SIDS.
- If you dress your baby in a kimono or sleep sack, you may not need to use a blanket. If you use a lightweight blanket, place your baby toward the foot of the crib, tuck the blanket around the mattress and pull the blanket up only to the baby's chest.

- Don't smoke or expose the baby to household smoke. Infants whose mothers smoke during and after pregnancy are three times more likely to die of SIDS than are infants of nonsmoking mothers.
- Keep the temperature in your baby's room at a level that's comfortable for you, not warmer than normal.

Some babies who sleep on their back may get a flat spot on the back of the head. For the most part, this flat spot will go away after the baby learns to sit up. You can help keep your baby's head shape normal by alternating the direction your baby lies in the crib — head toward one end of the crib for a few nights and then toward the other. This way, the baby won't always sleep on the same side of his or her head. You can also change the location of interesting objects, such as mobiles, so that your baby doesn't consistently look in one direction.

When your baby is awake and someone is watching, place the baby on his or her stomach for a little tummy time. This helps strengthen the baby's neck and shoulder muscles and reduces the likelihood of a flat spot on the head.

Clothing concerns

When you're buying clothes for your newborn, choose a 3-month size or larger so that the baby doesn't immediately outgrow them. In general, look for soft, comfortable clothing that's washable. Select sleepwear that's labeled flame resistant or flame retardant, which can be either a synthetic fiber or cotton treated with flame-retardant chemicals. Avoid buttons, which are easily swallowed, and ribbons or strings, which can cause choking. Don't buy garments with drawstrings, which can catch on objects and strangle a child.

Because you'll likely be changing your baby's clothing several times a day, or at least changing diapers, make sure the outfits are uncomplicated and open easily. Look for garments that snap or zip down the front and the legs, have loosefitting sleeves and are made of stretchy fabric.

During the first few weeks, babies are often wrapped in receiving blankets. This keeps them warm, and the slight pressure around the body seems to give most newborns a sense of security.

Dress for the weather

New parents sometimes overdress their infants. A good rule of thumb is to dress your baby in the same number of layers that you would feel comfortable wearing. Unless it's hot outside, you might put the baby in an undershirt and diaper, covered by pajamas or a dressing gown, and wrapped in a receiving blanket. In hot weather — over 75 F — a single layer of clothing is appropriate, but a cover is needed when the baby is in air conditioning or near drafts.

Remember that your baby's skin will sunburn easily. If you're going to be outside for any length of time, protect your baby's skin with clothing and a cap. Keep the baby in the shade to avoid overexposure to the sun. You can use sunblock after your baby is 6 months old, but don't rely on it as the baby's only sun protection. Babies don't sweat easily and can become overheated.

Diaper changing

To parents of young babies, life often seems to be an endless round of changing diapers. Indeed, the average child goes through 5,000 diaper changes before being toilet trained. That statistic is daunting, but it may help to think of this necessary task as an opportunity for closeness and communication with your baby. Your warm words, gentle touches and encouraging smiles help make your baby feel loved and secure, and soon your infant will be responding with gurgles and coos.

Because newborns urinate up to 20 times a day, it's important to change your baby's diapers every two or three hours for the first few months. But you can wait until your baby wakes up to change a wet diaper. Urine alone doesn't usually irritate a baby's skin. However, the acid content in a bowel movement can, so change a messy diaper soon after your baby awakens.

Get equipped

Make diaper changing more comfortable for you and your baby by being prepared with the basics:

- **Diapers.** Be sure to stock an adequate supply of diapers. You can buy cloth or disposable diapers, or you can use a diaper service, most of which offer a choice of cloth or disposable. You'll need 80 to 100 disposable or cloth diapers a week. If you plan to use disposable diapers, be sure to get the size corresponding to your baby's weight.

  If you plan to buy cloth diapers, the number you'll need depends on how often you plan to wash them. For example, if you have three dozen diapers, you'll probably need to wash them every other day. Even if you plan to use disposable diapers, you'll find it helpful to have a dozen cloth diapers on hand in case you run out of disposables. Cloth diapers are also handy to drape over your shoulder or to put on your lap while burping your baby.
- **Plastic pants, if you're using cloth diapers.**
- **Absorbent diaper liners, if you're using cloth diapers.**
- **Pre-moistened baby wipes.** Although a moistened cloth also works, it's hard to beat the convenience of pre-moistened baby wipes.
- **A diaper pail.** Various types of diaper pails are available. Look for a pail that is convenient, sanitary and holds in odors.

- **Baby lotion.** It's not necessary to use lotion at every diaper change, but it may come in handy if your baby develops diaper rash.
- **A baby wipes warmer.** Baby wipes warmers do just that — warm up the wipes to a temperature that's more comfortable for your baby.
- **A changing table.** Choose a table with a wide, sturdy base that has compartments for storing diaper-changing supplies. Putting the changing table near a wall reduces the chance of a fall.

How to change a diaper

When changing a diaper, use a flat surface — a changing table, a changing pad on the floor, or a crib. If you're using a changing table, be sure to use the safety belt or keep one hand on your baby at all times.

Your baby may urinate when you're changing the diaper. If your baby is a boy, you can avoid being sprayed by covering his penis loosely with a diaper or cloth while cleaning the rest of the diaper area.

Cleanup

After you've removed the soiled diaper, take time to thoroughly clean your baby's bottom:

- Hold the baby's legs at the ankles with one hand during the cleaning.
- Use either a cotton cloth dampened with warm water or a pre-moistened baby wipe to wipe your baby's diaper area. Use alcohol-free and fragrance-free wipes to avoid drying or irritating the baby's skin.
- When your baby has a bowel movement, use the unsoiled front of the diaper to remove the bulk of the stool.
- Wipe down and away from the genitals, folding the waste inside the diaper.
- Gently finish cleaning with a cloth or wipe, using a mild soap as needed. You needn't apply lotion, unless your baby tends to develop rashes.
- Lift your baby's lower body by the ankles and slide the new diaper underneath.

Disposable diapers

When changing a disposable diaper, lift the baby's legs and slide the diaper underneath with the tabs under the back. Bring the front of the diaper up through the legs, centering it on your baby. Fit the diaper snugly around your baby's waist and fasten the tabs on either side. For newborns, fold the top of the diaper down so that it doesn't rub against the umbilical cord.

Cloth diapers

If you use cloth diapers, you can fold them several ways. Experiment with different techniques for best absorbency and fit. Fold the side edges in, making shallow folds for a larger baby and deeper folds for a smaller baby. For boys, you may want to create extra padding in the front. Some people find that folding the front narrower than the back allows diaper pins to sit flatter on the stomach and brings the diaper around the legs more tightly.

If you're using diaper pins, you can avoid accidentally poking the baby by keeping the fingers of one hand between the diaper pin and your baby's body until the point of the pin is securely locked in the pin's hood. Cloth diapers should fit snugly because they tend to loosen as your baby moves around. Tuck the edges of the cloth into plastic pants to keep wetness inside.

Diaper rash

All babies get a red or sore bottom from time to time, even with frequent diaper changes and careful cleaning. Diaper rash may be caused by many things, including irritation from stools or from a new product, such as disposable wipes, diapers or laundry detergent. Sensitive skin, a bacterial or yeast infection, and chafing or rubbing from tightfitting diapers or clothing also can cause a rash.

Diaper rash is usually easily treated and usually improves within several days. The most important factor in treating diaper rash is to keep your baby's skin as clean and dry as possible. Thoroughly wash the area with water during each diaper change. While your baby has a diaper rash, avoid washing the affected area with soaps and disposable, scented wipes. Alcohol and perfumes in these products can irritate your baby's skin and aggravate or prolong the rash.

Allow the baby's bottom to air-dry before replacing the diaper, and do what you can to increase airflow to the diaper region:

- Let your child go without a diaper for short periods of time.
- Avoid using plastic pants or tightfitting diaper covers.
- Use larger-sized diapers until the rash goes away.

Use a soothing ointment such as Desitin, Balmex, or A and D any time pinkness appears in the diaper area. Many diaper rash creams and ointments contain the active ingredient zinc oxide. These products typically are applied in a thin layer to the irritated region several times throughout the day to soothe and protect the baby's skin.

Do not use talcum powder or cornstarch on a baby's skin. An infant may inhale talcum powder, which can be very irritating to a baby's lungs. Cornstarch can contribute to a bacterial infection.

To help prevent diaper rash, avoid using superabsorbent disposable diapers, because they tend to be changed less frequently. If you're using cloth diapers, be sure to wash and rinse them thoroughly, and select snap-on plastic pants, instead of those with elastic bindings, for better air circulation. In addition, try using absorbent liners with cloth diapers.

Check with your baby's health care provider if:
- The diaper rash doesn't improve in a few days.

Grooming your infant

Keeping your little one clean and taking care of his or her hair, nails and skin can be among the most enjoyable child-care tasks. Use a gentle touch and take the opportunity to talk and sing as you groom your baby.

Bathing

Your infant doesn't need much bathing. During the first week or two, until the stump of the umbilical cord falls off, give your newborn sponge baths. After that, a complete bath is necessary only one to three times a week for the first year. More frequent baths can dry out the baby's skin.

Once the umbilical area is healed, try placing your baby directly in the water. The first baths should be as gentle and brief as possible. If your infant resists baths, give sponge baths, cleaning the parts that really need attention, especially the hands, neck, head, face, behind the ears, under the arms and the diaper area. Sponge baths are a good alternative to a full bath for the first six weeks or so.

How to bathe your baby

Find a time for bathing your baby that's convenient for both of you. Many people give their baby a bath before bedtime, as a relaxing, sleep-promoting ritual. Others prefer a time when their baby is fully awake. You'll enjoy this time more if you're not in a hurry and not likely to be interrupted.

Most parents find it easiest to bathe a newborn in a bathinette, sink or plastic tub lined with a clean towel. Have all your bathing supplies ready and, if feasible, have the room warm — about 75 F — before you undress your baby. In addition to the basin of water, you'll need a washcloth, cotton balls, a towel, diaper-changing supplies and clothing. Plain water baths are fine most of the time. If needed, you can use mild baby soap and shampoo that are free of fragrances and deodorants.

Before filling the tub or basin, test the water temperature with your elbow or wrist. The water should feel warm, not hot. Fill the tub with just a couple of inches of warm water. Undress your baby, removing the diaper last. If the diaper is dirty, clean your baby's bottom before setting him or her in the bath. Use one hand to support your baby's head and the other to guide him or her in, feet first, then gently lower the rest of the body in. It's important to support the head and torso, to provide both safety and a sense of security.

It's not necessary to shampoo your baby's hair with every bath — once or twice a week is plenty. Massage the entire scalp gently. When you rinse soap or shampoo from the baby's head, cup your hand across his or her forehead so that the suds run toward the sides, not the eyes. Or tip your baby's head back a bit.

Use a soft cloth to wash your baby's face and hair with clear water. Use a damp cotton ball to wipe each eye from the inside to the outside corner. Gently pat the face dry. Wash the rest of the body from the top down, including the inside folds of skin and the genital area. For a girl, gently spread the labia to clean. For a boy, lift the scrotum to clean underneath. If he's uncircumcised, don't try to retract the foreskin of the penis. Let your baby lean forward on your arm while you clean his or her back and bottom, separating the buttocks to clean the anal area.

Be careful handling your infant when he or she is slippery and wet. As soon as you're done bathing, wrap the baby in a towel or a baby towel with a built-in hood and gently pat dry.

CRADLE CAP

Your baby may develop scaliness and redness on the scalp. This condition is called cradle cap (seborrheic dermatitis), which results when oil-producing sebaceous glands produce too much oil. Cradle cap is common in infants, usually beginning in the first weeks of life and clearing up over a period of weeks or months. It may be mild, with flaky, dry skin that looks like dandruff, or more severe, with thick, oily, yellowish scaling or crusty patches.

Periodic shampooing with a mild baby shampoo can help with cradle cap. Don't be afraid to wash the baby's hair more frequently than before. This, along with soft brushing, will help remove the scales.

Baby oil or mineral oil may not be helpful, as it allows scales to build up on the scalp. If you decide to try oil, rub a small amount of mild vegetable or olive oil into the scales, then shampoo and brush it out.

If cradle cap persists or spreads to your baby's face, neck or other parts of the body, especially in the creases at the elbow or behind the ears, call your baby's health care provider, who may suggest a medicated shampoo or lotion.

Nail care

Your baby's nails are soft, but they're sharp. A newborn can easily scratch his or her own face — or yours. To prevent your baby from accidentally scratching his or her face, you may need to trim the fingernails shortly after birth and then as often as a few times a week after that.

Sometimes you may be able to carefully peel off the ends with your fingers because baby nails are so soft. Don't worry — you won't rip the whole nail off. You can also use a baby nail clipper or a small scissors. Here are some tips to make nail trimming easier for you and your baby:

- Trim the nails after a bath. They'll be softer, making them easier to cut.
- Wait until your baby is asleep.
- Have another person hold your baby while you trim his or her nails.
- Trim the nails straight across, and keep them short.

Skin care

Many parents expect their newborn's skin to be flawless. More commonly, you'll see some blotchiness, bruising from birth and skin blemishes that are unique to newborns, such as baby acne (milia). Most young infants have dry, peeling skin, especially on their hands and feet, for the first few weeks. Some blueness of the hands and feet is normal and may continue for a few weeks. Rashes are also common.

Most rashes and skin conditions are treated easily or clear up on their own. If your baby has pimples, place a soft, clean receiving blanket under his or her head and wash the face gently once a day with a mild baby soap. If the baby has dry or peeling skin, try using an over-the-counter, unscented lotion.

Check with your baby's health care provider if:
- The baby has a rash or skin condition that's purple, crusty, weepy, has blisters or doesn't go away.

UMBILICAL CORD CARE

After your newborn's cord is cut, all that remains is a small stump. In most cases, it will dry up and fall off within 12 to 15 days after birth. Until then, keep the area as clean and dry as possible. It's a good idea to give sponge baths rather than full baths until the cord falls off and the navel area heals.

Traditionally, parents have been instructed to swab the cord stump with rubbing alcohol. But some research indicates that leaving the stump alone may help the cord heal faster, so some hospitals now recommend against this practice. If you're unsure about what to do, talk to your baby's health care provider.

Exposing the cord to air and allowing it to dry at its base will hasten its separation. To prevent irritation and keep the navel area dry, fold the baby's diaper below the stump. In warm weather, dress a newborn in just a diaper and T-shirt to let air circulate and help the drying process.

It's normal to see a bit of crusted discharge or dried blood until the cord falls off. But if your baby's navel looks red or has a foul-smelling discharge, call your baby's health care provider. When the stump falls off, you may see a little blood, which is normal. But if the navel continues to bleed, contact your baby's health care provider.

Every year, about 120,000 moms bring home more than one newborn — twins, triplets or higher-order multiples. Life changes for any new parent, but for parents of multiples the changes are also multiplied.

Having more than one new baby at once can be exciting. It's also extremely demanding. Sometimes just getting through the day can seem impossible. And multiples often are born early, so you may need to consult your pediatrician more frequently than you would with a single baby.

What are some of the changes you can expect with multiples? You'll be tired because you'll be getting a lot less sleep, and your household standards will probably have to relax for a few years. The financial impact is significant. If you have other children, the arrival of multiples can trigger more than the usual sibling rivalry. The babies require an enormous amount of your time and energy and attract extra attention from friends, relatives and strangers on the street.

You'll probably have some negative or difficult feelings from time to time. Having less time for each baby can make you feel guilty or sad, and those feelings become even more pronounced if you already have another child or children. Most parents of twins or other multiples have moments when they feel they aren't up to the job of caring for their babies.

While it's completely normal to feel stressed and overwhelmed, mothers of multiples are more likely to suffer from baby blues and postpartum depression than are other mothers. (See Complications: Postpartum depression, page 585.)

Here are some tips for dealing with the special challenges of caring for multiples:

- **Recruit help and accept all offers of help.** Even though this may be hard to do, it can make a big difference. Some families hire help, some rely on extended family, and some get help from friends, neighbors, places of worship or clubs for parents of multiples.
- **Establish a list of priorities.** These include babies' needs, such as feeding, bathing, sleeping and cuddling. Rest and breaks for you should also be on the list.
- **Recognize your babies as individuals from the beginning.** Select different-colored clothing for your babies, which helps you identify each one at a glance. Avoid referring to the babies as the twins or the triplets. Use their names. Be sure to take pictures of each child separately.
- **Use charts or checklists.** This is helpful for documenting feedings and keeping track of who has been cared for and when.
- **If you have older children, encourage them to be an active, helpful part of the experience.** Ask them to help with the baby chores. Make a special effort to set aside time regularly to spend alone with your other children.
- **Plan to use a diaper service or disposable diapers unless you have extra household help.** If you use disposable diapers, keep at least a dozen cloth diapers on hand for emergencies.
- **Gather practical advice, information and support.** Feeding, bathing and dressing multiples may require some special strategies. Consider attending a local support group for parents of twins or other multiples. You'll likely get many invaluable ideas from other parents. Read books, Web sites and magazines about parenting multiples.
- **Don't neglect your relationship with your partner.** Talk to each other about your feelings and problems. Try to give each other breaks when you can, and do what you can to keep some time as a couple.

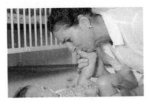

CHAPTER 15

postpartum care for moms

The period following labor and delivery is often exhausting, and you may be experiencing a wide range of aches and pains. You may wonder if your body will ever get back to normal.

It will take time to recover from the dramatic changes that occurred over the previous nine months. It's not realistic to expect to bounce back quickly after giving birth, but over time you'll start to feel better physically and get back in shape. This chapter offers a guide to some of the physical changes you can expect in the postpartum weeks.

Breast care

Your breasts may remain enlarged for a while after your baby's birth. To keep them comfortable, wear a good-quality, well-fitting bra. Clean your breasts and nipples daily with cotton balls and baby lotion or water, but avoid using soap. Soap strips away natural oils that keep the skin from drying and cracking and can aggravate sore or cracked nipples.

Engorgement

For the first few days after you have given birth, your breasts contain colostrum. Within a few days, they'll likely fill with milk — that is, your milk comes in. Your breasts may become larger and heavier, flushed, swollen and tender, whether or not you're planning to breast-feed. If you're not nursing your baby, your breasts may be engorged and hard until you're no longer producing milk. Even if you're breast-feeding, your breasts may at times overfill and become engorged. Engorgement usually lasts less than three days, but it can be uncomfortable.

To ease engorgement:
- Express a little milk, either manually or by feeding your baby.
- Stroke your breasts gently but firmly toward the nipple.

- Apply warm or cold washcloths or ice packs, or try a warm bath or shower.
- If you're not breast-feeding, avoid pumping or massaging your breasts, as this encourages milk production.

Leaking milk

If you're breast-feeding, don't be surprised if you leak milk during and between feedings. Milk may drip from your breasts anytime, anywhere and without warning. As many new mothers can attest, you might find yourself leaking when you think or talk about your baby, hear a baby cry or go for a long stretch between feedings. Milk may leak from one breast while you nurse from the other. Leaking is normal and common, particularly in the early weeks. Not leaking also is normal.

To deal with leaky breasts:
- Stock up on nursing pads. Avoid pads that are lined or backed with plastic because they can irritate your nipples. Change pads after each feeding and whenever they become wet.
- Place a large towel under you at night.
- Don't pump to prevent leaking — this may prompt more milk production.

Sore or cracked nipples

When you begin breast-feeding, your nipples may feel sore or tender. This is a common problem in the early weeks and can happen even if your baby is positioned perfectly and you're doing everything "right." Some women are surprised at how vigorously their babies suck — and how uncomfortable it can be. It takes some time to break in your nipples, but the tenderness usually disappears after a few days. A sore nipple that becomes cracked can be very painful and can lead to breast infection.

Follow these suggestions to prevent and treat sore or cracked nipples:
- Make sure your baby is latched on to your breast correctly, and take care when removing the baby from your breast. To help your baby get the nipple fully into his or her mouth, slip your hand between your breast and rib cage and push gently upward.
- Expose your nipples to air and sunlight. Let your nipples air-dry between feedings, and go topless occasionally, especially when resting.
- Avoid nursing pads with plastic linings and clothes made of synthetic fabrics. You might want to apply a drop of baby lotion to each breast pad.
- Try using a breast shield. The shield fits over the nipple, and the baby sucks through it.
- If a nipple becomes cracked, you may need to keep your baby off that breast for a few days and express milk to avoid engorgement.

BREAST SELF-EXAMINATION

Monthly breast self-examination can be more difficult during pregnancy and breast-feeding, but it's no less important. The key is to find a convenient time and establish a routine. If you're breast-feeding, it's best to do the self-examination right after you've fed your baby, when your breasts are emptier and any abnormalities may be more obvious.

Blocked ducts

In the early weeks of breast-feeding, a milk duct may become blocked as a result of engorgement, a too-tight bra or a blocked nipple opening. If you get a blockage, your breast may feel tender and lumpy and the skin may be red. To clear a blocked duct, start feedings with the affected breast and gently massage it while feeding.

Call your health care provider if:
- You have pain and feel sick or have a fever, as you may have mastitis.

Healing from an episiotomy or tear

If you received stitches after delivery due to an episiotomy or tear, the stitches will dissolve and you'll be feeling more comfortable about two weeks after delivery. As with any surgical wound, the tissue around an episiotomy or a tear wound can take about six weeks to regain its natural strength. If you've had an extensive tear, the tenderness may continue for a month or more. Those weeks may be tough because it can be painful to walk or sit while the episiotomy or tear heals. View the pain as a reminder to rest and pamper your body.

To ease your discomfort:
- You may want to squat rather than sit when you use the toilet. A squirt bottle of water is helpful for rinsing afterward. You can also try pouring warm water over yourself as you're passing urine, to reduce the sting.
- Gently cooling the wound with ice can decrease swelling. You could try placing ice in a washcloth or rubber glove or using an ice pack.
- Special perineal pads that fit between a sanitary napkin and the wound are soothing. Chilled witch hazel pads also may help.
- Keep the wound clean. Warm baths and showers may be soothing.
- You may find it more comfortable to sit on hard surfaces because soft surfaces allow your bottom to stretch and pull on the stitches. Squeeze your buttocks together when you lower yourself to sit on a soft surface.
- Do Kegel exercises frequently. You can start about a day after birth.
- When you move your bowels, the pressure can stretch your tissues and cause pain around the wound. To prevent stretching, hold a clean pad firmly against the stitches and press upward while you bear down.

- Ask your health care provider for a pain relief spray or a ring to sit on.
- If your wound becomes hot, swollen and painful or produces a pus-like discharge, you may have an infection. Call your health care provider.

Fatigue

During the first weeks of caring for a newborn baby many mothers feel a fatigue that never seems to let up and an almost total lack of energy. After the tiring work of labor, you're hit with the round-the-clock rigors of taking care of the baby. Night after night of interrupted sleep and the energy required for breast-feeding and carrying around a baby can add to your exhaustion. Fatigue may be even more pronounced if you have other children, if your baby was premature or has health problems, or if you had multiple babies.

Over time, your fatigue will probably lessen as your body adjusts to the demands of motherhood, you gain experience in dealing with your baby and the baby sleeps through the night.

You most likely won't be able to completely avoid being tired, but these tips may help keep fatigue from depleting you:

- Try to rest whenever you can. Take advantage of your baby's daytime naps to get some sleep yourself.
- Avoid heavy lifting.
- Enlist your partner to share the work of baby care and household chores. Accept offers of help from other people, too.
- Try not to do too much. Cut back on less important tasks, such as housework. Limit the number of guests you have.
- Exercise regularly to increase your energy level and help you fight fatigue. Eating well also is important, but don't eat too much late at night because digestion can interfere with your sleep.
- Go to bed early and unwind by listening to music or reading.
- Have your partner help with nighttime feedings. If you're breast-feeding, express milk for this purpose.
- If your fatigue doesn't seem to improve over time, check with your health care provider.

Bowel and urination problems

Hemorrhoids

You may have developed hemorrhoids during pregnancy, or you may discover them after giving birth. If you notice pain during a bowel movement and feel a swollen mass near your anus, you probably have a hemorrhoid. To prevent constipation and the need to strain, which contribute to hemorrhoids, eat a fiber-rich diet, including fruits, vegetables and whole grains, and drink plenty of water. You may also find comfort by soaking in a bath or by applying chilled witch hazel pads to the area. If your stools are still hard, try using stool softeners (Colace, Surfak, others) or fiber laxatives (Citrucel, FiberCon, others).

For other suggestions for relieving the discomfort of hemorrhoids, see page 453. If you continue to have problems, talk to your health care provider, who might suggest a prescription medicine.

Leaking urine

About 20 percent of women who give birth vaginally experience urinary incontinence, compared with about 10 percent of women who haven't had a baby. Women who've had a Caesarean birth are more likely to pass urine inadvertently than are those who haven't had a baby, though not as likely as those who delivered vaginally. Incontinence is more common during and after pregnancy because pregnancy and birth stretch the base of the bladder and may cause nerve and muscle damage to the bladder or urethra. You're most likely to leak urine when coughing, straining or laughing.

Fortunately, this problem usually improves within three months. In the meantime, wear sanitary pads and do your Kegel exercises.

Bowel movements

You may not have a bowel movement for a few days after delivery. That's because of the lack of food during labor and because the muscle tone in your intestines is temporarily decreased. After delivery, your abdominal muscles are relaxed and stretched, which can slow the passage of feces through your bowels. This slowing can lead to constipation. In addition, you may find yourself holding back from passing stools out of fear of hurting your perineum or aggravating the pain of hemorrhoids or an episiotomy wound.

Another potential problem for new moms is fecal incontinence — the inability to control bowel movements. This may be caused by the stretching and weakening of pelvic floor muscles, tearing of the perineum or nerve injury to the muscles around the anus. You're more likely to experience fecal incontinence if you had an unusually long labor and vaginal delivery. Kegel exercises can help return tone to your anal muscles. Talk to your health care provider if you're having persistent trouble controlling bowel movements.

To prevent constipation and help keep your stools soft and regular:
- Drink plenty of fluids.
- Increase your intake of fiber-rich foods, including fresh fruits and veg-

etables and whole grains. Dried prunes and figs are good choices, as are prune, pear and apricot juices.
- Remain as physically active as possible.
- Try using stool softeners (Colace, Surfak, others) or fiber laxatives (Citrucel, FiberCon, others).

Difficulty urinating

After giving birth, you may sometimes experience hesitancy or a decreased urge to urinate. This may be the result of swelling or bruising of the perineum and the tissues surrounding the bladder and urethra, perineal pain or fear of the sting of urine on your tender perineal area.

To encourage your urine to start flowing:
- Contract and release your pelvic muscles.
- Increase your intake of fluids.
- Place hot or cold packs on your perineum.
- Try straddling the toilet saddle style when you urinate.
- Pour water across your perineum while you urinate.

The problem usually resolves over time. However, if you experience intense burning after urination or an intense, painful and unusually frequent urge to urinate, you may have a urinary tract infection. Contact your health care provider if you have these signs and symptoms or you suspect you aren't emptying your bladder.

Afterpains

After your baby's birth, your uterus begins shrinking immediately, decreasing to its normal size over about six weeks. As the uterus shrinks (contracts), you may feel contractions — called afterpains — for several days. Afterpains are often mild after the birth of your first baby. They're usually more noticeable and painful if you've had a child before.

Afterpains tend to be more intense when you're breast-feeding, because the baby's sucking triggers the release of the hormone oxytocin, which also causes your uterus to contract. Medications used to control hemorrhaging also can increase cramping.

You may find some relief from afterpains by breathing slowly and relaxing. If your cramps are causing a lot of discomfort, your health care provider may prescribe a pain medication. Many medicines are safe even if you're breast-feeding. See your health care provider if you have a fever or the pain persists for more than a week, as these signs and symptoms could indicate a uterine infection.

Other postpartum changes

Vaginal discharge

As your uterus sheds its lining and returns to its normal size after birth, you'll have a vaginal discharge known as lochia. It varies widely in amount, appearance and duration, but it typically starts off as a bright red, heavy flow of blood. After about four days, it gradually diminishes and becomes paler, changing to pink or brown and then to yellow or white after about 10 days. The vaginal discharge can last from two to eight weeks.

To reduce the risk of infection, use sanitary napkins rather than tampons. Don't be alarmed if you occasionally pass blood clots — even if they're as large as a golf ball.

Call your health care provider if:

- You're soaking a sanitary pad every hour for more than a few hours or you feel dizzy.
- The discharge has a foul odor.
- Your abdomen feels tender, or your bleeding increases and you're passing numerous clots.
- You pass clots larger than a golf ball.
- The flow suddenly becomes bright red again after fading in color.
- You have a temperature of 100.3 F or higher.

Hair and skin

You may notice some changes in your hair and skin after the birth of your baby.

Hair loss. For some women, one of the most noticeable changes after delivery is hair loss. During pregnancy, elevated hormone levels keep you from losing hair at the usual rate of 100 hairs a day — which probably gave you an extra-lush head of hair. After the birth, your body sheds all that excess hair. Don't worry — the hair loss is temporary, and by the time your baby is six months old, your hair will probably be back to normal.

To keep your hair healthy, eat well and continue taking a vitamin supplement. Ask your hairdresser for a cut that's easy to maintain. Shampoo only when necessary, use a conditioner and keep your use of blow-dryers or curling irons to a minimum. You may want to put off coloring or relaxing your hair or having a perm until your hair seems back to normal.

Red spots. Small red spots on your face after the birth are caused by small blood vessels breaking during the pushing stage of labor. The spots usually disappear in about a week.

Stretch marks. Stretch marks won't disappear after delivery, but over time they usually fade from reddish purple to silver or white.

Skin darkening. Skin that darkened during pregnancy, such as the line down your abdomen (linea nigra) and the mask of pregnancy (skin darkening on the face), fade over several months. They rarely go away completely.

Weight loss

After you give birth, you'll probably feel pretty flabby and out of shape. In fact, you may look in the mirror and feel like you're still six months pregnant. But don't berate yourself — this is perfectly normal, and no woman is going to slip back into a tight pair of jeans a week after having a baby. Realistically, it will probably take three to six months or longer to lose the weight you gained while pregnant.

You'll probably lose about 10 pounds during birth, including the weight of the baby, the placenta and amniotic fluid. During the first week after delivery, you'll lose additional weight from leftover fluids. After that, the amount of weight you lose will depend on your diet and how much exercise you get. Look for a gradual reduction in your weight — about half a pound a week — if you maintain a healthy eating plan and exercise regularly.

A healthy diet

Good nutrition is important to your well-being — and your baby's if you're breast-feeding. Instead of cutting back significantly on how much you eat, skipping meals or going on a fad diet, focus on eating healthy foods, including vegetables, fruits, whole grains and low-fat sources of protein.

Exercise

Regular daily exercise can help you recover from labor and delivery, restore your strength and get your body back to its pre-pregnancy shape. In addition, exercise can increase your energy level and help you fight fatigue, and can improve your circulation and help prevent backaches. Physical activity also brings important psychological benefits. It can boost your sense of well-being and improve your ability to cope with the stresses of being a new parent.

If you exercised before and during pregnancy and had an uncomplicated vaginal delivery, it's generally safe to resume exercising as early as 24 hours after delivery or as soon as you feel ready. About a day after you give birth, you can start doing Kegel exercises and gradually work up to 25 or more repetitions several times a day. If you had a Caesarean or complicated birth, talk to your health care provider about when and how to start an exercise program.

Even if you had an easy delivery, you'll need to start off slowly and carefully. Don't try to do too much too soon or expect to return immediately to your pre-pregnancy level of exercise. Walking and swimming are excellent activities to help you get back in shape. Begin slowly and pick up the pace and distance as you feel up to it. Some new moms enjoy postpartum exercise classes.

Here are some tips for exercising after giving birth:

- Exercises to tone and strengthen your abdominal and pelvic floor muscles are especially important after giving birth. They restore abdominal strength, tone and flatten the abdomen and help you maintain good posture. Exercise also can help heal an episiotomy, prevent incontinence and re-establish control of the anal muscles.
- If you didn't exercise much during your pregnancy, you'll need to start slowly and gradually work your way into more vigorous activity.
- Start with a series of small, achievable fitness goals — aim for moderate rather than high-intensity workouts. Exercise a few times a day in brief sessions rather than for one long period.
- Choose activities you can do with your baby, such as walking with a stroller or baby carrier, dancing with the baby and jogging with a jogging stroller. Some postnatal fitness tapes even show you how to include your baby in your workout.
- Wear a supportive bra and comfortable clothing.
- If you're breast-feeding, you'll probably feel more comfortable if you feed your baby right before you exercise.
- Avoid jumping and jerky, bouncy or jarring motions during the first six weeks postpartum. Also avoid rapid changes of direction, deep flexion or extension of joints, knee-to-chest exercises, full sit-ups and double leg lifts.
- Don't overdo it. Stop before you feel tired, and skip your workout if you're feeling particularly exhausted. Stop exercising immediately if you experience pain, faintness, dizziness, blurred vision, shortness of breath, heart palpitations, back pain, pubic pain, nausea, difficulty walking or a sudden increase in vaginal bleeding.
- Drink plenty of liquids before, during and after exercising.
- Stick with it. Even after you lose your pregnancy weight, physical activity brings many physical and mental health benefits.

The postpartum checkup

Your health care provider will probably schedule you for a checkup four to six weeks after the birth. This can include a pelvic exam to check your vagina and cervix and assess the size and shape of your uterus. Your health care provider may also examine your episiotomy site or other incisions. He or she may do a breast exam and check your weight and blood pressure.

Your health care provider may ask about how you're feeling emotionally and how you're coping. He or she may discuss the method of birth control you plan to use and offer you a prescription or other help in making your plan work.

Your postpartum checkup is a good opportunity to bring up any questions or problems you're having. Bring a list of your questions and concerns.

The next scheduled visit after this checkup might be in six to 12 months for appropriate health maintenance, which may include renewing contraception and evaluating your method of contraception.

Emotional and lifestyle changes

The physical changes and complaints of the postpartum period are only part of life after having a baby — and, some women would say, the easy part. As you and your partner get to know your baby and begin to bond as a family, your feelings will probably be more intense and fluctuating than you expected, and the stresses may be more overwhelming than anticipated. Caring for a new baby is a demanding and exhausting job that can turn your life upside down.

During the postpartum weeks, most women are nervous about their ability to deal with the new responsibilities. You may have concerns about losing your pre-baby freedom and identity, finding time for yourself, bonding with your baby, juggling all of your other responsibilities and maintaining a good relationship with your partner. Mood swings are common, as are the baby blues and feelings of depression. Exhaustion, lack of sleep and hormone changes can contribute to your emotional struggles.

It may help if you accept the reality that your life is going to be chaotic or topsy-turvy for the foreseeable future. You probably won't be getting a good night's sleep for a while, and showers, sit-down meals and time alone may be rare treats at first. But even though your first year as a new mother is likely to be challenging, it will probably also be more joyful and energizing than you ever imagined. The demands on your time, energy and emotional resources can be difficult, but you and your partner can take steps to make this time easier.

RECOVERING FROM A CAESAREAN BIRTH

If you had a Caesarean birth, you can expect a few additional discomforts and precautions during the postpartum period. See Chapter 12, "Caesarean birth," page 187, for information about recovering from a Caesarean birth.

Stress

Besides the challenges of round-the-clock baby care, many other factors can leave you feeling stressed, overwhelmed or depressed during the postpartum weeks. Many new parents will experience some of these situations and feelings:

- If you're used to feeling in control and organized, you may be dismayed when your orderly lifestyle flies out the window after you give birth. Rather than the serene family life you envisioned, it may be chaotic.
- If your baby's birth didn't go as expected — for example, you had an unexpected Caesarean delivery or a very long labor — you may feel disappointed, resentful or like a failure.
- If you had a premature baby or more than one baby, you're dealing with extra responsibilities.
- For parents who have been working full time, the transition from being a competent worker to a novice caregiver may be difficult.
- You may face feelings of inadequacy and self-doubt as you figure out by trial and error how to take care of your baby — and you realize that it doesn't just come naturally.
- You may find it hard to adjust to limited time spent with adults. After all, a newborn doesn't provide conversation. You may miss your friends.
- Financial worries are common to most parents. No matter what your income level, having a child may strain the budget.
- It may be difficult to embrace your role as a new parent. Many women feel a sense of mourning for their old identity as a carefree, possibly career-oriented person. You may feel ill at ease with your new identity as "mother" or with the shift from center stage to backstage as your baby becomes the focus of attention.
- You may feel guilty or worried if you don't bond immediately with your baby or don't have overwhelming feelings of love at first sight.
- The dynamics of your relationship with your partner may change after the birth. You have to figure out how to divide work, child care and household duties and how to balance having time with the baby, time as a couple and time alone.
- Many couples experience a significant change in sexual activity after the birth of a baby. Because of fatigue, physical discomfort, hormonal changes, lack of desire or dissatisfaction with how they look following the birth, most women feel less interested in sex for a while after having a baby.

Tips for when you're feeling overwhelmed

When you bring your baby home, there will probably be times when you feel exhausted, stressed or overwhelmed. One of the most important ways to minimize stress is to take good care of yourself by continuing to eat as well as you did throughout your pregnancy, drinking plenty of fluids, staying physically active and getting as much rest as you possibly can.

In addition, the following suggestions can help you survive the postpartum period:

- **Get help.** Accept offers of help from friends and family members, and don't be afraid to ask for help. Keep a list of jobs that need to be done so that you'll have a specific task for someone who offers to help. Most people are glad to help out with cooking, housework, errands or watching the baby while you run errands. Many communities have services for new mothers. Check with your hospital nurse, with your local health department or in the Yellow Pages.

- **Get out of the house.** Being housebound with a crying newborn day after day can make anyone stir-crazy. Take your baby out for a walk or find someone to watch the baby for a few hours while you get out. Consider swapping child care with other new moms or joining a child-care cooperative.

- **Simplify.** Keeping the house clean doesn't have to be your priority right now. Getting enough rest and taking care of your baby are more important than having a spotless house. Accept some clutter in your life. During mealtimes, use shortcuts such as paper plates, frozen dinners or takeout foods. Don't feel guilty for bowing out of some commitments or turning down others.

- **Avoid guilt.** Many moms seem to be experts at feeling guilty. Remember that you can only do your best. There's no such thing as the perfect parent or the perfect child. Learn from any mistakes and try to do better next time.

- **Establish some routines.** Even though your baby's eating and sleeping patterns will change frequently during the first year, try to find ways to adapt your life to his or her daily routine. Try to have your baby eat and sleep at the same times every day.

- **Take time to nurture yourself.** It's easy to get caught up in the never-ending demands of baby care, but you'll be better able to meet those demands if you arrange to have at least a few hours to yourself every week. Make an arrangement with your partner, a friend or a relative to watch the baby while you pursue one of your own interests, have lunch with a friend or go on a special outing. In addition, try to do something you enjoy every day. For example, go for a walk, read a book, write, draw or listen to music. Treat yourself to a massage or bath. Talk with people you find uplifting.

- **Take time to nurture your relationship or marriage.** Find ways to spend time together both with and without the baby. See "Nurturing your relationship" on page 266.

- **Share your feelings.** Talk about all of your feelings — including feelings of anger, frustration and sadness — with someone you trust. Be sure to keep communicating with your partner.
- **Connect with other parents.** Make friends with other parents. Keep in touch with the people you met at prenatal class, or take a parenting class at a local school, child-care center, community center, health clinic, hospital or house of worship. You could also join a support group with other mothers and new babies or participate in an online bulletin board or mailing list for women who gave birth the same month you did.

The baby blues

Most new mothers feel depressed to some degree after giving birth. The abrupt drop in levels of estrogen and progesterone following childbirth is thought to be a cause of baby blues and postpartum depression.

But hormonal changes aren't the only factor. If you're sleep deprived and overwhelmed, it's natural to feel depressed. Other possible contributing factors include the many physical changes you go through after delivery, difficulties during your pregnancy or labor, the letdown after an exciting event, changes in your family's finances, unrealistic expectations of childbirth and parenting, inadequate emotional support, and relationship and identity adjustments.

Some men experience symptoms of depression after their babies are born. Men whose partners have postpartum depression are at particular risk of experiencing depression themselves.

As many as 80 percent of new mothers experience what's called the baby blues, a mild form of depression. Signs and symptoms include episodes of anxiety, sadness, crying, headaches and exhaustion. You may feel unworthy, irritable and indecisive. After the initial excitement of having the baby wears off, you may find that the reality of motherhood seems difficult to cope with. The baby blues usually occur about three to five days after the birth and last about a week to 10 days.

You can help recover more quickly if you get extra rest, eat a healthy diet and get regular exercise. In addition, try to express your feelings by talking about them, particularly with your partner. If these measures don't help, you may have a more severe form of depression. For more information on postpartum depression and postpartum psychosis, see page 585. Talk with your health care provider if your symptoms are severe or last longer than a few weeks.

Bonding with your baby

As soon as babies are born, they need and want you to hold, stroke, cuddle, touch, kiss and talk and sing to them. These everyday expressions of love and affection promote bonding and recognition. They also help your baby's brain develop. Just as an infant's body needs food to grow, his or her brain needs positive emotional, physical and intellectual experiences. Relationships with other people early in life have a vital influence on a child's development.

Some parents feel an immediate connection with their newborn, and for others, the bond takes longer to develop. Don't worry or feel guilty if you aren't overcome with a rush of love at the beginning. Not every parent bonds instantly with a new baby. Your feelings will almost certainly become stronger over time.

It also takes time to learn how to interpret your baby's cries and signals and to figure out what he or she likes and needs. Even as a newborn, each baby has a distinct personality. If you have other children, they'll also be learning how to relate to their new sister or brother.

At first most of your baby's time is likely to be spent eating, sleeping and crying. Your warm, loving responses to the baby's needs form the foundation of nurturing and bonding. When babies receive warm, responsive care, they're more likely to feel safe and secure. Routine tasks present an opportunity to bond with your baby. For example, as you feed your baby and change diapers, gaze lovingly into his or her eyes and talk gently to him or her.

Babies also have times when they're quietly alert and ready to learn and play. These times may last only a few moments, but you'll learn to recognize them. Take advantage of your baby's alert times to get acquainted and play.

To bond with and nurture your baby:

- Don't worry about spoiling your newborn. Respond to your child's cues and clues. Among the signals babies send are the sounds they make — which will be mostly crying during the first week or two — the way they move, their facial expressions and the way they make or avoid eye contact. Pay close attention to your baby's need for stimulation as well as quiet times. See "How to tell when your baby needs a break" on page 265.

- Talk, read and sing to your baby. Even infants enjoy music and being read to. They don't grasp the meaning of words, but these early "conversations" help your baby's language capacity grow and provide an opportunity for closeness. When you talk to your baby, remember that high-pitched voices are most appealing to babies. Baby talk isn't silly — babies actually prefer soft, rhythmic sounds. You can try various sounds to see if your baby shows preferences for some sounds over others. Even though a baby may not turn toward a sound, you may notice that your voice can cause your baby to settle down or become quiet.

- Cuddle and touch your baby. Newborns are very sensitive to changes in pressure and temperature. They love to be held, rocked, caressed, cradled, snuggled, kissed, patted, stroked, massaged and carried.

- Let your baby watch your face. Soon after birth, your newborn will become accustomed to seeing you and will begin to focus on your face. Babies prefer the human face over other patterns or colors. Allow your baby to study your features, and provide plenty of smiles.
- Give your baby an opportunity to imitate you. Choose a simple facial movement such as opening your mouth or sticking out your tongue. Slowly repeat the gesture a few times. Your baby may or may not attempt to mimic your gesture.
- Give your baby simple toys that appeal to sight, hearing and touch. These include unbreakable crib mirrors, rattles, textured toys and musical toys. Choose toys and mobiles with strong contrasting colors, such as black and white or black and red.
- Play music and dance. Put on some soft music with a beat, hold your baby's face close to yours and gently sway and move to the tune.
- Avoid overstimulating your baby. Offer your baby one toy or stimulus at a time. Too many play activities at once can lead to confusion and overstimulation.
- Establish routines and rituals. Repeated positive experiences provide children with a sense of security.

HOW TO TELL WHEN YOUR BABY NEEDS A BREAK

Your baby may give you very direct signals when playtime is over. Watch for these clues to let you know the baby is tired and needs a break:
- Closing eyes
- Turning away or dropping arm and shoulders away from you
- Stiffening or clenching fists
- Becoming irritable
- Beginning deep, rhythmic breathing
- Tensing up, arching back
- Avoiding your gaze

Take your time

Be patient with yourself in these first weeks with your new baby. Remember that you and your family have undergone a tremendous change. It can be daunting, discouraging, thrilling and perplexing, all in the same hour. In time, you'll grow stronger physically. And your skills as a parent will grow, too, day by day, as you explore with this new person in your world.

This month, you may also be interested in:
- **"Complications: Postpartum conditions," page 579**

Nurturing your relationship

As you and your partner begin to bond with the baby and form a family, it's important to make time for yourselves as a couple. The postpartum period is a time of major adjustment for a couple as you work out how to share parenting duties and relate to each other in your new role as parents. Here are some tips for coping with the changes in your relationship and nurturing your partnership:

- **Keep the lines of communication open.** Being a new parent can be scary for both people. It helps to talk about these feelings with your partner. Share your feelings about what's happening in your sexual relationship, too.
- **Share the job and experiences of parenting.** Being a parent is easier for both of you if you share the work. Both parents should be ready to respond to the baby's cries, give the baby baths and change diapers. The dad can help out with feedings. If the mom is breast-feeding, she can pump some milk for dad's use at nighttime feedings. In addition, take time to do fun things together as a family. Young babies are very portable, so you can include the baby in your social life and continue your lifestyle to a large degree. Allow your shared love for your baby to bring you closer together as a couple.
- **Make decisions together.** If you disagree about how to take care of the baby, work it out. Getting comfortable with this process can help you make tougher decisions later.
- **Spend time alone together.** Even though you're both busy with the baby and other responsibilities, finding time in your daily routine when you and your partner can be alone together is an important way to maintain your relationship. At home, continue small rituals you may have together, such as doing a crossword puzzle together or chatting at the end of the day. Plan dates on a regular basis. Turn to someone you trust for baby-sitting and get some time together away from the baby.
- **Take turns giving each other breaks.** Each parent needs some time away from the baby.
- **Be patient and ease back into sex.** Many couples experience a decrease in sexual activity in the first year after childbirth — for many reasons. You may be too exhausted and sore to even think about sex in the first weeks and months after the birth. Many women feel less attractive in the postpartum period and experience a lack of libido or inability to achieve orgasm. Intercourse may be painful, due to hormonal changes and breast-feeding.

  Whether you've given birth vaginally or had a Caesarean birth, your body can need several weeks to heal. Most women wait three to six weeks before resuming intercourse. If you had a Caesarean birth, your health care provider may advise you to wait six weeks. You can gain confidence about resuming intercourse when you no longer feel pain as you press on your vaginal opening or episiotomy.

  During the weeks when you're not having intercourse, aim to maintain emotional and sexual intimacy. Lovemaking without intercourse can resume soon after birth if you wish. This can reaffirm your affection for each other.

  When you do resume intercourse, lubricating creams or gels may be necessary because lower hormone levels cause vaginal dryness. Try different positions to take pressure off the sore area and control penetration. Be honest with your partner and tell him if sex causes you discomfort or pain. Finally, unless you want to become pregnant again immediately, use birth control.

Part 2

decision guides for pregnancy, childbirth and parenthood

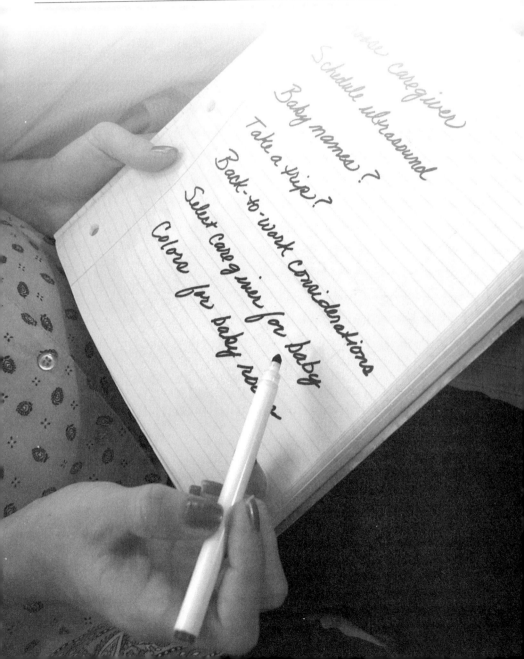

"How do I choose a health care provider for pregnancy? Should I undergo pre-natal testing? What are my options for pain relief during labor and childbirth?"

During pregnancy, you're likely to be faced with these and many other important questions. This section, "Decision Guides for Pregnancy, Childbirth and Parenthood," offers information to guide you toward the answers that are right for you and your situation.

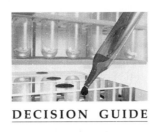

understanding genetic carrier screening for prospective parents

Although most babies are born healthy, having a baby means taking a risk. There are no guarantees that a child will be born healthy.

Some people have a genetic makeup that increases their risk of having a child with health problems. Today, tests are available that offer parents-to-be an opportunity to explore some of the risks that genetics may pose for their unborn children.

These tests are called genetic carrier screening tests. They're designed to identify people who carry one copy of an altered gene that leads to a specific disease. Although these people carry the altered gene, they aren't affected by it, because two altered copies of the gene must be present before the disease develops. Genetic carrier screening can be done on prospective parents before a baby is conceived. It can also be done during pregnancy to help determine whether further testing during the pregnancy may be considered. With this information, potential parents can weigh the risks and make decisions.

This decision guide explains what kinds of tests are available to examine potential health risks that may be included in your genetic code. It explains what those tests can — and can't — tell you.

Issues to consider

It's up to you to decide if you want to pursue genetic carrier screening. Consider these questions as you make that decision:
- Is there a family history of any certain condition?
- Are you in a racial or ethnic group that puts you at higher risk of being a carrier for a certain condition?
- How often does the condition occur in the higher-risk population?
- How severe is the condition likely to be?

- Will you use the information if you find that you and your partner are carriers of the same genetic condition? If yes, how?
- How might you respond emotionally to the testing process?
- Will the test be covered by your insurance? If not, will you be able to afford the testing? Be aware that tests used for purposes other than diagnosing a condition may not be covered by insurance.
- Will the time it takes to complete the test give you adequate time to make decisions regarding beginning or continuing a pregnancy?
- Would discussing the options and issues related to genetic carrier screening with a genetic counselor or other health care provider be of benefit to you?

WHAT'S THE DIFFERENCE BETWEEN A CONGENITAL DISORDER AND A GENETIC DISORDER?

A congenital disorder is a disorder that a baby is born with. A genetic disorder is one that's inherited, passed from one generation to the next through the family's genetic makeup.

A baby may be born with a disorder that's both present at birth (congenital) and caused by his or her genetic makeup (genetic). However, not all congenital disorders are genetic. For example, cerebral palsy is a congenital disorder that affects the nervous system's ability to control motion. Because it's a congenital disorder but not a genetic one, cerebral palsy can't be identified through genetic carrier screening.

Genetic disorders — such as Tay-Sachs disease, cystic fibrosis and others discussed in this decision guide — can be identified through genetic carrier screening tests. It's important to understand that genetic testing can uncover some, but not all, possible birth defects.

Who might consider genetic carrier screening?

With few exceptions, screening everyone for even the most common disorders isn't possible or practical. In the United States, several criteria must be met for widespread screening to be justified:

- A simple, accurate test is available
- The population — usually a certain ethnic or racial group — has a high incidence of carriers
- Reproductive or treatment options are available to people identified as carriers

You might consider undergoing genetic carrier screening if:

- You're part of a population group in which a genetic disease is known to be more common
- You or your partner has a family history of a particular health condition

Population-based screening

Certain racial and ethnic groups are more at risk than are others for certain disorders, some of which are listed below. If you belong to one of these groups, talk to your health care provider or a genetic counselor about your risks of being a carrier and the screening process.

Racial or ethnic group	Genetic disorder
Ashkenazi Jew	Tay-Sachs disease, cystic fibrosis, Canavan disease, Niemann-Pick disease (type A), Fanconi anemia (group C), Bloom syndrome, Gaucher disease, familial dysautonomia
French Canadian, Cajun	Tay-Sachs disease
Black	Sickle cell disease
Mediterranean	Beta-thalassemia
Chinese and Southeast Asian (Cambodian, Filipinos, Laotian, Vietnamese)	Alpha-thalassemia
White (European)	Cystic fibrosis

Population-based genetic carrier screening is available for people who are part of a group at risk of certain disorders. Screening can be done for:
- **Autosomal recessive disorders.** Your DNA is made up of paired sets of genes, one set received from your mother, one set from your father. With an autosomal recessive genetic disorder, if you carry a single altered gene for a disease, you don't have the signs and symptoms of it. If two people carry a recessive gene for the same disease, there's a 25 percent chance that their child will have the disease, a 25 percent chance that a child wouldn't be a carrier or affected, and a 50 percent chance that the child wouldn't have the disease but would be a carrier of the altered gene, like the parents (see visual, page 272).

Autosomal recessive disorders include Canavan disease, cystic fibrosis, sickle cell disease and thalassemias, among thousands of others.

Family history screening

If a certain disease runs in your family, you may wish to be tested to determine whether you carry the genetic alteration that causes it. For instance, if you have a sibling with an autosomal recessive condition, there's a 50 percent

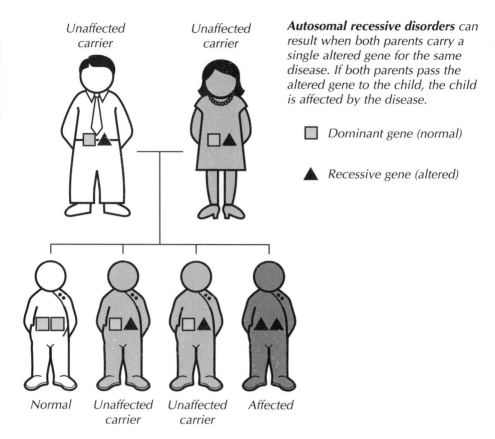

Unaffected carrier

Unaffected carrier

Autosomal recessive disorders *can result when both parents carry a single altered gene for the same disease. If both parents pass the altered gene to the child, the child is affected by the disease.*

☐ *Dominant gene (normal)*

▲ *Recessive gene (altered)*

Normal   Unaffected carrier   Unaffected carrier   Affected

chance that you're a carrier. There's also a 50 percent chance that you're not. If you're not a carrier, you can't pass the disease on to your children.

Sometimes, when testing for a familial disorder, several people in your family may be tested, including those with the condition. The tests can be complicated. It's best to discuss the testing with a knowledgeable health care provider, such as a genetic counselor.

Directed genetic carrier screening can be done in families where a member has received a diagnosis of a certain condition. This is an effective technique for detecting autosomal recessive disorders. Directed genetic carrier screening tests can also look for:

- **X-linked disorders.** This type of disorder results from an altered gene residing on the X chromosome. A woman who carries two X chromosomes may be a carrier of an X-linked disorder but not be affected by it because her normal X chromosome provides the needed function for that gene. She has a 50 percent chance of passing the altered chromosome on to her child. If the child who receives the altered gene is a boy, who has only one X chromosome, the effects of the altered gene will be seen, meaning the boy

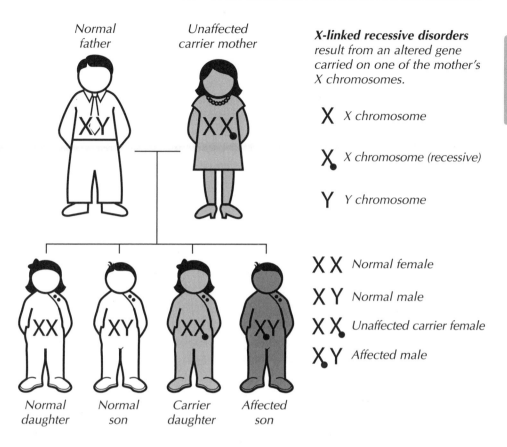

Normal father

Unaffected carrier mother

X-linked recessive disorders *result from an altered gene carried on one of the mother's X chromosomes.*

X *X chromosome*

X *X chromosome (recessive)*

Y *Y chromosome*

X X *Normal female*

X Y *Normal male*

X X *Unaffected carrier female*

X Y *Affected male*

Normal daughter

Normal son

Carrier daughter

Affected son

WHAT'S A GENETIC COUNSELOR?

A genetic counselor's role is to help you make decisions if you're concerned about the risks of an inherited disease. The genetic counselor can help you:

- Understand if your potential future child is at risk of birth defects or hereditary disorders
- Decide whether to be screened
- Interpret any related test results
- Understand how a specific disease may affect your child
- Make decisions about test results that are consistent with your values and beliefs

Certified genetic counselors (C.G.C.s) have completed special training in human genetics and counseling. Medical doctor (M.D.) geneticists are also specially trained in genetics and counseling. In addition, other doctors or nurses may have training on the subject.

To find a genetic counselor in your area, talk with your health care provider. You can also contact your local March of Dimes office, the National Society of Genetic Counselors *(www.nsgc.org)* or the American College of Medical Genetics *(www.acmg.net)*.

will have signs and symptoms of the disease. If the child who received the altered gene is a girl, she, like her mother, will be a carrier of the disorder.

X-linked disorders include Duchenne's muscular dystrophy, fragile X syndrome and hemophilia, among others.

- **Chromosome rearrangements.** In some families, babies are born with birth defects caused by the presence of too much or too little genetic material. This can happen if a parent carries a chromosome rearrangement. These rearrangements may also lead to the occurrence of more miscarriages than expected in a family. If you have a family member with a chromosome disorder or birth defects or if a number of miscarriages have occurred, talk to your health care provider about whether chromosome studies are indicated.

- **Mitochondrial disorders.** Some disorders are caused by errors in a separate set of genes in each cell. These separate genes are in each mitochondria, the energy-producing organs of the cell. Mitochondrial disorders can have many different signs and symptoms, such as low blood sugar, muscle problems, seizures and other conditions. If you have a family member who's been diagnosed with a mitochondrial disorder, discuss this with your health care provider or a geneticist to decide whether testing might be right for you.

When it's done

Genetic carrier screening performed before conception gives you the most options in terms of family planning. It may also be done during pregnancy to determine if the pregnancy is at increased risk.

How it's done

A simple blood sample contains enough white blood cells to either do a DNA study or analyze white blood cell proteins, depending on the test being done. Doing the study on both future parents will make it possible to see if the pregnancy is at increased risk.

Interpreting the results

Deciding how to use information from genetic carrier screening tests may be challenging. It's important to talk with someone experienced in genetics and disease before and after testing.

If test results indicate you're not a carrier, no special precautions with pregnancy are necessary, unless they're related to a separate condition. However, the test results shouldn't be taken as a guarantee that your child will be healthy. Although genetic carrier screening is accurate most of the time, it doesn't identify all carriers. Some diseases, such as cystic fibrosis, have many mutations. The test may focus only on the most common ones. Even if the test says you're not a carrier, it's possible that you do, in fact, carry a little-known or unknown mutation of the disease.

When discussing the genetic carrier screening test results, your genetic counselor or health care provider may review your probability of being a carrier. For example, whites have a four or five in 100 (4 percent to 5 percent) chance of carrying a cystic fibrosis gene alteration. If the cystic fibrosis carrier test is negative, that chance is reduced to one in 240 (0.4 percent) for those of Northern European descent.

The test may tell you that you're a carrier of a specific altered gene, but it may not reveal how severe the disease may be if it occurs in one of your

EXPLAINING THE CONDITIONS

Alpha-thalassemias result in a deficiency of red blood cells (anemia). The most severe form results in fetal or newborn death. Most cases are much less severe.

Beta-thalassemias also result in anemia. In its most severe form (thalassemia major), children require regular blood transfusions. With proper treatment, most people with this condition live into adulthood. Less severe forms cause varying degrees of complications related to the need for more red blood cells.

Canavan disease is a severe condition of the nervous system that's usually diagnosed soon after a child's birth. Death usually occurs in early childhood.

Cystic fibrosis affects the respiratory and digestive systems, causing severe chronic respiratory disease, diarrhea, malnutrition and exercise limitation. Recent treatments enable most affected people to live into adulthood.

Duchenne's muscular dystrophy (MD) affects the muscles of the pelvis, upper arms and upper legs. It occurs in young boys and is the most common form of MD that affects children. It can lead to muscle weakness and, in severe cases, death.

Fragile X syndrome is the most common genetically inherited cause of mental retardation, caused by alterations on the X chromosome.

Sickle cell disease prevents blood cells from moving smoothly through the body. Affected infants have an increased susceptibility to infection and slow growth rates. The disease can cause bouts of severe pain and damage to vital organs. With early and consistent medical treatment, complications can be minimized.

Tay-Sachs disease is a condition in which the enzyme needed to break down certain fats (lipids) is absent. These substances build up and gradually destroy brain and nerve cells until the central nervous system stops working. Death usually occurs in early childhood.

For in-depth information on these and other genetic diseases, see the National Center for Biotechnology Information web site at *www.ncbi.nih.gov/omim.*

children. If an increased risk of a specific disease is indicated, you may wish to talk with your health care provider, a geneticist or a genetic counselor about the implications of the disease.

If the test indicates that you're a carrier, your genetic counselor will help you assess the options available to you. These may include:

- Foregoing conception
- Adopting a child
- Using a donor egg or donor sperm
- Using pre-implantation genetic diagnosis (see page 295)
- Using diagnostic tests such as amniocentesis (see page 299) or chorionic villus sampling (see page 304) during pregnancy to determine if your baby has the disease

If you're pregnant, a genetic counselor can help you consider the next steps in your pregnancy. The genetic counselor's goal is to help you make decisions consistent with your own values, so don't be afraid to ask questions or to request that information be repeated.

If you and your partner plan a pregnancy in the future and have reasons to be concerned about genetic disorders, you may want to talk with a genetic counselor now to see if any new tests or treatment options are available now or will be soon. Remember that genetic screening information pertains to a unique couple. If, in the future, you plan a pregnancy with a different partner, he or she may wish to be screened as well.

Possible concerns

You may wish to consider other issues. For example, if you test positive as a carrier for a particular condition, it's possible that others in your family also may carry it. This may be difficult news to share with family members. In addition, genetic carrier screening may reveal previously unknown information about a child's biological parents, such as whether the man is not a child's biological father (nonpaternity).

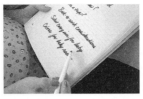

choosing your health care provider for pregnancy

Pregnancy is a journey. Whether it's a new venture for you or you're an old hand at it, finding the right health care provider and thinking through the type of childbirth you want can make a big difference in your experience.

Plenty of options are available for obstetrical care, birth locations and birth plans. The nature of your pregnancy and your own personal preferences serve as your guides to choosing your care. This decision guide is designed to help you get to know the different types of care and health care providers that may be available to you.

Throughout your pregnancy and childbirth, remember that you chose your health care provider for a reason. You trust his or her abilities to safely guide you and your baby through the birthing process. Allow your provider to give you the best possible care.

Where to start

Finding the right health care provider for your pregnancy and childbirth can be a daunting process. Use this information to help you make this important decision.

Look for help in identifying potential obstetrical health care providers:
- Ask family and friends for recommendations.
- Consult with your regular doctor and other medical professionals.
- Contact your county medical society for a list of the providers in your area.
- Check your local Yellow Pages for a list of providers by area of specialty.
- Contact the hospital you prefer and find out who its maternity care providers are.
- Contact the labor and delivery unit at the hospital you prefer and ask the nurses for a recommendation.

- Use the Internet. If you don't have access to the Internet, try your local library. Most libraries offer Internet access to the public. The following Web sites offer search tools that give you a list of providers in your area:
    - American Medical Association, "Doctor Finder"
      www.ama-assn.org
    - American College of Obstetricians and Gynecologists, "Find a Physician"
      www.acog.org
    - American College of Nurse-Midwives, "Find a Midwife"
      www.midwife.org
    - Society for Maternal-Fetal Medicine, "Physician Locator"
      http://smfm.org
    - National Association of Childbearing Centers, "Find a Birth Center"
      www.birthcenters.org

You can also use the Internet to check a doctor's certification. Visit the Web site of the American Board of Medical Specialties at *www.abms.org* and click on "Who's Certified." Currently, you need to be registered to use this service — registration is free. Or you can call toll-free (866) ASK-ABMS, or (866) 275-2267.

As you study your options, consider these questions:
- Is the health care provider's office a convenient distance from your home or work?
- Is the health care provider going to be able to deliver your baby in the place you want to give birth — at a particular hospital or birthing center?
- Does the health care provider work in a solo or group practice? If it's a group practice, how often will you see your health care provider? How often will you see others from the practice?
- Who will replace your health care provider if he or she isn't available in an emergency or when your labor begins?
- Is the health care provider available to answer questions in between your scheduled appointments?
- How much do the health care provider's services cost? Is the cost covered by your insurance company?
- What level of expertise do you feel your pregnancy demands? Will your health care provider meet that need?
- How much do you value the opportunity for your health care provider to serve the entire family?

As you meet a potential health care provider, think about these issues:
- Does the health care provider listen to your concerns and provide helpful answers to your questions?
- Does the health care provider seem open to and comfortable with your philosophy regarding pregnancy and childbirth?
- Will the health care provider keep you informed and allow you to participate as you wish in medical decisions affecting you and your baby?

Types of health care providers

Obstetrical care is offered by family physicians, obstetricians-gynecologists, maternal-fetal medicine specialists and midwives.

Family physicians

Family physicians provide care for the whole family through all stages of life, including pregnancy and birth.

Training for family physicians:
- Medical school followed by at least three years in training at a hospital or another patient setting (residency).
- Study and work in various fields of medicine, including obstetrics, pediatrics, internal medicine, gynecology and surgery.
- Certification by the American Board of Family Practice, for which they must pass an extensive exam.
- Training and experience that allows them to manage most pregnancies, including minor surgical procedures for vaginal delivery. Some perform Caesarean deliveries, but most do not.

Practice. Family physicians may work solo, or they may be part of a larger group practice that includes other family physicians, nurses and other medical professionals. They're usually associated with a hospital where they can perform deliveries.

Advantages. If you've been going to your family doctor for a while, he or she will probably know you well. Your doctor will probably be familiar with your family and medical history. Thus, a family doctor is likely to treat you as a whole person. Your pregnancy is seen as part of the larger picture of your life. Also, a family doctor can continue to treat you and your baby after birth.

Issues to consider. Family physicians can cover most of the range of obstetrical care. But if you've had problems with pregnancy before, your family physician may refer you to a specialist in obstetrics or use a specialist as a consultant or backup. The same may be true if you have diabetes, high blood pressure, heart disease or another medical problem that may complicate your pregnancy. If you have a family history of a genetic problem, your doctor may refer you to a geneticist or genetics counselor.

It's possible that your family physician may not be available at the time of your delivery. If so, you may be giving birth with a doctor you don't know. One way to get around this is to meet your doctor's backup before your due date.

You might choose a family physician if:
- You and your doctor don't foresee any problems with your pregnancy.
- You want your doctor to be involved with all members of your family.
- You want continuity in care from prenatal appointments throughout childhood and beyond.

WHO'S MAKING DELIVERIES?

According to the Centers for Disease Control and Prevention, here's who delivered America's babies in 2001:
- Physicians (including family physicians and ob-gyns) delivered 91 percent of all births, which is down from 99 percent in 1975.
- Midwives attended 8 percent of births, which is up from 1 percent in 1975.
- Almost 95 percent of midwife-attended births were by certified nurse-midwives.

And here's where the deliveries occurred:
- 99 percent of births were in hospitals.
- Of the 1 percent out-of-hospital births, 65 percent were in a residence, and 28 percent were in a free-standing birthing center.

(Source: Centers for Disease Control and Prevention, "Births: Final Data for 2001.")

Obstetricians-gynecologists

Doctors of obstetrics and gynecology are commonly referred to as ob-gyns. They specialize in the care of women during pregnancy and in general, including care of a woman's reproductive organs, breasts and sexual function. Because of their emphasis on women's health, ob-gyns serve as the main health care provider for many women.

Training for obstetricians-gynecologists
- Medical school followed by a four-year residency.
- Focus on obstetrics, gynecology, infertility and surgery.
- Preparation to handle all phases of pregnancy, including before conception, during pregnancy, labor and childbirth, and postpartum.

- Training in preventive medicine, which includes regular checkups and exams to detect problems before you become sick.
- Training in diagnosing and treating menstrual and hormonal disorders, gynecologic infections, vulvar and pelvic pain problems, as well as in performing pelvic surgery.
- In many cases, certification by the American Board of Obstetrics and Gynecology. To be certified, a doctor must pass written and oral tests.
- In some cases, a role as a teacher and researcher at a medical school or teaching hospital.

Practice. Ob-gyns often work in a group practice consisting of various medical professionals, including recent graduates from medical school (residents), nurses, certified nurse-midwives, physician assistants, dietitians and social workers. Ob-gyns may work in a clinic or hospital setting.

Advantages. If you already see an ob-gyn you like for your general health care, he or she may be a natural choice for continuing to provide care during your pregnancy and childbirth. Many women choose an ob-gyn for obstetrical care because if a problem or complication arises during pregnancy, they won't have to switch health care providers. An ob-gyn can, if necessary, perform an episiotomy, forceps delivery or Caesarean delivery.

Issues to consider. An ob-gyn can meet all the needs of most pregnant women, except perhaps for those with extremely high risk pregnancies. In such a case, your ob-gyn may refer you to a maternal-fetal medicine specialist, while ideally remaining involved in your overall care.

As with a family physician, your ob-gyn may not be available when you're ready to give birth. For this reason, you may wish to meet the other health care providers who may deliver your baby if your doctor isn't available.

You might choose an ob-gyn if:
- You have a high-risk pregnancy. You may be high risk if you are over the age of 35 or you develop diabetes during pregnancy (gestational diabetes) or high blood pressure during pregnancy (preeclampsia).
- You're carrying twins, triplets or more.
- You have a pre-existing medical condition, such as diabetes, high blood pressure or an autoimmune disorder.
- You want the reassurance that if a problem does arise, such as the need for an operative vaginal or Caesarean delivery, you won't need to be transferred to a different care provider.

Maternal-fetal medicine specialists
Maternal-fetal medicine specialists are trained in the care of very high-risk pregnancies. They concentrate exclusively on pregnancy and the unborn child, dealing with the most severe complications that arise.

Training for maternal-fetal medicine specialists
- Medical school followed by four years of residency.
- Three-year fellowship focusing on obstetrical, medical and surgical complications of pregnancy.
- Preparation to provide care for women with high-risk pregnancies.
- Training to provide consultation for family physicians, ob-gyns, certified nurse-midwives and other specialists.
- In some cases, a role as a teacher and researcher at a medical school or teaching hospital.

Practice. Similar to other doctors, maternal-fetal medicine specialists often work as part of a group practice. They may be part of a group of obstetrical consultants. They're often associated with a hospital, university or clinic.

Advantages. This highly specialized doctor will be familiar with the complications of pregnancy and adept at recognizing abnormalities. When women with major medical problems become pregnant, their physicians often consult with maternal-fetal medicine specialists in order to optimize care for both the mother and her fetus.

Issues to consider. Maternal-fetal medicine specialists concentrate solely on the problems that occur with pregnancy. Most women don't need their services because most pregnancies are fairly routine. In addition, these specialists tend to be less directly involved with their patients than are family physicians, ob-gyns and midwives. However, this isn't true for all maternal-fetal medicine specialists. Don't let it stop you from seeking one out if you need the type of care he or she can provide.

A maternal-fetal medicine specialist rarely serves as the primary health care provider for a pregnant woman. This specialist is brought in at the request of another health care provider, such as an ob-gyn or a certified nurse-midwife.

You might choose a maternal-fetal medicine specialist if:
- You have a severe medical condition complicating your pregnancy, such as an infectious disease, heart disease, kidney disease or cancer.
- You've previously had severe pregnancy complications or had recurrent pregnancy losses.
- You plan on having prenatal diagnostic or therapeutic procedures, such as comprehensive ultrasound, chorionic villus sampling, amniocentesis, or fetal surgery or treatment.
- You're a known carrier of a severe genetic condition that may be passed on to your baby.
- Your baby has been diagnosed before birth with a medical condition, such as spina bifida.

Midwives

Midwives provide preconception, maternity and postpartum care for women at low risk of complications during pregnancy. Throughout much of the world, midwives are the traditional care providers for women during pregnancy. In the United States, the use of midwives is steadily increasing.

In general, midwives follow a philosophy that builds on the view that women have been having babies for millennia, and that they don't always need all of the technologic intervention that's available.

Training for midwives

Midwives don't have a medical degree. But most receive formal training in midwifery and in well-woman care. Midwives are often classified according to the training they've received:

- **Certified nurse-midwives** are registered nurses who have completed advanced training in obstetrics and gynecology and have graduated from an accredited nurse-midwifery program. They are certified by the American College of Nurse-Midwives (ACNM), for which they must pass several exams. Certified nurse-midwives are licensed in all 50 states and the District of Columbia. Some can prescribe medications. Most can recommend diet, exercise and lifestyle changes.
- **Direct-entry midwives** don't have a nursing degree but may be trained in other areas of health care. They may have training through self-study, apprenticeship, a midwifery school or a college- or university-based program separate from nursing. They may be licensed, certified or neither. Different states have different licensing requirements. Some states have very strict standards. Others don't regulate midwives at all.
- **Certified midwives** are direct-entry midwives who have been certified by the American College of Nurse-Midwives and have met the same standards required by the college as certified nurse-midwives. This is a fairly new certification and is currently licensed only in the state of New York. However, other states and midwifery organizations may use the same designation for individuals whom they have licensed. Although this may sound confusing, most certified midwives are happy to explain to you where they got their certification.
- **Certified professional midwives** are direct-entry midwives who have been certified by the North American Registry of Midwives, an international certification agency created by the Midwives Alliance of North America.
- **Lay midwives** are uncertified or unlicensed midwives who generally have had more-informal training.

Most midwives in the United States today are certified nurse-midwives or certified midwives.

Practice. Midwives may work in a hospital setting, in a birthing center or in your home. They may practice solo but often are part of a group practice, such as a team of obstetric care providers. Most midwives are associated with an ob-gyn in case problems occur. The majority of certified nurse-midwives attend births in a hospital or birthing center, although some may attend a birth in a home. Direct-entry midwives are more likely to deliver at home.

Advantages. Midwifery care may offer a more natural, less regimented approach to pregnancy and childbirth than does standard care. If you give birth attended by a midwife in a hospital, you'll still have access to pain relief medications.

In many cases, a midwife is able to provide greater individual attention during pregnancy and is more likely to be present during labor and delivery than is a doctor. Various studies have found no significant differences in outcome between having a midwife attendant who's integrated with an existing health care system and having a doctor attendant for women with low-risk pregnancies.

Issues to consider. When considering a midwife for your primary obstetrical care, check to see that she or he has a backup arrangement with a hospital so that you can have access to obstetrical skills and equipment in case of pregnancy or birthing problems.

If you're not giving birth in a hospital, create an emergency plan with your midwife. Include details such as the name and number of your midwife's back-up doctor, the hospital you'll be taken to, how you'll get there, the name and number of the persons who need to be alerted and contingency plans for your other children, if you have any. This can reduce stress later if you need to be transferred during labor. Birthing centers often do this as a matter of policy.

If you're thinking of working with a midwife but aren't sure about his or her credentials, ask him or her about training and certification and licensure in your state. The American College of Nurse-Midwives suggests asking the following questions:

- Do you have a college degree?
- Did you graduate from a nationally accredited midwifery program?
- Did your midwifery education require preparation in core sciences such as biology, chemistry, anatomy and physiology, and others?
- Have you passed a national certification examination?
- Are you licensed to practice?
- How will you determine if I am an appropriate candidate for midwifery care? What will happen if I need the care of a doctor?
- Are you prepared to provide well-woman and gynecological care, including screening for common health problems and writing prescriptions?
- Are you certified by the American College of Nurse-Midwives Certification Council?

You might choose a midwife if:
- You're free of health problems and you expect to have a low-risk pregnancy.
- You want someone who can spend a significant amount of time discussing your pregnancy with you.
- You prefer a more personalized approach to the birthing process.
- You desire a less regimented birthing process.
- You desire fewer interventions.

Choosing a birthing location

You have a choice about where to have your baby. This decision is often closely tied to your choice of a health care provider and where he or she has practicing privileges. Most women in the United States — around 99 percent — have their babies in a hospital. Others choose to give birth at a birthing center or in their own home.

Hospital

Today, hospitals treat childbirth less like a medical procedure and more as a natural process. Many hospitals offer a relaxed setting in which to have your baby, with options such as:
- **Birthing rooms.** These are suites with a homelike decor, and sometimes a bath, where you can labor and deliver. The father or other labor partner can be an active part of the birthing team. In some cases, you may be able to recover in the same room after having your baby.
- **Rooming-in.** In this arrangement, the baby stays with you almost all of the time instead of being taken to the nursery. An experienced nurse is available to help you get used to feeding and caring for the baby. Other family members are encouraged to take part in the baby's care.
- **Nursery.** If you choose to have your baby taken to the nursery, you can still see him or her whenever you want. Having the hospital staff care for your baby for a few hours each day can give you some much-needed rest before you go home.
- **Family-centered maternity care.** This option combines the advantages of rooming-in and the nursery. A single nurse is assigned to both you and the baby. During the day, the nurse cares for you and the baby at the same time and can teach you how to care for a newborn. At night, the nurse can take your baby to the nursery if you wish.

If you have a vaginal delivery in a hospital, you'll probably stay for 48 hours. That's the time health insurers are required to cover in most states. If you have a Caesarean birth, you may stay up to four or five days. Health insurers are required to cover 96 hours for a post-Caesarean stay.

Possible advantages of delivering in a hospital:
- It provides the people, equipment and blood supplies needed in case of an emergency.
- Pain management options are available if you want them.
- Fetal monitoring is offered to help ensure your baby's safety.

Possible down sides of delivering in a hospital:
- You may have more medical interventions than you want — such as fetal monitoring or episiotomy — and more than you would in a birthing center or at home. However, most of these interventions are for your benefit.
- You may at times be separated from your baby.
- It may be more expensive.

Before your due date, you may wish to find out about the kind of maternity services your hospital offers and the flexibility of its policies.

Birthing center

Birthing centers can be free-standing facilities or part of a hospital. The goal of a birthing center is to separate routine pregnancy, labor and delivery care from the more intensive care required for high-risk pregnancies and births. In this way, birthing centers can reduce their costs because of the diminished need for personnel and equipment. They also strive to provide a natural birthing experience and avoid overuse of medical intervention.

Most birthing centers are run by certified nurse-midwives or teams of obstetrical health care providers. Staff often includes an ob-gyn doctor available for consultation and referral of at-risk pregnancies. Birthing centers try to be as much like home as possible.

Possible advantages of delivering in a birthing center:
- You labor and deliver in the same room. Your whole family is invited to be with you, including your children.
- You may be offered amenities such as a whirlpool tub, plenty of room to walk about, and the opportunity to eat and drink as you wish.
- You are encouraged to have input in your delivery.
- You usually go home sooner than if you were in a hospital, although postpartum care is available through office or home visits.

Possible disadvantages of delivering in a birthing center:
- Though many birthing centers have the equipment necessary to initiate an emergency response, if complications arise, you'll likely be transferred to a hospital, and that takes time. If you're considering a birthing center, find out its emergency management policies. Look into whether your midwife or doctor will be able to accompany you to a different facility.

- Your insurance may not cover delivery at a birthing center. Call and check.
- Your opportunity to use a birthing center may be limited. Most states have only a few accredited birthing centers, and some states have none. Still, close to 10,000 women in the United States had their babies at birthing centers in 2001.

Home

Just over 23,000 women had their babies at home in 2001. This trend has been fairly stable among American women, but still remains somewhat controversial. Midwives are almost always the health care providers for home deliveries. You usually rely on your own methods for coping with pain.

Possible advantages of delivering at home:
- You're in a comfortable, familiar environment.
- Anyone you wish can be involved with the delivery.
- Financial costs are kept to a minimum.

Possible disadvantages of delivering at home include:
- If you need medical intervention, you'll have to be moved to a hospital. A review of a number of studies comparing home-like settings for labor and delivery with hospital settings showed that substantial numbers of women — ranging from 19 percent to 67 percent — who started out in home-like settings transferred to standard care before or during labor because they were no longer appropriate for a home-like delivery.
- If you haven't received proper prenatal care, emergency care may be more difficult.

One of the interesting findings of these studies is that the atmosphere and decor of the birthing locations were less important than the quality of support provided by the health care provider throughout the birthing process. Whereas too much focus on risk and technology on the part of the health care provider might lead to unnecessary medical intervention, excessive focus on normality might lead to a delay in recognizing complications and taking action. Although many births would be very safe at home, no one knows that until the birth is over. Selecting home delivery and then having a common complication may result in loss of life.

Creating a birth plan

A birth plan encourages you to think about your labor and delivery before it happens. You can record your preferences regarding labor, delivery and postpartum care. You can use the list to talk about your preferences with your doctor, midwife or other support persons. This type of plan isn't set in stone because no one can predict how the birth will go. But it does help ensure the experience will come as close to your expectations as reasonably possible.

Your health care provider may ask you to fill out a form stating your preferences. Or you may create a birth plan on your own or as part of a childbearing class. Be sure to communicate your wishes to your health care provider so that you both understand how you feel.

Remember to be flexible. You may think you don't want any pain relief medication. But you may change your mind during labor. If you're flexible, you won't be setting yourself up for worry if things don't go as you planned.

YOUR BIRTH PLAN

Your birth plan may include details such as:

❑ When to come to the hospital or birthing center.
❑ What to bring with you — your favorite nightgown, personal items, music CDs, breast cream, contact phone numbers.
❑ Concerns you may have regarding giving birth.
❑ Things you look forward to during birth.
❑ Your support person(s) during labor and delivery.
❑ Preferences for nonmedicated pain relief — shower, birthing ball, music, dim lights, walking, rocking chair.
❑ Preferences for medicated pain relief — epidural or other.
❑ Your goals in terms of medication use — no medications, some medications, wait and see.
❑ Hydration methods — do you wish to sip water during labor, have unrestricted access or have no oral intake?
❑ Positions for pushing and delivery — sitting up in bed, lying on your back and using stirrups, lying on your side, squatting.
❑ Episiotomy preferences — although your doctor may do what he or she considers best under the circumstances.
❑ Preferences regarding the delivery — Do you want to observe with a mirror? Do you want to have your family observe?
❑ Preferences for what happens right after birth — Do you want the baby handed directly to you or wrapped in a blanket and then handed to you?
❑ Circumcision preference.
❑ How you plan to feed your baby.
❑ Rooming-in or nursery preferences.
❑ Mom and baby follow-up care.
❑ Preferences regarding being present at the baby's first bath and exams.
❑ Caesarean birth preferences.

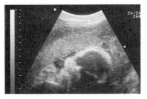

DECISION GUIDE

understanding prenatal testing

Pregnancy is often a time of great anticipation. You may be wondering about a number of things concerning your baby. Will you have a girl or a boy? Will he have blue eyes or brown eyes? Will she be funny like her dad and smart like her mom? How will it feel to finally hold your baby in your arms?

Along with feelings of excitement and joy, you may have moments of doubt and anxiety. What if something goes wrong with the pregnancy? Will your baby be healthy? These are completely normal feelings experienced by most pregnant women. It may reassure you to know that most pregnancies — more than 95 percent — are healthy and result in the safe delivery of a healthy baby.

Still, in some instances you may wish to know specific information about your baby's health before his or her birth. Maybe your weight gain or the size of your uterus suggests that you're carrying more than one baby. Perhaps because of your age or family history you're at increased risk of carrying a baby with a chromosomal problem or some other genetic disorder. Whatever the reason, certain tests can help determine the health of your baby while still in your womb. These are called prenatal tests.

Basically, two types of prenatal tests are available:

- **Screening tests.** These are safe, relatively inexpensive tests that are offered to large groups of people. These tests try to identify those who are more likely to be at risk of certain conditions. Their purpose is to indicate who might benefit from more narrowly focused diagnostic tests. Screening tests aren't required, but your health care provider will probably ask whether you want to be tested.
- **Diagnostic tests.** These tests are usually done when a screening test has indicated a possible problem or when you or your baby is at high risk of a certain condition. They can provide your health care provider with enough information to diagnose a medical condition while the baby is still in the uterus. These tests generally are more invasive, more expensive and slightly riskier than screening tests. Again, the choice of whether to have these tests is largely yours, although your health care provider may offer one or more.

Issues to consider

Before undergoing prenatal testing, think about what it can do for you. Many women choose to undergo basic ultrasounds and blood tests. But not all do. Most women don't undergo the more detailed diagnostic tests because most pregnancies don't carry a high risk of complications.

Before scheduling a prenatal test, you and your partner may wish to consider these questions:

- *What will you do with the information once you have it? How will it affect decisions regarding your pregnancy?*
  Most results from prenatal testing come back normal, which can help ease your anxiety. If a test indicates that your baby may have a birth defect or another health condition, how will you handle it? You may be faced with decisions you never expected to have to make, such as whether to continue the pregnancy. On the other hand, knowing about a problem ahead of time may give you the option of planning for your baby's care in advance.

- *Will the information help your health care provider to provide better care or treatment during pregnancy or delivery?*
  At times, prenatal testing can provide information that affects your care. Testing may uncover a problem with the baby that health care providers can treat while you're pregnant. It may alert health care providers to a problem that requires a specialist to be on hand to treat your baby right after he or she is born.

- *How accurate are the results of the test?*
  Prenatal tests aren't perfect. Even if the result of a screening test is negative — meaning that your fetus is at low risk of having a certain condition — there's still a small chance that the condition is present. If this is the case, the initial results are a false-negative. Even if a screening test has a positive result, placing you in a higher-risk group, it's possible, or even likely, that no disease exists. This result is called a false-positive. The proportion of false-negative and false-positive results varies from test to test, as noted in the following information on each individual test.

- *Will undergoing a test be worth the anxiety it may cause?*
  Screening tests identify women at risk of certain conditions. Even if a test indicates a risk, the majority of women won't have an affected baby. Thus, a screening test may cause anxiety unnecessarily.

- *What are the risks of the procedure?*
  You may want to weigh the risks of the test — such as pain, worry or possible miscarriage — against the value of learning the information.

- *How much does the test cost? Is it covered by your insurance company?*
  Tests that aren't medically necessary usually aren't covered by insurance. In some cases, a social worker or genetic counselor may help you get information about financial assistance, if necessary. If financial help isn't available, are you willing and able to cover the cost of the test?

Prenatal tests

The following guide to prenatal tests will help you become better informed about common prenatal tests. In addition, talk to your doctor, midwife or a genetic counselor about the benefits and risks that each test may have for you.

Triple test

What it is
The triple test consists of three screening tests that can assess your risk of having a baby with certain defects. It looks at levels of three substances normally present in the bloodstream of a pregnant woman. The tests measure:
- Maternal serum alpha-fetoprotein (MSAFP), which evaluates the levels of alpha-fetoprotein (AFP) in your blood. AFP is a protein produced by your baby's liver. Small amounts of the protein cross through the placenta and amniotic fluid and show up in your blood.
- Human chorionic gonadotropin (HCG), a hormone produced by the placenta.
- Estriol, an estrogen produced by both the baby and the placenta.

The triple test, also known as the multiple marker screen, is used to screen for:
- Chromosomal disorders, such as Down syndrome (trisomy 21)
- Spinal abnormalities (neural tube defects), such as spina bifida

When it's administered
These tests may be offered to you between the 15th and 22nd weeks of your pregnancy. Levels of these chemicals change substantially as your baby continues to develop, so it's critical that the calculated age of your baby is correct. The MSAFP test is most accurate when done between the 16th and 18th weeks of gestation.

How it's done
The substances to be evaluated can be measured from a sample of your blood. To obtain a sample, a nurse or technician will probably draw blood from a vein inside your elbow or the back of your hand.

What the results may tell you
Low levels of MSAFP and estriol along with high levels of HCG may indicate the possibility of Down syndrome. Use of all three tests combined can detect 60 percent to 70 percent of babies with Down syndrome.

Some laboratories use another protein produced by both mother and baby (inhibin A) in addition to the triple test or instead of estriol. In one study, use of the inhibin A test increased the detection rate of Down syndrome to 85 percent. The overall risk of having a baby with Down syndrome is one in 1,000, but this risk increases with the age of the mother.

Low levels of all three substances may indicate trisomy 18, a chromosomal abnormality characterized by three number 18 chromosomes. Trisomy 18 typically causes severe deformity and mental retardation. Most babies with trisomy 18 die within their first year. The risk of having a baby with trisomy 18 is very low — only one in 6,000 live births.

By itself, the MSAFP test screens for spinal abnormalities such as spina bifida. High levels of MSAFP in your blood may indicate the presence of a neural tube defect, most commonly spina bifida or anencephaly. Spina bifida occurs early during fetal development when tissue fails to close over the spinal cord, leaving an opening in the baby's body. Anencephaly occurs when tissue fails to cover over the baby's brain and head. The rate at which these defects occur is low. Out of 1,000 women who undergo MSAFP screening, between 25 and 50 women have results that are higher than normal. Only about two of the 1,000 have babies with a neural tube defect, roughly half with spina bifida and half with anencephaly.

About 93 percent of women who undergo MSAFP screening have normal results. Of the pregnancies showing abnormal MSAFP levels, only about 2 percent to 3 percent result in birth defects.

Abnormal MSAFP levels may occur for several other reasons, including:
- **Miscalculation of how long you've been pregnant.** If the gestational age of your baby has been calculated incorrectly, the interpretation of MSAFP levels may be affected. MSAFP levels normally increase during the first 20 weeks of pregnancy. If you're later in your pregnancy than you thought, your blood will contain higher levels of MSAFP than expected. If earlier, MSAFP levels may be lower than expected.
- **A multiple birth.** Two or more babies will produce more MSAFP than one.
- **Problems with the placenta.** A defect in the placental wall that allows the baby's blood to enter your circulation will allow additional MSAFP

into your bloodstream. This may happen occasionally in pregnant women who have high blood pressure or who have another illness that affects the placenta.

- **Failure to account for other factors.** Your age, weight, race and whether you have type 1 diabetes (formerly called juvenile or insulin-dependent diabetes) each may affect MSAFP levels.
- **Other defects.** Any area that hasn't closed completely, such as with an abdominal wall defect, will increase the levels of MSAFP in the amniotic fluid and, eventually, your blood. Other reasons for elevated MSAFP include certain skin conditions, kidney problems and loss of the fetus.

Possible concerns

The biggest concern for most mothers is the anxiety caused by waiting for the results of the test, which take a few days. Most of the time, results come back negative, meaning no increased risk of abnormalities has been found. That doesn't mean your risk of having a baby with a problem is zero, but rather that your risk is about the same as that found in the general population (3 percent).

About 7 percent of the time, results will be positive, and additional, more-invasive and riskier tests will be offered. Still, most women within this positive group have normal babies.

Reasons to have it done

If you're concerned about your baby's health, negative results may provide you with reassurance. If you receive positive results, you can talk to your health care provider or a genetic counselor about your options. Knowing about possible problems before birth can give you time to make any necessary arrangements. You may plan to give birth at a hospital with the resources to care for your newborn. Some women faced with a severe abnormality in the fetus may choose to end the pregnancy.

What happens next

If you have negative results, no further testing is needed. If your results come back positive, you'll likely be offered additional testing. Occasionally, it makes sense to repeat the test. In most cases, further evaluation will take place in any event.

Most likely, your health care provider will recommend an ultrasound exam. This helps to establish the correct duration of the pregnancy and stage of development of your baby. It may also determine whether you're carrying twins or other multiples. Your health care provider can also examine the fetus for visible defects or other structural problems, which can often be seen during an ultrasound.

If your triple test indicates a high risk of chromosomal abnormality, amniocentesis may be used to obtain fetal cells to check for Down syndrome or another abnormality.

If a baby has spina bifida, 95 percent to 97 percent of the time the defect will be visible on ultrasound at 18 weeks. If your MSAFP levels are high and the ultrasound is normal, amniocentesis may be offered to check the amniotic fluid levels of MSAFP. If the amniocentesis indicates that MSAFP levels are high, the chances that your baby has a neural tube defect are very high. Measuring a chemical in the fluid called acetylcholinesterase can confirm the presence of a neural tube defect. Your health care provider may recommend another ultrasound. It may help determine the location and extent of the defect so that you can have more accurate counseling about the problems your baby may have.

Accuracy and limitations of the test
The triple test can detect Down syndrome 60 percent to 70 percent of the time, with a false-positive test result rate of about 5 percent. The MSAFP test can detect spina bifida about 80 percent of the time and anencephaly about 90 percent of the time.

WHAT'S NEW IN PRENATAL TESTING?

Efforts to improve prenatal testing have opened the door to earlier diagnosis, which many women seek. Data suggests two tests — first-trimester proteins and nuchal translucency — may be helpful in providing early pregnancy screening. A third test, pre-implantation genetic diagnosis, offers testing for parents using in vitro fertilization (IVF). Availability of these tests may be limited, but it's likely to increase.

Like all screening tests, these two tests require confirmation with a diagnostic test such as chorionic villus sampling (CVS) or early amniocentesis.

First-trimester proteins

Two proteins appear in the first trimester: free beta-human chorionic gonadotropin (beta-HCG) and pregnancy-associated plasma protein-A (PAPP-A, or PA). The proteins can be detected through a blood test. Abnormal levels of them have been associated with an increased risk of Down syndrome. These proteins aren't related to one another, so measurement of each reveals independent information. The result of one can confirm or cast doubt on the other.

These values, along with your age at delivery, yield an estimated risk of Down syndrome similar to that of the triple test. And they do so earlier because the triple test is given in the second trimester.

This test has a few limitations. The best time to measure free beta-HCG is after 12 weeks of gestation. PAPP-A begins to lose its testing accuracy after about 13 weeks. This leaves a small window of time to perform the tests. In addition, the length of the pregnancy must be known as accurately as possible to avoid error.

It's important to remember that these tests are screening tests. They can't uncover any actual problems or defects, only the risk of them. They aren't reliable screening tests for many other diseases. If results are normal, there still remains a chance that your baby will have a health problem. Even if the screening test results aren't normal, most babies will be healthy. This potential for false-negative and false-positive results may be a consideration in your decision about whether to be screened.

Ultrasound

What it is

The ultrasound exam may be the prenatal test you've heard the most about. Your health care provider can use ultrasound imaging to get a picture of your unborn baby and determine how your pregnancy is progressing. Usually, you're able to watch the screen and see images of your baby while the test is being done. Ultrasound can also be used to diagnose some types of birth defects, such as a spinal abnormality (neural tube defect) or, in some cases, a heart defect.

Nuchal translucency

Using ultrasound, this first-trimester test measures the size of a specific region under the skin behind your baby's neck. An increase in the size may be an indication of Down syndrome, a birth defect of the heart (congenital heart disease) or other abnormalities. Health care providers aren't exactly sure why this is. They suspect that it may be because of a buildup of lymph fluid due to underdevelopment of the lymphatic ducts. A rigorous approach to standardizing this measurement is needed for the test to be as accurate as was reported in early studies.

Pre-implantation genetic diagnosis

A third option in prenatal testing is called pre-implantation genetic diagnosis. If you choose to have your eggs fertilized outside of your body — a procedure called in vitro fertilization (IVF) — doctors can perform genetic tests on the embryo before implanting it in your uterus. The procedure is complex. First, fertilization of the harvested eggs occurs in the laboratory, creating several embryos. A single cell is removed from each embryo, and genetic analysis is done. Only the embryos without evidence of genetic disease are selected for implantation.

To use this test, the couple must be at an increased risk of having a child with a testable condition. Both parents must be tested for genetic problems so the health care provider knows what problems to look for (see "Genetic carrier screening" on page 269). The test is designed to look for genetic defects that are more likely to occur, such as genetic mutations or balanced chromosome rearrangements. It may become useful in finding conditions such as sickle cell disease or cystic fibrosis.

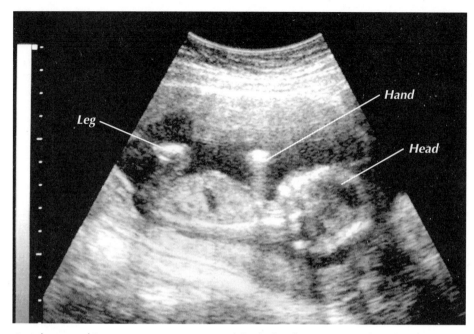

An ultrasound image creates a picture of the baby that can provide information about your pregnancy.

The ultrasound exam works by directing sound waves of very high pitch at the tissues in your abdominal area. These sound waves, which you can't hear, bounce off the curves and variations in your body, including the baby in your uterus. The sound waves are visually translated into a pattern of light and dark areas. The waves create an image of the baby on a monitor. This is similar to shouting into the Grand Canyon and being able to hear the echoes come back to you as they bounce off the peaks and valleys of the canyon.

Several different types of ultrasound examinations are available:

- **Standard ultrasound.** This ultrasound creates two-dimensional (2-D) images that can give your health care provider information about your pregnancy. It may show the gestational age of your baby, how he or she is developing, and the relationship between your body and the baby. It usually lasts about 20 minutes.

- **Advanced ultrasound.** This is also called a targeted ultrasound. It's often used to explore a suspected abnormality found during a standard ultrasound or a triple test. The exam is more thorough and may use more sophisticated equipment. It's also longer, taking from 30 minutes to several hours. Your health care provider may recommend an advanced ultrasound if you're considered to have a high-risk pregnancy. Advanced ultrasound is a noninvasive approach that may add further information where the only alternative is genetic amniocentesis. This type of ultrasound can be used to view your baby's head and spine in detail, and it's 95 percent effective at diagnosing neural tube defects.

- **Transvaginal ultrasound.** In early pregnancy, your uterus and fallopian tubes are closer to your vagina than to your abdominal surface. If you have an ultrasound during your first trimester, your health care provider may opt for a transvaginal one. It'll provide a clearer picture of your baby and the structures around it. A transvaginal ultrasound uses a slender, wand-like device that's placed inside your vagina. It sends out sound waves and gathers the reflected information.
- **Three-dimensional (3-D) ultrasound.** This newer type of ultrasound offers 3-D images with details similar to those of a photograph. It's used in selected medical centers to enhance the understanding of images from an advanced ultrasound.
- **Doppler ultrasound.** Doppler imaging measures minute changes in the frequency of the ultrasound waves as they bounce off moving objects, such as blood cells. It can measure the speed and direction at which blood circulates. With it, health care providers can determine how much resistance there is to the flow of blood through various tissues.

   If you have high blood pressure, a Doppler ultrasound may help determine whether blood flow is being limited for the baby or the placenta. This may help inform your health care provider about the effect of high blood pressure or other stresses on the baby.
- **Fetal echocardiography.** This type of exam uses ultrasound waves to provide a more detailed picture of your baby's heart. It focuses on the heart's anatomy and function. It may be used to confirm or rule out a congenital heart defect.

When it's administered

An ultrasound exam can be done at any time during your pregnancy. Most health care providers obtain an ultrasound between the 18th and 20th weeks. By this time, the fetus is big enough to be evaluated yet not so big that gestational age assessment is inaccurate. And your baby has developed enough so that structural problems can be detected and all four chambers of the heart can be seen.

   In some situations, such as a high-risk pregnancy, ultrasounds may be repeated throughout the pregnancy. They're used to monitor the health of both the mother and the baby and to track the baby's growth.

How it's done

You'll probably be asked not to empty your bladder before the exam, especially if the ultrasound is done early in your pregnancy. A full bladder eliminates pockets of air between the uterus and the bladder, which can distort the sound waves and produce an unclear image. If you're having a transvaginal ultrasound or if it's late in your pregnancy, a full bladder isn't necessary.

A gel is applied to your abdominal area. (You may want to wear a two-piece outfit to make it easier to expose your abdomen.) The gel acts as a conductor for sound waves and helps to eliminate air bubbles between the transducer and your skin. The transducer is a small plastic device that both sends out the sound waves and records them as they bounce back.

During the exam, the ultrasonographer moves the transducer back and forth over your abdomen, directing sound waves into the uterus. The sound waves reflect off bones and tissue. As the transducer captures the reflected sound waves, they're digitally converted into black, white and gray images on a screen. The images may be somewhat hard for an untrained observer to decipher, so don't worry if you can't see your baby. Ask your health care provider or technologist to help explain what's on the screen.

Depending on your baby's position, you may be able to make out a face, tiny hands and fingers, or arms and legs. Throughout the exam, your health care provider will stop to measure the baby's head, abdomen and thigh bone, among other structures, to record growth. He or she may also take some pictures to document important structures. You'll probably be given copies of some of these scans. Some clinics may also offer you a videotape of the ultrasound.

What the results may tell you
Based on the images produced by the ultrasound exam, your health care provider can determine a number of things about your pregnancy and your baby, including:
- The fact that you are indeed pregnant.
- How many weeks it has been since conception (baby's gestational age).
- How many babies you're carrying.
- Your baby's growth rate and development.
- Your baby's movement, breathing and heart rate.
- The sex of your baby. Being able to determine what sex your baby is depends on the baby's position in the uterus and the position of the umbilical cord. Decide in advance if you want to know this information.
- Structural variations or abnormalities in your baby, such as spina bifida.
- The location and development of the placenta. Sometimes a pregnancy develops outside the uterus (ectopic pregnancy), usually inside a fallopian tube.
- Whether you've had a miscarriage.
- Assessment of the cervix and the tendency toward preterm delivery.
- Measures of fetal well-being such as urine output, muscle tone and activity.

Possible concerns

Ultrasound examination doesn't involve radiation. Forty years of experience suggests that it's a safe exam for both you and your baby.

Reasons to have it done

Ultrasound is used so often with pregnancy that you may assume it's a routine part of prenatal care. But researchers have found that for most healthy women with normal pregnancies, a routine ultrasound doesn't seem to make a difference in the outcome of the pregnancy. It may not be cost-effective if there aren't any questions of normal fetal development.

If concerns do develop, those concerns are often best addressed by an ultrasound. If you're not sure when you became pregnant, an ultrasound can determine the baby's gestational age. If blood tests indicate an abnormality, an ultrasound may be able to identify it. If there's any bleeding or a concern about the baby's growth rate, an ultrasound is the best initial test. In addition, ultrasound imaging can be used to guide your health care provider while performing other prenatal tests, such as amniocentesis or chorionic villus sampling.

Many women and their partner look forward to an ultrasound because it gives them a first glimpse of their baby. Some parents value an ultrasound for finding out the sex of their baby. Although this is often possible, it's not recommended as the sole purpose of an ultrasound. Talk to your health care provider about your need for an ultrasound.

What happens next

If results of the ultrasound are normal, no additional ultrasounds may be required. If your health care provider suspects abnormalities, he or she may recommend further testing. An advanced ultrasound, amniocentesis or other studies may be used to confirm or rule out a diagnosis. In many higher-risk pregnancies, ultrasounds are used frequently to monitor the pregnancy.

Accuracy and limitations of the test

Although ultrasound is a very useful imaging tool, it can't detect all fetal abnormalities. If an ultrasound can't offer an explanation for a perceived problem, your health care provider may recommend other diagnostic testing, such as amniocentesis or chorionic villus sampling.

Amniocentesis

What it is

With amniocentesis, your doctor uses a thin needle inserted into your abdomen to take a small sample of amniotic fluid from the sac surrounding your baby. The two common types are genetic amniocentesis and maturity amniocentesis:

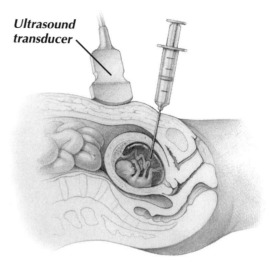

Ultrasound transducer

- **Genetic amniocentesis.** It can give you and your doctor information about your baby's genetic makeup before your baby is born.
- **Maturity amniocentesis.** With this test, the fluid is analyzed to find out if the baby's lungs are mature enough to function normally at birth.

The amniotic fluid is a clear liquid that envelops your baby in the uterus and provides a cushion against everyday bumps and jars. The fluid consists mostly of urine from your baby. It also contains cells that your baby has shed.

During amniocentesis, an ultrasound transducer shows on a screen the positions of your fetus and the needle, enabling your doctor to safely withdraw a sample of amniotic fluid for testing.

With genetic amniocentesis, a sample of these cells can be collected and grown in a laboratory. From that sample, the chromosomes and genes can be checked for abnormalities, such as Down syndrome. The amniotic fluid sample can also be tested for signs of neural tube defects, such as spina bifida.

When it's administered

Genetic amniocentesis is usually performed between the 15th and 19th weeks of gestation. At this point, your uterus generally contains enough amniotic fluid, and your baby is still small. It can be done earlier, but that may increase the risk of a pregnancy loss.

Maturity amniocentesis is done when there may be a reason to deliver the baby before the due date. It indicates whether the baby's lungs are ready for birth. It's usually done from 32 to 39 weeks of gestation.

How it's done

Amniocentesis can be done in your doctor's office. It doesn't require a hospital stay. Before the procedure begins, your doctor or genetic counselor will likely discuss the test with you and help you consider what a positive or negative result might mean. An ultrasound is performed to show the exact location of your baby in the uterus. Together, the discussion and preliminary ultrasound take about 45 minutes to an hour.

After the baby's position is determined, the amniocentesis begins. Your abdomen is cleaned with an antiseptic. Then, guided by ultrasound images, your doctor inserts a thin, hollow needle through your abdomen and into your uterus. About 2 to 4 teaspoons of amniotic fluid are withdrawn into a syringe. The procedure is over when the needle is removed.

Many women find that the procedure isn't as painful as they had anticipated. You'll notice a stinging sensation or a prick when the needle enters your skin and some menstrual-like cramping during the procedure. The discomfort is usually about the same as having blood drawn.

The sample is sent to a laboratory. Some results may be available within a few hours or days. Chromosomal assessment may take seven to 14 days, because the fetal cells must be allowed to multiply until there are enough to be tested. For information on a rapid 24- to 36-hour preliminary test result, see "FISH: Speeding up genetic analysis," on page 304.

What the results may tell you

Genetic amniocentesis is often used to identify various genetic defects. Some of the information an amniocentesis may provide includes:

- **Chromosomal abnormality.** Amniocentesis allows the lab to look at the number and structure of each of your baby's 23 pairs of chromosomes. It allows your doctor to check for chromosomal abnormalities such as Down syndrome, trisomy 13 and trisomy 18.
- **Neural tube defects.** The sample of amniotic fluid can be assessed for abnormally high levels of alpha-fetoprotein (AFP). Elevated levels of AFP may indicate a neural tube defect, such as spina bifida.

  Amniocentesis is a definitive diagnostic test for neural tube defects, although the development of advanced ultrasound offers a noninvasive alternative.
- **Genetic disorders.** The genetic material from cells collected during amniocentesis can be examined for many hereditary disorders. These conditions are relatively rare. They include defects in the body's chemistry (metabolic disorders) such as cystic fibrosis, Tay-Sachs and sickle cell disease; disorders that are passed by the mother to a male infant (X-linked disorders), such as some types of muscular dystrophy and hemophilia; and disorders that are passed from either the mother or father to the baby, such as Huntington's disease. There are so many genetic disorders that it's not practical to look for all of them. These diseases are assessed only if you have a specific reason to look for the problem, such as a family history of a particular genetic disorder.

Maturity amniocentesis is used to determine your baby's lung maturity:

- **Lung maturity.** Testing the amniotic fluid can tell your doctor whether your baby's lungs are developed enough to function outside of the uterus. This is important if you need to deliver the baby early.

Other, less common uses of amniocentesis include:
- **Rh incompatibility.** If you don't have a type of protein called Rhesus (Rh) factor in your blood (that is, you're Rh negative) but your baby does have it (he or she is Rh positive), you have a condition called Rh incompatibility. Although it's not likely to cause a problem during your first pregnancy, it's possible that your immune system may produce antibodies against the Rh factor in your baby's blood in subsequent pregnancies. This can lead to mild or severe damage or death. Amniocentesis can be used to determine whether and how much your baby is affected.
- **Intrauterine infections.** In order to determine whether you have an infection caused by a viral agent or parasite such as toxoplasmosis, your doctor may require a sample of the amniotic fluid for analysis.

Possible concerns
Although amniocentesis is a relatively safe test, it carries a few risks:
- **Miscarriage.** Amniocentesis done before 24 weeks of gestation carries a risk of miscarriage of about one in 200 (0.5 percent). Amniocentesis performed early in the pregnancy, before 14 weeks, carries a risk of miscarriage of about two to five in 100 (2 percent to 5 percent). Most of these losses occur because of rupture of the amniotic sac. When amniocentesis is used later in pregnancy to assess lung maturity, a rupture of the amniotic sac is much less likely to cause a fatal complication to the baby because it may be safe to deliver the baby at that point.
- **Post-procedural complications.** You may have cramping, bleeding or leaking of amniotic fluid after the procedure. Bleeding occurs in 2 percent to 3 percent of cases. Amniotic fluid leakage occurs in about 1 percent of cases. These problems usually go away with no treatment, but call your health care provider if you have bleeding or leakage. Infection rarely occurs, but if you develop a fever following an amniocentesis, contact your health care provider.
- **Rh sensitization.** In a few cases, amniocentesis may cause an influx of fetal blood into the maternal bloodstream. If this happens and your blood type is Rh negative and your baby's is Rh positive, it may lead to Rh disease. Rh disease can be fatal to the baby. Generally, if you have a negative blood type, you're given a drug called Rh immunoglobulin (RhIg) after the procedure, which can prevent the condition.
- **Needle injury.** There's a slight chance that the baby may be punctured by the needle, though use of the ultrasound for guidance makes this rare.

Reasons to have it done

The most common reason women have an amniocentesis is their age. If you'll be 35 years or older when your baby is born, your baby has an increased risk of chromosomal abnormalities. As with most prenatal tests, this test is voluntary. The decision to have a genetic amniocentesis is a serious one. Talk to your health care provider or a genetic counselor about your options, no matter what your age. Other reasons you and your health care provider may consider genetic amniocentesis include:

- A previous pregnancy complicated by a chromosomal abnormality or neural tube defect.
- Abnormal results from a screening test, such as a triple test.
- Either parent carries a chromosome rearrangement that doesn't immediately affect him or her but may affect the child.
- Either parent has a central nervous system defect such as spina bifida or a close relative with such a problem.
- Either parent has a chromosomal abnormality such as Down syndrome or a close relative with such a problem.
- Parents are known carriers of a genetic mutation that causes a disease such as cystic fibrosis, Tay-Sachs disease or another single-gene disorder.
- The mother has a male relative with muscular dystrophy, hemophilia or some other X-linked disorder.

What happens next

Most tests come back normal. If there is a problem, you and your health care provider or genetic counselor need to carefully discuss the next step.

Chromosomal problems can't be corrected, and very few treatments for hereditary disorders can be done before birth. This can be a difficult time. It's important to seek out and receive support from your medical team, your family, your spiritual advisers and any others whom you trust and who care about you.

Terminating a pregnancy is never an easy decision. The fact that your child may have a serious or even fatal condition doesn't make that choice any less difficult. Many women decide to continue the pregnancy, and their health care team can refer them to medical and child-care specialists who can help them plan for the future. Adoption is another option. Organizations that specialize in adoption of children with special needs are readily available.

Accuracy and limitations of the test

Although amniocentesis is accurate in identifying certain genetic disorders, such as Down syndrome, it can't identify all birth defects. For example, it can't detect a heart defect, clubfoot or cleft lip and palate. A normal result from an amniocentesis may provide reassurance regarding certain congenital problems, but it doesn't guarantee that your baby is free of all defects.

Chorionic villus sampling

What it is

Like amniocentesis, chorionic villus sampling (CVS) can detect chromosomal and other genetic abnormalities in your unborn baby. But instead of sampling amniotic fluid, CVS examines tissue from the placenta. Because no amniotic fluid is collected, CVS can't test for neural tube defects, such as spina bifida.

Part of the placenta is a membrane layer called the chorion. Tiny, hair-like projections called villi extend out of the chorion and act as routes for nutrients, oxygen and antibodies from you to your baby. These chorionic villi contain fetal cells complete with your baby's DNA.

During a CVS procedure, your doctor takes a sample of chorionic villus cells from the placenta. This is done by inserting either a thin tube through

FISH: SPEEDING UP GENETIC ANALYSIS

A method of genetic analysis that is faster than traditional techniques is now available. It's called fluorescence in situ hybridization (FISH), and it can deliver results in as little as 24 hours. In contrast, it will take from several days to two weeks to get results from a standard approach.

With amniocentesis, there aren't enough fetal cells collected in the sample to immediately perform a reliable comprehensive chromosomal analysis. Lab technicians must wait for sample cells to divide and multiply (culture). They then capture them at the phase of cell division when chromosomes can be seen as separate structures (metaphase). Once this occurs, the cells can be studied. The cell's chromosomes are then stained, revealing a unique pattern that allows them to be counted and analyzed under a fluorescent microscope.

FISH uses a technique that relies on short sequences of DNA called probes. These probes, which have a fluorescent tag attached to them, are designed to seek out and attach (hybridize) to specific genetic sequences in a cell sample.

Normally, a baby has two of every chromosome, totaling 23 pairs of chromosomes. Occasionally, a chromosomal abnormality occurs. This is the case with Down syndrome, which is characterized by three number 21 chromosomes. Abnormal numbers of chromosomes are called aneuploidies. Along with Down syndrome, other common aneuploidies that can be identified by FISH include:

- Trisomy 18
- Trisomy 13
- Extra or missing X (female) or Y (male) sex chromosomes

With FISH, for example, a red-labeled chromosome 21 probe will seek out all the number 21 chromosomes in a cell sample and mark them as red. When the sample is viewed under a fluorescent microscope, the red markers are easy to see and count. FISH analysis can be used on cells that aren't in the division process (interphase stage) so culturing isn't needed. This allows a much faster evaluation.

your cervix or a needle through your abdomen, guided by ultrasound views of the uterus. The sample is then sent to a laboratory for analysis.

When it's administered
CVS is usually performed between the ninth and 14th weeks of gestation. That's earlier in the pregnancy than amniocentesis is generally done. If you wish to have a diagnostic test early in your pregnancy, your doctor will probably recommend CVS over early amniocentesis because of the increased risk of miscarriage that early amniocentesis carries.

How it's done
A chorionic villus sample may be taken transcervically or transabdominally. Both approaches are considered equally safe. Which is used depends on the

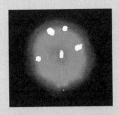 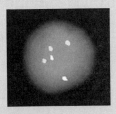

The FISH test can determine the sex of the fetus and any numeric chromosomal problems that include the chromosomes X, Y, 13, 18 and 21. Unlike the reproductions here, actual FISH tests include colors that indicate the results.

Using FISH for rapid diagnosis often lets you know the results of your test much sooner than if conventional chromosomal analysis is used. That may give you more time to make decisions regarding your pregnancy.

Detection of common aneuploidies using FISH is generally very accurate. It has false-positive and false-negative rates of less than 1 percent.

But the technique has some limitations. Although accurate, FISH only identifies the problems listed above. And, although the number of chromosomes for 13, 18, 21, X and Y may be readily apparent during FISH analysis, the actual structure of the chromosome isn't apparent. Thus, structural abnormalities, which can indicate a problem, aren't evident with FISH, but they are with the conventional genetic analysis used with amniocentesis. In addition, FISH can't tell the difference between maternal cells and fetal cells. If maternal cells have contaminated the sample, the results may not truly reflect the genetic status of the baby. For this reason, most health care providers use FISH as a supplement to diagnosis, not as the sole basis for prenatal decisions.

position of the placenta and your doctor's experience. In general, placentas on the back side of the uterus are easier to sample through the cervix. Placentas in the front allow either approach.

An ultrasound is done before the procedure to determine the position of the placenta. Both variations of the procedure are done with ultrasound guidance.

- **Transcervical CVS.** This type of CVS procedure may feel similar to a Pap test with just slightly more cramping. You lie on your back with your feet in stirrups. After cleansing your vagina and cervix with antiseptic, your doctor inserts a thin, hollow tube (catheter) through your vagina and cervix into the chorionic villi. Gentle suction is then used to obtain a small placental cell sample. Some women have noticeable discomfort, and some don't.

- **Transabdominal CVS.** This procedure is similar to amniocentesis in that it uses a long, thin needle to obtain the cell sample. A safe entry site for the needle is determined using ultrasound, and your abdomen is

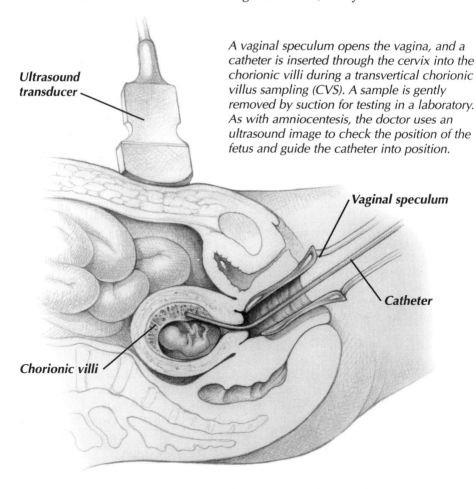

Ultrasound transducer

A vaginal speculum opens the vagina, and a catheter is inserted through the cervix into the chorionic villi during a transvertical chorionic villus sampling (CVS). A sample is gently removed by suction for testing in a laboratory. As with amniocentesis, the doctor uses an ultrasound image to check the position of the fetus and guide the catheter into position.

Vaginal speculum

Catheter

Chorionic villi

cleansed with antiseptic. Then your doctor inserts the needle through your abdomen into the chorionic villi and removes the sample.

The procedure takes about 45 minutes. The needle is in place only for a small part of that time. With CVS, generally a larger sample of cells is collected than with amniocentesis, so results of CVS are available sooner — within two to seven days, depending on the complexity of the laboratory analysis.

What the results may tell you
As in amniocentesis, analysis of fetal cells in the sample can reveal whether your baby has a chromosomal abnormality, such as Down syndrome, or another genetic disorder, such as Tay-Sachs disease, if there's reason to look for them.

Possible concerns
If you have a cervical infection, such as chlamydia or herpes, transcervical CVS isn't recommended. CVS requires more expertise than amniocentesis, so it's important to have an experienced obstetrician perform the procedure. In general, the risks of CVS are similar to those of amniocentesis:

- **Miscarriage.** The risk of miscarriage with CVS is slightly higher than with amniocentesis — about one in 100 (1 percent).
- **Post-procedural complications.** Vaginal bleeding occurs in about 7 percent to 10 percent of transcervical procedures, but rarely in transabdominal procedures. Cramping also may occur. Call your health care provider if you experience any of these problems. Infections are rare, but contact your health care provider if you develop a fever.
- **Rh sensitization.** As in amniocentesis, it's possible that some of your blood may mix with the baby's blood. If you're Rh negative, your health care provider will probably give you an injection of RhIg after the procedure to prevent you from producing antibodies against your baby's blood cells.

Several years ago, there was some controversy about whether CVS causes an increased incidence of limb defects. Reports at that time showed a slight increase (one in 3,000) in limb malformations with CVS. Since that time, other studies have detected no increase. Based on existing evidence, researchers have generally concluded that there's no association between these types of defects and CVS performed after 10 weeks of gestation.

Reasons to have it done
Both CVS and amniocentesis can provide genetic information about your baby. The advantage of CVS is that it's available earlier in pregnancy. CVS can also detect a few extremely rare genetic disorders in families with known risk that can't be found with amniocentesis.

What happens next

If the results are normal, no further testing may be required. If there's evidence of a chromosomal abnormality or other genetic disorder, you and your health care provider or genetic counselor can discuss the next step. In about 1 percent of cases, CVS results are unclear and amniocentesis may be necessary to confirm the diagnosis.

If ending the pregnancy is a consideration for you, the early availability of a CVS diagnosis may be an advantage. Ending the pregnancy sooner rather than later is generally safer and has fewer complications.

Early diagnosis can also be helpful in the treatment of certain disorders. For example, if a female baby has congenital adrenal hyperplasia, a condition in which excessive amounts of male hormones are produced, hormone therapy may be given to the mother to prevent the baby from developing male characteristics.

Accuracy and limitations of the test

CVS has less than a 1 percent chance of yielding false-positive results. A false-positive means that the test indicates the baby has an abnormality when there really is none. If you get negative results, you can be fairly certain that no chromosomal abnormalities are present in your baby. But CVS can't be used to check for all conditions. For example, it can't be used to test for neural tube defects, such as spina bifida.

Percutaneous umbilical blood sampling

What it is

With percutaneous umbilical blood sampling (PUBS), a sample of blood is taken from your baby through the vein in the umbilical cord. This diagnostic procedure can detect chromosomal abnormalities, some genetic problems and the presence of infectious disease. PUBS is also known as umbilical vein sampling, fetal blood sampling and cordocentesis.

Your health care provider may offer this procedure if other prenatal diagnostic tests, such as amniocentesis, ultrasound and CVS, have been unable to uncover sufficient information. In the past, PUBS offered the fastest way to gather a sample for chromosomal analysis. New laboratory techniques, such as FISH (see page 304), allow chromosomal evaluation to be completed within a day or two and provide rapid analysis of samples obtained through amniocentesis or CVS. Still, sampling the baby's blood has the potential to revolutionize diagnosis, just as blood tests became so key in adult medicine for helping health care providers in making diagnoses.

In addition, PUBS may be performed to diagnose certain blood disorders and infections and to supply blood transfusions to the baby.

WHEN TEST RESULTS INDICATE A PROBLEM

The unthinkable is happening: Your prenatal test results suggest that your baby may have a problem. Amid the shock, worry and fear, one question surfaces: What now?

To answer that question, start by scheduling a meeting with your health care provider. Talk about the findings and what they might — and might not — mean to you and your baby. If your baby may have a genetic condition, you might want to ask for an immediate referral to a genetic counselor or medical geneticist.

Before meeting with your health care provider, make a list of your questions. Some you might consider:

- How accurate are the test results? Is it possible there's a mistake?
- Can my baby survive this condition? If so, how long is she or he likely to live after birth?
- What problems might be caused by this condition? How might the baby be affected physically? How might the baby be affected mentally?
- Is it likely that my child will need surgeries or other medical treatments to manage the condition? If so, will they be painful? If my baby is in pain, how can the pain be recognized and treated?
- Are there other health care professionals who can give us more information?
- What is involved in caring for a child with this condition?
- Are special programs available to help my child's mental and physical development?
- Is there a support group in our community for families who have a child with this condition? How can we contact parents of children who have a similar condition?
- What are the chances that this condition will affect our next pregnancy?
- What resources are available to us if we decide to end the pregnancy? What counseling services or support groups are available?

Once you've gathered the information, you'll need to make a decision based on your personal circumstances. Consider the emotional and physical aspects of your decision, along with your personal and financial resources.

Here are your options:

- **Continue the pregnancy.** Make plans for how best to manage the rest of the pregnancy, your labor and delivery, and your baby's treatment after birth. Think about how the baby will affect your family and lifestyle, and, as much as possible, make plans accordingly. Consider seeking out a counselor or support group to help you learn about and meet your child's needs.
- **End the pregnancy.** The decision to end a pregnancy is never an easy one, even if your baby has a condition that is incompatible with life. Counseling and support groups, both before and after making the decision, can be invaluable in helping you sort out your feelings. Remember, only you can decide if this is the right decision for you. Counselors, health care providers and community resources can provide information, but this most serious of decisions is one you must make.

    If you want to consider this option, it's likely that you'll need to gather information quickly. Your health care provider or genetic counselor can help you explore your options.

When it's administered
PUBS is usually done later in the pregnancy, after 18 weeks. Before this point, the umbilical vein is still fragile.

How it's done
As with amniocentesis, for this procedure you lie on your back with your abdomen exposed. Gel is spread over your abdomen and advanced ultrasound is used to locate the umbilical cord. This area on your abdomen is cleansed with antiseptic. With the help of the ultrasound images, your doctor inserts a thin needle through your abdomen and uterus into the umbilical cord vein and withdraws a sample of blood. The sample is then sent to the laboratory for analysis. The entire procedure lasts about 45 minutes to an hour, with the needle in place for only a fraction of the time. Depending on the test, results may be back in as little as two hours.

What the results may tell you
PUBS may provide the following information:
- **Chromosomal or other genetic abnormalities.** PUBS can detect some of the same chromosomal abnormalities and genetic disorders as can amniocentesis and CVS, such as Down syndrome, and can more directly test for sickle cell disease and hemophilia.
- **Blood disorders.** The baby's blood sample can be analyzed for signs of anemia and Rh disease. PUBS can also determine the severity of the condition. If the condition is severe, a blood transfusion can be done at the same time. More recently, Doppler ultrasound, which measures the speed of blood flow, may be used as a less risky alternative to diagnosing moderate to severe anemia.
- **Infections.** If you have an infection, such as toxoplasmosis or rubella, PUBS can determine whether the baby has acquired the infection. However, recent genetic techniques enable health care providers to detect viruses or bacteria directly from amniotic fluid, which is safer.
- **Restricted growth.** In cases of severe intrauterine growth restriction, PUBS can help determine why your baby isn't growing as he or she should.

Possible concerns
PUBS carries about a 2 percent risk of fetal death. This risk is more than twice that of CVS or amniocentesis. Other risks associated with PUBS include bleeding from the needle entry site — which usually goes away on its own — temporary slowing of the baby's heart rate, infection, cramping and fluid leakage. Call your health care provider if you notice fever, bleeding or leakage of fluid after this procedure.

Reasons to have it done

Because PUBS is somewhat riskier than other prenatal tests, your health care provider will probably offer you other diagnostic options before PUBS. But if you're Rh negative, your baby is Rh positive and a blood test indicates high levels of antibodies against your baby's blood cells, then amniocentesis may be performed to determine whether your baby is developing anemia. When the problem is severe, PUBS can provide a route to deliver a transfusion to your baby.

A few other circumstances might make PUBS the method of choice, for example, if your baby needs a blood transfusion or an infusion of medication.

What happens next

If results are normal, no further testing is usually required. If chromosomal abnormalities are present, you and your health care provider or genetic counselor can discuss your options and arrange for any medical support you'll need.

If your baby has severe anemia, your health care provider may induce early delivery if your baby is mature enough to live outside the uterus. Your baby may be given a blood transfusion through the umbilical cord.

If your baby has an infection, your health care provider will let you know the treatment options available.

Accuracy and limitations of the test

Having an experienced health care provider perform the procedure is critical to the test's success. Thanks to the development of FISH and more sophisticated forms of genetic analysis, the use of PUBS to rapidly diagnose genetic conditions has decreased. However, the procedure still plays an important role in assessing fetal blood disorders and delivering blood transfusions and medication to the baby in the uterus. In the future, this procedure may have other uses.

At times, your health care provider may think it's a good idea to check in on how well your baby is doing. Tests that give you and your health care provider a sneak peek at baby's well-being include electronic fetal nonstress and stress tests and biophysical profile scoring.

Electronic fetal nonstress and stress tests

What they are
Fetal nonstress and stress tests assess your baby's well-being by looking at the baby's heart rate. They're typically performed during the last trimester of pregnancy. A baby is considered in good health if his or her heart rate increases after moving and the heart rate is constantly adjusting for the baby's condition. This is what nonstress testing is all about.

Contraction stress tests evaluate the baby's health by monitoring the baby's heart rate in response to contractions induced by medication. Babies in good health will generally tolerate contractions without a significant change in heart rate.

These tests can help your health care provider evaluate the overall health of your baby and verify that continuing the pregnancy doesn't present a significant threat to the baby. One or both may be done, particularly if you have a high-risk pregnancy or if you're past your due date.

When it's administered
These tests are best performed after 28 weeks of gestation.

How it's done
The nonstress and contraction stress tests are performed in the following manner:

- **Nonstress test.** During this test, a belt with transducers attached to it is placed on your abdomen. The transducers are part of the Doppler ultrasound equipment, which measures your baby's heart rate through the use of sound waves. Your health care provider may ask you to push a button each time you feel your baby move, or he or she may record your baby's movement. The heart rate measurement shows up as a graph. Each time the button is pushed, a little arrow shows up on the graph to indicate when the baby has moved.

  If your baby doesn't seem to be moving, he or she may be asleep. Your health care provider may wait a few minutes until your baby wakes up or use a buzzer to wake the baby. The test takes about 20 to 40 minutes.

- **Contraction stress test.** The contraction stress test is performed in much the same way as the nonstress test, using the Doppler ultrasound equipment. During this test, the fetal heart rate is measured while mild contractions are induced. These contractions aren't nearly as uncomfortable as those of labor.

  If the contractions aren't occurring on their own, your health care provider may give you an infusion of oxytocin. To be considered adequate, the test usually requires three contractions within a 10-minute period. This test may take one to two hours to complete.

What the results may tell you
About 85 percent of nonstress test results are normal (reactive), which means that your baby's heart rate increased as expected. Abnormal results are termed nonreactive, which means the baby's heart rate didn't accelerate as expected. A

nonreactive test result isn't necessarily a reason to worry. The most common reason for a nonreactive result is that the baby was asleep during testing. Occasionally, abnormal results indicate an oxygen deficiency in your baby.

Results of a contraction stress test are normal (negative) if the baby's heart rate doesn't slow down after contractions. Results are abnormal (positive) if the heart rate consistently slows down after contractions. This may mean your baby isn't getting enough oxygen and may be in danger of dying in the womb. Only 3 percent to 5 percent of contraction stress test results are positive. As scary as this sounds, many positive tests occur in babies who will be normal.

Possible concerns
The nonstress test carries virtually no risk and is safe for both you and your baby. But if you're at risk of premature labor, such as if you're carrying twins, your health care provider may not recommend the contraction stress test.

Reasons to have it done
Your health care provider may recommend a nonstress test if you notice a marked decrease in your baby's movement or if your baby's growth rate seems abnormally slow. Your health care provider may also suggest monitoring your baby's health with a nonstress test once or twice a week after 28 weeks of gestation if you have one of the following conditions:
- Diabetes
- A disease that may harm your baby, such as kidney or heart disease
- High blood pressure during pregnancy (preeclampsia)
- A history of stillbirth
- Prolonged gestation (You're past your due date.)
- Multiple gestation (You're carrying two or more babies.)
- An abnormal amount of amniotic fluid, indicated by ultrasound examination

Contraction stress testing is usually performed if the results from a nonstress test are abnormal.

What happens next
If results of the nonstress test are nonreactive, the test may be prolonged or repeated, or a contraction stress test performed. In one study, about 80 percent of nonstress tests that were nonreactive in the morning became reactive when the test was repeated later in the day.

If a contraction stress test is positive, this doesn't necessarily mean there's a problem. Your health care provider may repeat the test in 24 hours or combine it with other tests, such as biophysical profile scoring (see page 314), to verify whether your baby is in danger. If so, you and your health care provider may decide to induce labor if your baby is old enough to survive. A Caesarean birth may be an option.

Accuracy and limitations of the test
Both tests have very high false-positive rates. A false-positive means the test indicates a problem when there actually is none. Most of the time, abnormal results will be normal when the test is repeated. Because the tests are safe and can be repeated with no harmful effects, they're often the best tools to monitor your baby's health during the last few weeks of pregnancy.

Biophysical profile scoring

What it is
Biophysical profile scoring is another means of monitoring your baby's health during the last trimester. It combines an ultrasound exam with a nonstress test. The tests usually assess five different aspects of your baby's health, including:
- Heart rate
- Breathing movements (Your baby doesn't breathe air inside the uterus, but breathing movements move small amounts of fluid in and out of the lungs.)
- Body movement
- Muscle tone
- Amount of amniotic fluid

Each of these factors is given a score of 0 or 2, and the scores are added together to achieve a total from 0 to 10.

When it's administered
This test may be used as early as the 26th week of gestation.

How it's done
Your baby's heart rate is measured using a nonstress test. The other four factors — breathing, movement, muscle tone and amniotic fluid — are evaluated with ultrasound. If a factor is normal, it receives an individual score of 2. If it's absent or less than expected, it receives a score of 0.

What the results may tell you
A score of 6 or less may indicate your baby is suffering from a lack of oxygen. The lower the score, the greater the cause for concern. In a large study of over 26,000 high-risk pregnancies, almost 97 percent had biophysical profile scores of 8 or more.

Possible concerns
Both the nonstress test and ultrasound are considered to be very safe. Some medications may reduce the biophysical profile score.

Reasons to have it done
The reasons for having a biophysical profile done are similar to those for having the nonstress and stress tests. It helps you and your health care provider keep track of your baby's health before delivery, particularly if you have a high-risk pregnancy.

What happens next
Depending on your score, your health care provider may recommend one of several courses of action. If you have diabetes or are past your due date and the score is 8 or above, testing may be repeated once or twice a week. If the score is 6 or below, the test may be repeated to confirm the score. If necessary, your health care provider may recommend that the baby be delivered ahead of your due date.

Accuracy and limitations of the test
The false-positive rate for any individual factor of the biophysical profile is high, but when all factors are combined, the false-positive rate decreases. Having a low score doesn't necessarily mean that your baby is in trouble. It may just mean that you need special care throughout the rest of your pregnancy.

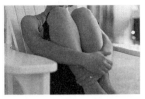

trying again after a pregnancy loss

A pregnancy loss can be an extremely difficult experience. You may feel as if your hopes for the future have been taken from you. These feelings can occur even if the pregnancy was only a few weeks along.

There's no set of rules about what you will or will not feel after a pregnancy loss. You may even feel simply numb for a while. Allow yourself to have your feelings. Try to work through them.

Grieving a pregnancy loss takes time. Some couples think that they must try to conceive again right away in order to fix the problem or replace the hurt. Unfortunately, it's unlikely that a subsequent pregnancy will carry the same feelings of innocence and bliss. A pregnancy after a loss can be highly stressful because of anxiety and fear that something may go wrong.

Although a pregnancy loss can be extremely difficult, it doesn't mean you won't be able to have another baby. In most cases, your chances of having a normal, healthy pregnancy are still excellent, even if you've had more than one or two losses. Your decision on whether and when to try again rests on the type of pregnancy you had, as well as your physical and emotional recovery.

Issues to consider

There is no perfect time to try to conceive again. Most experts advise that you give yourself the necessary time to heal both physically and emotionally before trying another pregnancy. In general, health care providers recommend waiting at least one menstrual cycle before trying again. In some cases, you may wish to consult a specialist before attempting to conceive again.

Emotional recovery

Losing a child is one of the most difficult things in life, and losing one before birth can be no less difficult. If you find yourself grieving deeply after a

CAUSES OF PREGNANCY LOSS

Pregnancy loss may occur because of a miscarriage, cervical incompetence, an ectopic pregnancy or a molar pregnancy.

A *miscarriage* is the loss of an embryo or fetus, usually because of genetic abnormalities in the developing cells. With *cervical incompetence,* the cervix begins to open before the pregnancy has come to term, which can result in a miscarriage.

In an *ectopic pregnancy,* the fertilized egg attaches itself to a place other than the uterus, usually a fallopian tube. A *molar pregnancy* is characterized by the development of an abnormal mass of cells in the uterus after fertilization.

pregnancy loss, allow yourself the time to do so. Emotional recovery can, and usually does, take much longer than physical recovery.

Some may wonder why you mourn for a child you've never known. But in many ways you may have already bonded with the baby growing inside of you. You and your partner may have shared many moments imagining the days when you would hold your baby in your arms. The missed opportunity of watching your child grow and develop may be especially poignant. Even if no embryo was ever present, you will still grieve when your dreams and expectations were to have a baby. Grieving is the process of letting go of the emotional attachment you've developed.

Stages of grief

No one goes through the grieving process the same way. But certain emotional stages are common to people who've had an important loss. They include:

- **Shock and denial.** Immediately after a traumatic event, people often feel numb and devoid of emotion. This is normal and doesn't mean you're uncaring. As reality sets in, these feelings often change.
- **Guilt and anger.** After a pregnancy loss, you may be tempted to blame yourself for what has happened. But a pregnancy loss is rarely preventable. It's highly unlikely that anything you did or could have done contributed to the pregnancy loss. You may also feel angry — with yourself, family, friends or simply with the circumstances. This is to be expected. It may help to just let yourself be angry for a while.
- **Depression and despair.** Depression isn't always easy to recognize. You may find that you feel profoundly tired or you lose interest in things you used to enjoy. Your appetite or sleeping patterns may change. Or you may find yourself crying over things that might otherwise seem minor.
- **Acceptance.** Although you may not think this now, eventually, you'll come to terms with your loss. This doesn't mean you'll be free from hurt, but it'll become easier to function.

These stages have no timetable. Some may take longer than others. Even after you've come to accept your loss, feelings of sorrow and pain may recur on an important date, such as the day you had your miscarriage or surgery, your baby's due date or the day you found out you were pregnant. During these times, the loss may feel fresh in your mind.

If you find that your feelings are so overwhelming that you can't function or that they make you hostile or violent or interfere with your relationships with loved ones, talk with your health care provider or seek the help of a mental health professional. He or she can help you deal with some of the issues you're facing. Even if you're not overwhelmed, talking to a counselor or therapist can help you realize that your feelings are normal. Support groups may also be helpful.

Your partner

You and your partner may deal with a pregnancy loss in different ways. It may not always be easy to recognize that the other person is hurting. You may wish to talk things out, and your partner may prefer to stay silent. Or one may feel the need to move on before the other is ready.

Now more than ever you need to rely on each other for support. Try to listen and respond to each other while accepting the other person's feelings. You may wish to consider seeing a counselor or therapist for help in expressing your emotions and expectations in more neutral territory.

Your children

If you have other children, they may be affected by the loss. They may have shared in your anticipation. They may even feel that what happened is somehow their fault. It's important to talk openly with them and explain to them that no one is to blame. Children are quick to pick up on the feelings of their parents, so be honest about feeling sad or confused. But reassure them that they are loved nonetheless.

Physical recovery

Miscarriage

Physically speaking, it generally takes one normal menstrual cycle for a woman to recover from a miscarriage. It's usually four to six weeks before your period comes back. It's possible to conceive in those weeks between the miscarriage and your first menstrual cycle. During this time, you may wish to use a mechanical form of birth control, such as a condom or diaphragm.

If you and your partner feel ready to become pregnant again, there are several issues to consider. Before conceiving, talk to your health care provider about your plans. He or she can help you come up with a strategy that will optimize your chances of a healthy pregnancy and delivery. If you had a single miscarriage, your chances of a subsequent healthy pregnancy are virtually the same as someone who has never had a miscarriage.

Your health care provider may suggest that you wait longer or have additional testing or monitoring if you've had recurrent miscarriages, an ectopic pregnancy or a molar pregnancy.

Recurrent pregnancy losses

If you've had three or more pregnancy losses, you may wish to see a doctor with expertise in this area. Most ob-gyns can address this issue, or they may refer you to a maternal-fetal specialist or a reproductive endocrinologist. Your health care provider can help you find the appropriate person.

Because recurrent pregnancy loss has various causes, you may go through several tests and evaluations. In addition, your health care provider may recommend that you see a geneticist or genetic counselor to look for potential chromosomal problems. However, even with additional testing, you may not have an explanation about why the pregnancy losses have occurred.

If a cause is found, there may or may not be a treatment for it. For example, a weak (incompetent) cervix can be temporarily held closed during the first and middle stages of pregnancy to prevent it from opening before the baby is ready to be born. But if the cause is a chromosomal problem, there may not be a treatment.

TIPS FOR FUTURE PREGNANCIES

Although it's very unlikely that you can prevent a pregnancy loss, you can do things to give yourself the best chance for a healthy pregnancy. Here are some tips to consider:
- Eat a healthy diet and exercise regularly.
- Get your daily dose of folic acid, either in a supplement or multivitamin.
- Get preconception and prenatal care.
- Don't smoke, drink alcohol or use illicit drugs while you are trying to conceive or are pregnant.
- Get checked and, if necessary, treated for sexually transmitted diseases.
- Limit caffeine consumption.
- Work with your health care provider. Together you can keep yourself and your baby as healthy as possible.

The good news is, even women who have had three losses have a 75 percent chance of going on to have a successful pregnancy.

A previous ectopic pregnancy

Your chances of having a successful pregnancy outcome are a bit lower after having had an ectopic pregnancy, but they're still good — between 60 percent and 80 percent if you have both fallopian tubes. Even if one fallopian tube has been removed, you still have more than a 40 percent chance of having a successful pregnancy outcome. But your chances of having another ectopic pregnancy increase — around 15 percent — so your health care provider should monitor you closely the next time you conceive.

A previous molar pregnancy

After a molar pregnancy, there's a slight risk of further abnormal tissue growth. These growths are usually noncancerous (benign), but in rare cases they may be cancerous (malignant). This tissue growth is usually marked by high levels of the pregnancy hormone human chorionic gonadotropin (HCG). Your health care provider will likely want to measure your levels of HCG on a regular basis until it has dropped back to normal. It's important that you not become pregnant for a full year because the rising levels of HCG that occur with conception may be confused with recurrent disease. The risk that a molar pregnancy will develop in a future pregnancy is between 1 percent and 2 percent. Your health care provider may recommend that you undergo ultrasound early in your next pregnancy to make sure that the pregnancy is normal.

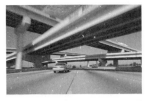

managing travel during pregnancy

It's usually safe to travel while you're pregnant, as long as you're in good health and observe basic safety precautions. Generally speaking, the best time to travel is during the second trimester, when you're likely to have less morning sickness, your body is more adjusted to carrying a baby, and you have less chance of a miscarriage or premature labor. By the third trimester, you may find it more difficult to move around.

However, if you have a medical problem or obstetrical condition, such as heart or blood vessel disease or a history of problems with pregnancy, your health care provider may advise you to stay close to home in case an emergency arises.

Always talk to your health care provider before setting out on an extended trip, as your mode of travel and destination may have implications for your pregnancy. Your doctor may want to review your medical history and give you a physical exam before you leave. If you travel often, such as for business, tell your health care provider about your schedule. Together you may find ways to make your trips more comfortable.

Issues to consider

Here are some tips for traveling during your pregnancy that may increase your level of safety and comfort.

Car travel

When traveling by car, remember to:
- **Stop regularly to stretch.** Avoid staying in a sitting position for more than two hours at a time. Limit total car time to six hours a day, if possible. Walking around for a few minutes every couple of hours will keep blood from pooling in your legs. This activity will reduce the risk of a blood clot forming.

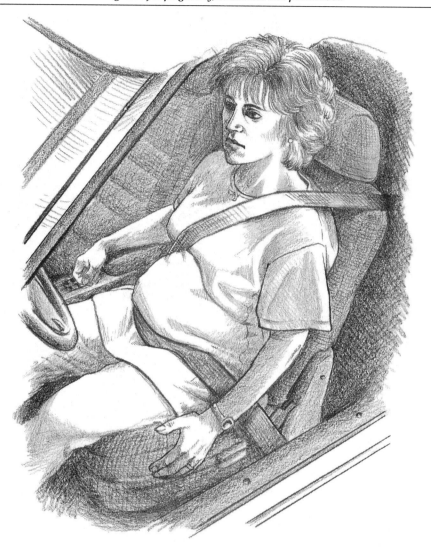

- **Wear your seat belt.** Now more than ever, it's important to wear your seat belt. Trauma to the mother-to-be is the leading cause of fetal death, and vehicular accidents are to blame for most severe trauma to pregnant women. Wear the lap belt below your abdomen and over your upper thighs, and wear the diagonal shoulder strap between your breasts.

Air travel

Traveling in an airplane usually doesn't pose any more risk when you're pregnant than it does when you're not. However, you may be at increased risk of problems if you have a history of blood clots, severe anemia, sickle cell disease or problems with the placenta. As with any major air travel, talk with your health care provider before flying.

Airport security devices aren't harmful to you or your baby. Remember, though, that most airlines won't allow you on board if you're past your 36-week mark, and most foreign airlines stop admitting pregnant passengers at 35 weeks. You may wish to take along a note from your health care provider stating your due date.

To minimize discomfort and danger while flying, consider the following:

- **Wear your seat belt.** As long as you're seated, wear your seat belt in case of unexpected turbulence. Position the belt low around your hips to avoid injury to the baby.
- **Move around.** Get up and walk around periodically, especially if the flight is long. This will minimize your risk of swelling and blood clots. You might consider wearing support stockings. In addition, try flexing and extending your calves while you're seated.
- **Choose your seating.** If possible, request an aisle seat or a seat in the bulkhead or exit row, which offers the most room. A seat over a wing offers the smoothest ride.
- **Stay hydrated.** Drink plenty of nonalcoholic fluids before you board and during your flight. The low humidity in the cabin has a dehydrating effect. Consuming adequate fluids also minimizes jet lag. This good advice can also cause a problem, so plan to empty your bladder before the seatbelt sign comes on.

Sea travel

Ships and cruise liners are just as safe for pregnant women as are other forms of travel, and many vessels have medical facilities onboard. Most cruise liners accept women through the seventh month of pregnancy. Realize that the movement of the ship may increase problems with nausea and vomiting. In addition, be careful walking on deck so that you don't slip or lose your balance and fall.

International travel

When traveling abroad, issues to consider include where you're going, vaccinations, and quality and availability of medical care at your destination. If you're going to a developing country or a place where the risk of a disease or an infection is high, your health care provider may recommend that you get immunized or postpone your trip.

In general, vaccines aren't recommended during your first trimester, and avoid live vaccines throughout your pregnancy. Live vaccines are made from weakened but not dead microorganisms. In theory, they may pose a risk to your baby, although no such cases have been reported.

To avoid traveler's diarrhea, don't use tap water in high-risk areas. Don't drink it, brush your teeth with it, or use ice cubes made from it. Your safest bet is to stick with bottled drinks. In addition, stay away from street food and fruits and vegetables that you can't peel or that you haven't peeled yourself. If you get diarrhea, be sure to drink plenty of liquids to avoid dehydration.

Consider creating a pregnancy kit to take with you on an overseas trip. Items that may come in handy include:

- **Copies of your medical records.** If you require medical care abroad, these will give your health care provider a head start.
- **Supplemental medical insurance.** If your health insurance doesn't provide coverage where you're going — many policies don't cover care abroad — you may wish to obtain additional coverage.
- **Drugs for diarrhea and vomiting.** Ask your health care provider for anti-diarrheals that are appropriate for pregnant women. If you're traveling to a place with lower levels of sanitation, your health care provider may prescribe antibiotics to take with you in case you need them.
- **Acetaminophen (Tylenol, others).** Take this for pain relief. Avoid nonsteroidal anti-inflammatory drugs (NSAIDs), such as ibuprofen (Advil, Motrin, others).
- **Packets of rehydration salts.** In case you do get diarrhea and become dehydrated, a solution created from one of these packets will help you re-hydrate.

To obtain information about specific countries and how to find medical assistance abroad, try the following resources.

Centers for Disease Control and Prevention: Traveler's Health
www.cdc.gov/travel

Obgyn.net: Country Pages
www.obgyn.net/country/country.asp

International Association for Medical Assistance to Travellers
Phone: (716) 754-4883
www.iamat.org

International SOS
Phone: (800) 523-6586
www.internationalsos.com

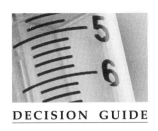

understanding pain relief choices in childbirth

What type of pain management is best during labor? That answer largely depends on your preferences and on how your labor progresses. No two women have the same tolerance for pain. No two labors are exactly the same. Some women need little or no pain medication. Others find that pain relief gives them a better sense of control over their labors and deliveries. Ultimately, you need to choose what's right for *you*.

The decision of whether to use medication during labor and delivery is mostly yours. However, it may also depend on your health care provider's recommendations, what's available at your hospital or birthing center, and the specific character of your labor.

Sometimes, you won't know what kinds of pain relief you want until you're in labor. Each woman's labor is unique to her. Your perception of labor pain will differ from that of other women in labor. In addition, your capacity to deal with pain during childbirth can be affected by factors such as the length of your labor, the size and position of your baby, and how rested you are as labor begins. No one can predict how you'll cope with the pain of your first labor, and subsequent labors often don't follow the same pattern.

When making your decision, keep in mind that birth isn't a test of endurance. You won't have failed if you ask for a pain relief drug. Keep in mind, too, that the contractions of labor have a purpose. Labor pains are a sign that your body is working hard to open your cervix and move the baby down the birth canal.

Before that first contraction kicks in, it's a good idea to think about the method — or methods — of pain relief you might prefer and to discuss your preferences with your health care provider. Whatever birth plan you ultimately devise, keep an open mind about it. Labors often don't go according to plan.

Choices in pain management

Today, women have more options for managing the discomforts of childbirth than ever before. These options fall into two categories:

Pain medications
Medications to relieve pain are known medically as *analgesics*. A common pain medication used in labor is nalbuphine (Nubain), which is given either intravenously or by injection. *Anesthetics* are medications that cause loss of sensation. Two examples of anesthetic techniques used in childbirth are epidural blocks and spinal blocks.

Natural pain relief methods
Natural childbirth means labor and delivery without the use of pain medications. Natural (nonpharmaceutical or nonmedicinal) methods of pain relief take many forms, some dating back centuries. Relaxation and massage are two examples of pain relief options of natural childbirth.

Many options are available within these broad categories. Learning about these categories of pain management ahead of time will help you make an informed decision about pain relief during labor and delivery. Education itself is a form of pain relief. Having to deal with fear in addition to discomfort dramatically worsens pain. If you know what to expect during labor and delivery and you've reviewed your choices for pain relief, you'll likely get through labor and delivery more smoothly than will someone who is tense and fearful.

Issues to consider

To help you choose the pain relief method or methods that are right for you, keep these questions in mind as you review your options. Ask yourself:
- What's involved in the method?
- How will it affect me?
- How will it affect my baby?
- How quickly will it work if I decide to use it?
- How long will the pain relief last?
- Do I need to organize or practice the method in advance, or is it done by the health care provider?
- Can I combine it with other methods of pain relief?
- Can I use it before I come to the hospital?
- When during labor is the method available?

Pain medications

Pain medications, in addition to natural pain relief methods, may be valuable aids to you in labor and delivery. They help reduce pain, usually quickly. They allow you to rest between contractions. Sometimes, the relaxation seems to lead to accelerated opening (dilation) of your cervix.

You're free to request or refuse pain medications during your labor and delivery. But remember that medications may have different benefits and risks at different times during labor. You always need to take into account the course and progress of your labor when choosing a pain relief method.

Discuss pain medications with your health care provider well before the start of your first contractions. Once you're in labor, your provider may make suggestions about pain medications depending on the specific character of your labor. But they're only suggestions. Weigh the advice of your provider alongside your own preferences for pain relief.

The debate continues about whether some medical approaches to pain relief affect the progress of labor. Some methods have been implicated in slowing labor. Yet when labor is moving slowly, pain relief is more likely to be needed. It's clear that being tense, fearful and miserable doesn't help you to make progress. In the end, your need for relief is the best determinant of when a technique should be used.

When you take narcotic medications can be as important as *what* you take. A baby is affected by medication taken by the mother, but the extent of that effect depends on the type of medication, the dose and how close to delivery it's administered. If enough time passes between when you receive a narcotic pain medication and when your baby is born, your body will process the drug, and your baby will have minimal effects from the medication at birth. If not, the baby may be sleepy and unable to suck. Less frequently, the baby may experience breathing difficulties. Any such effects on the newborn are generally short-lived and can be treated, if necessary.

Your health care provider is with you during labor and delivery to ensure that your baby arrives safely and in good health. He or she is familiar with each medication option and can share this knowledge with you. Trust your provider to tell you when it's safe — and when it's not safe — to take medications during labor and delivery. Understand that you may not always be able to have a medication when you feel you need it.

Several types of pain medication can be used during labor and childbirth.

Tranquilizers and barbiturates

These medications are not pain relievers. They're used only to relieve the mother's anxiety and promote rest.

Barbiturates
Amobarbital (Amytal), pentobarbital (Nembutal), secobarbital (Seconal)

Tranquilizers
Diazepam (Valium), promethazine (Phenergan), propiomazine (Largon)

When they're administered
Tranquilizers or barbiturates are occasionally given in early labor.

How they're administered
They're given by mouth, injected into a muscle in your thigh or buttocks, or injected into an intravenous (IV) catheter.

How they affect you
These medications have a relaxing effect, but they don't eliminate pain. They last four to eight hours, depending on the type used.

Possible concerns
Tranquilizers or barbiturates will make you drowsy. They may interfere with your ability to remember the details of labor later. Barbiturate medications may suppress a baby's activities at birth. Tranquilizers such as diazepam may diminish a baby's muscle tone at birth. These medications are used infrequently.

Analgesics and narcotics

These medications include butorphanol (Stadol), fentanyl (Sublimaze), meperidine (Demerol), nalbuphine (Nubain).

When they're administered
Narcotics can be given anytime in labor, but they're favored in earlier labor — when you're dilated less than 7 centimeters (cm) if you're a first-time mom or less than 5 cm if you've given birth before.

How they're administered
The medications are injected into a muscle in your thigh or buttocks or injected into an IV catheter. In some instances, you may be able to control your dosage by pressing a button that injects a fixed dose of the medication into your IV.

How they affect you
Depending on the dose, these medications decrease the perception of pain and make it easier to rest. They usually don't diminish your ability to push. They last from two to six hours, depending on the type used.

Possible concerns
These medications can cause sleepiness. At high doses, they can cause depressed respirations in the mother and baby. These effects are reversible. More frequently, these medications can decrease your memory of labor.

Local anesthetics

These medications include chloroprocaine, lidocaine and other "caine" drugs.

When they're administered
Local anesthetics are given shortly before or after delivery.

How they're administered
These medications are injected directly into tissue at the opening of the vagina before a cut to enlarge the opening (episiotomy) is made or a tear is repaired.

How they affect you
These medications numb the opening of the vagina specifically to allow a brief procedure to be done. They provide only temporary pain relief in a small area of the body. They don't lessen the pain of contractions, and there's no use for them during labor.

Possible concerns
Used properly, these medications have no negative effects on you or your baby. Very rarely, injecting such medications into the mother's vein can cause falling blood pressure and fainting. Some people are allergic to substances in this family of medications.

Pudendal block

These medications include chloroprocaine, lidocaine and other "caine" drugs.

When it's administered
A pudendal block may be given shortly before delivery.

How it's administered
This medication is injected into the wall of your vagina at a specific location marked by a bony landmark in your pelvis.

How it affects you
Just as a dentist can block pain from a group of your teeth by giving an injection at a specific location, your health care provider can use an injection

to block pain in the area between your vagina and anus (perineum). It provides numbness that lasts for several minutes up to an hour. It's useful if a forceps-assisted delivery or vacuum extraction becomes necessary. It provides pain relief if you need an episiotomy or if you tear during your delivery. It doesn't lessen the pain of contractions.

Possible concerns
Use of this technique may result in a slightly decreased urge to push. Allergies to the medication occur occasionally, and injecting it into a blood vessel can cause problems. Generally, it has no negative effects on you or your baby.

Epidural blocks

An epidural block is an anesthetic and narcotic mixture. Anesthetics used include chloroprocaine, lidocaine and other "caine" drugs. Narcotics used include fentanyl (Sublimaze), meperidine (Demerol), morphine and nalbuphine (Nubain).

When it's administered
The epidural block is used during active labor. It can also be used for Caesarean births.

How it's administered
The medication is injected into a space surrounding the spinal nerves. It takes about 20 minutes to administer, and it can take another 20 minutes for the pain relief to begin working. It can be administered continuously or off and on throughout labor.

How it affects you
Depending on the balance of anesthetic and narcotic, the epidural temporarily blocks pain in the lower body or alters your perception of the pain. In either case, it's a highly effective pain relief method that may be used continuously for several hours. A form called walking epidural provides pain relief but leaves you with enough muscle strength to walk during labor. Epidural techniques allow you to remain awake and alert. After dilation to 10 cm, the balance of medications may be altered to ensure perception of pushing.

Possible concerns
Occasionally, due to variations in a person's anatomy, the block may work better on one side than the other. The most common side effect that causes concern is a decrease in your blood pressure. Very rarely, this is enough of a

drop to make you feel faint or nauseated. More often, the drop is enough to decrease blood flow to the placenta, which may cause your baby to experience some temporary drops in heart rate. Scientific studies don't support that it causes a significant slowing of labor.

If too much medication is used, the block may affect the muscles of your chest, making it hard to perceive breathing. It's a scary side effect, but very manageable. It's also rare. Allergies to medications also may occur.

In rare cases, the needle perforates the membrane that holds the spinal fluid around the spinal canal. Occasionally, such a perforation leaks for a short time, which can give you a severe headache (spinal headache) when you're sitting up or standing.

RECEIVING AN EPIDURAL BLOCK

To receive an epidural block:
1. You lie on your side in a curled-up position or sit on the bed with your back rounded.
2. The doctor numbs an area of your back with a local anesthetic.
3. The doctor inserts a needle into the epidural space just outside the membrane that encloses the spinal fluid and spinal nerves.
4. A thin, flexible tube (catheter) is threaded through the needle, and the needle is removed. The catheter is taped in place.
5. The medication is injected through the catheter. The medication flows through the catheter to surround the nerves, blocking the pain.

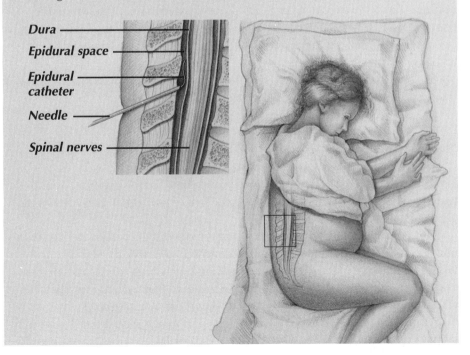

Dura
Epidural space
Epidural catheter
Needle
Spinal nerves

Spinal block

This technique offers an anesthetic and narcotic mixture. Anesthetics used include chloroprocaine, lidocaine and other "caine" drugs. Narcotics include fentanyl (Sublimaze), meperidine (Demerol), morphine, nalbuphine (Nubain).

When it's administered
A spinal block is given during active labor or, if necessary, shortly before a Caesarean birth.

How it's administered
The medication is injected into the fluid-filled space around the spinal nerves. It takes effect in seconds.

How it affects you
The technique provides complete pain relief from the chest down for labor, vaginal delivery or Caesarean birth. It provides relief for up to two hours and allows you to remain awake and alert.

Possible concerns
Side effects for you may include spinal headache or low blood pressure. Spinal headaches are somewhat more frequent in this technique than with epidural blocks because the perforation of the membrane that holds the spinal fluid is intentional. A smaller needle is used than that used with an epidural, though, so temporary leakage isn't common. You may need a catheter for your bladder because you'll lack bladder control.

As with epidural anesthesia, this method can cause low blood pressure in the mother, which may cause problems for the baby.

Natural pain relief methods

Natural birth refers to a childbirth experience in which the mother avoids the use of drugs for pain relief and favors the use of natural and complementary types of pain relief.

Stress during labor increases tension and reduces your ability to cope with pain. Natural (nonpharmaceutical or nonmedicinal) methods of pain relief work in a variety of ways. They may stimulate your body to release its own natural painkillers (endorphins). Most distract you from your pain. They can all soothe and relax you, allowing you to stay more in control of the pain.

Natural pain relief methods will help you manage pain, but they won't stop it entirely. You may choose to go for a completely nonmedicated childbirth or to combine it with pharmaceutical pain relief. Before considering other options, many women will try nondrug measures first to relieve pain during labor.

Methods of natural pain relief can be particularly useful both in early and active labor. It's during transition, when your cervix opens (dilates) the final centimeters to a full 10 cm, and during pushing that women who choose natural childbirth typically feel the greatest discomfort.

Natural pain relief methods include relaxation, massage, guided imagery, meditation, positive affirmation, breathing techniques, and others.

Relaxation techniques

Relaxation is the release of tension from the mind and body through conscious effort. By reducing muscle tension during labor and delivery, you can short-circuit a fear-tension-pain cycle. Relaxation allows your body to work more naturally, helping you conserve energy for the work ahead. Relaxation and patterned breathing are mainstays of the self-comforting measures women use for labor. These methods and others are usually taught in childbirth classes.

Relaxation doesn't mean fighting the pain, which would actually create more tension. It means allowing the pain to roll over you while you concentrate on tension-relieving and distracting exercises.

Relaxation is actually a learned skill and one that will be most effective if you practice it before the onset of labor. The more proficient you become at it, the more self-confident you'll be during labor. Here are some tips for mastering self-relaxation:

- Choose a quiet environment to practice.
- Turn on soft music, if desired.
- Assume a comfortable position with pillows to support you.
- Use slow, deep abdominal breathing. Feel the coolness of the air as you breathe in. Feel the tension carried away as you breathe out.
- Become aware of areas of tension in your body and concentrate on relaxing them.

With a natural pain relief technique called progressive relaxation, you relax groups of muscles in a series between or during your contractions or at periodic times during labor when you feel yourself becoming tense. Beginning with your head or feet, relax one muscle group at a time, moving toward the other end of your body. If you have trouble isolating the muscles, first tense each group for a few seconds, then release and feel the tension melt away. Pay particular attention to relaxing your jaw and hands; many women unconsciously tense up their faces and make fists during contractions.

Touch relaxation is a method similar to progressive relaxation. But your cue for releasing each muscle group is when your labor coach presses on that area of your body. He or she should apply firm pressure or rub using small circular movements for five to 10 seconds, then move on to the next spot. For example, your labor coach could start by rubbing your temples and then move on to touching the base of your skull, and then points on your back and shoulders, your arms and hands, and finally, your legs and feet.

Relaxation techniques can help you detect tension during labor and delivery so that you can better release it. But not everyone likes to be touched during labor. If you prefer not to be touched, have your labor coach give you verbal, rather than tactile, direction. For example, he or she may say to you in a calm, soothing voice, "I want you to relax your jaw muscles now." During your pregnancy, have your labor coach practice touch relaxation with you until your response to touch or command becomes automatic.

Massage

Various massage techniques — light or firm rhythmic stroking over your shoulders, neck, back, abdomen and legs; firm kneading, friction or pressure on your feet and hands; fingertip massage of your scalp — may help relax

WHAT'S A DOULA?

A doula is a woman who is specifically trained to be a labor coach. Women have been assisting one another through labor for centuries, but the role of the doula is a more formal and modern interpretation of the assisted birth. As you make decisions about pain relief, you may want to consider hiring a doula as part of your birth plan.

What do doulas do? A doula's main role is to help a pregnant woman through childbirth. A doula won't take the place of your labor coach or the medical experts caring for you during your labor and delivery. She is there to offer additional support and expertise. Most doulas are mothers themselves. In addition, doulas receive many hours of professional training in childbirth.

Some doulas become involved early on in your pregnancy, helping to educate you on what to expect during labor and delivery and to create a birth plan. If you request it, your doula can come to your home during early labor to coach you through your beginning contractions.

But the real work of doulas becomes evident at the hospital or birthing center. A doula can offer you — and your partner — continuous support once your labor has started. She can lend an extra hand, bringing you ice chips or massaging your back. She can help you with your breathing and relaxation techniques. She can advise you on labor positions. Most important, doulas provide both you and your partner with welcome words of encouragement and reassurance.

A doula can also serve as a mediator, helping you make educated decisions during labor. She can explain medical terms and procedures. She can indicate your wishes to your health care provider for you. However, doulas don't perform medical exams or assist in the actual birth.

you during labor. You can do some yourself, such as circular stroking over your abdomen during contractions. But most are better done by your labor coach, doula, midwife or nurse.

Massage can soothe aching and tense muscles, as well as stimulate your skin and deeper tissues. It can be used at any time during labor. The more skilled the massager is, the more likely that you'll find it soothing. If done properly, the effects of massage can last for a considerable time.

In addition to encouraging relaxation, massage blocks pain sensations. Some women feel most of the pain of labor in their backs, and for them a back massage given by a labor coach can really help. You may find yourself requesting that your labor coach push hard on your lower back, because counterpressure can be a very effective natural pain relief method for back labor.

Here are some back-massage techniques your labor coach might try:
1. Begin on the lower back, with hands on either side of the spine, and slowly move up to the shoulders. Slide hands across the shoulders, then down along the sides of the back. Gradually increase pressure, at the instruction of the recipient.

Doulas provide expectant parents with extra attention and care as they bring their new babies into the world. Doulas give emotional support, which may be important to the mother during childbirth. In fact, studies have shown that women who have the support of doulas tend to have fewer complications and fewer medical interventions during birth.

How do you find a doula? Your doctor or the hospital or birthing center where you plan on delivering may be able to provide you with a list of names. Some hospitals and birthing centers offer doula services. You can also contact Doulas of North America, an organization that promotes and trains doulas, at *www.dona.org* or at the group's toll-free number (888) 788-DONA, or (888) 788-3662. Most doulas charge a one-time fee for their services, and many base their fees on a sliding scale.

Before hiring a doula, meet with her to make sure that you're compatible. Ask her about her training and what her philosophies are about childbirth. Doulas shouldn't encourage or discourage pain relief during childbirth. The doula's role is to help you have the kind of birth experience you want to have, and one that's safe and satisfying. Some doulas even offer postpartum care, so you may want to ask whether that's included.

Doulas can be an especially good idea for first-time parents and single mothers. An alternative to a doula is to have a trusted friend or family member who has gone through labor be with you in the delivery room.

2. Move hands to the lower back. With fingers pointing outward and wrists about an inch apart, inhale. Exhale and gently press down. Inhale again and move the hands slightly lower on the back. Repeat, pressing with the exhale. Continue moving down the back.

3. Place thumbs about a half-inch to either side of the spine, at the small of the back. Press firmly, making small, slow, circular motions. Slowly move up the back to the neck. Then place the index finger at either side of the spine and draw a firm line down the back to the buttocks. Repeat.

4. To massage the neck and shoulders, rest the hands on the shoulders. Make circular motions — not squeezing or grasping motions — with the thumbs in the area between the upper back and lower neck. Then use gentle sweeping motions, hand over hand, from the arm to the neck.

Give your labor coach the following suggestions:
- Use oil or lotion to reduce friction against the skin.
- First warm the area to be massaged, for example with a hot pack.
- Try to keep one hand resting on the skin, even while changing massage techniques or while reaching for more oil or lotion. Moving the hands totally off and then back on the body may cause tension.

Before labor, you and your labor coach may want to work together to establish the kinds of massage you prefer. But keep in mind that things will go much better if everyone remains flexible during labor. You may assume that you'll want to be massaged in labor only to find it surprisingly uncomfortable.

Guided imagery

Guided imagery is a drug-free method of pain relief that helps laboring mothers create an environment with a feeling of relaxation and well-being. Sometimes called daydreaming with a purpose, this method can be used anytime during your labor to help you relax. It involves imagining yourself in a comfortable and peaceful place. For example, you may picture yourself sitting on a warm, sandy beach or walking through a lush, green forest. Your chosen place can be real or imaginary. As you relax, allow the details of this special place to unfold: the sounds, the smells, the feeling of wind on your face. Feel your body growing heavier and enjoy the sensation. Sometimes, you can enhance the imagery by playing tapes of surf, rain, waterfalls, birds in the woods or any soft music you enjoy.

Meditation

A type of meditation that involves focusing on a calming object, image or word can help relax you during labor and reduce the amount of pain you experience. Focus on a single point. This can be something in the room, such as a picture you have brought along, or it can be a mental image or a word you repeat to yourself over and over. When distracting thoughts come into your consciousness, allow them to pass by, without dwelling on them, and bring your focus back to your chosen focal point.

Positive affirmation

Remaining positive is important during the trials of labor and delivery. You may find it helpful and comforting to say positive, encouraging things to yourself, out loud or silently, as a means of coping with pain. You can also ask your labor coach, doula or partner to say them to you.

Some examples include:
- My body knows what to do.
- I'm relaxed and focused.
- I'm in rhythm with my body.
- I'm calm and confident.
- I'm strong, and I can push my baby out.
- I have the energy I need to get my baby out.

Breathing techniques

Breathing techniques, like other natural pain relief options, don't involve drugs or require medical supervision. You're in control. They involve the use of practiced, paced breathing during contractions and are another mainstay of self-comforting measures for labor.

Concentrating on your breathing during labor and delivery helps distract you from the pain and relaxes your muscles so that tension, which heightens pain, is eased. Deep, controlled, slow breathing can also reduce nausea and dizziness during childbirth. Most important, perhaps, concentrated breathing helps bring oxygen to you and your baby.

It's best to learn about and practice breathing techniques before you go into labor. Breathing methods, such as Lamaze, are taught in childbirth classes. Take your labor coach with you to class so that he or she can help you with the techniques during labor. The more you practice, the more natural it will be for you to use these methods once contractions begin.

Breathing exercises can work immediately, should you choose to use them during labor. Many women do. However, these methods aren't always successful because they depend on your reaction to labor pains, which can't be predicted, and on your ability to concentrate on something other than your labor pains. Breathing techniques can be combined with other types of pain relief.

Lamaze method

Lamaze is both a philosophy of childbirth and a breathing technique used in labor. The Lamaze philosophy holds that birth is a natural, normal, healthy process and women should be empowered through education and support to approach childbirth with confidence.

Lamaze classes focus on relaxation techniques, but they also encourage you to condition (program) your body's response to pain through training and practice. For example, you're taught controlled breathing exercises, which are a more constructive response to pain than are holding your breath and tensing up.

Lamaze instructors teach expectant mothers to take a deep, cleansing breath to begin and end each contraction: Inhale through your nose, imagining cool, pure air. Exhale slowly through your mouth, imagining tension blowing away. The deep breath signals to everyone in the labor room that a contraction is beginning or ending and is a signal for your body to relax.

Different levels of Lamaze breathing are used in labor and delivery, as outlined below. When you're using this method, start with the first breathing technique and use it as long as it works for you, then move on to the next level. Again, these methods are taught in childbirth classes:

Lamaze level 1: Slow-paced breathing
This is the type of breathing you use when you're relaxed or sleeping. Take in slow, deep breaths through your nose and exhale through your mouth at about half the speed of your normal rate. If you like, repeat a phrase with the breathing: "I am (inhaling) relaxed (exhaling)," or "In one-two-three (inhaling), out one-two-three (exhaling)." Or breathe in rhythm while walking or rocking.

Lamaze level 2: Modified-pace breathing
Breathe faster than your normal rate but shallowly enough to prevent hyperventilation: "In one-two (inhaling), out one-two [exhaling], in one-two [inhaling], out one-two (exhaling)." Keep your body, particularly your jaw, relaxed. Concentrate on the rhythm, which may be faster at the height of the contraction, then slower as it fades.

Lamaze level 3: Pattern-pace breathing
Use this type near the end of labor or at the height of strong contractions. The rate is a little faster than normal, as with modified-pace breathing, but now you use a pant-blow rhythm such as "ha-ha-ha-hoo" or "hee-hee-hee-hoo" that forces you to focus on the breathing rather than the pain. Repeat the pattern. Start slowly. Increase the speed as each contraction peaks and decrease as it fades. Keep in mind that when you increase the rate, the

breathing should become shallower so that you don't hyperventilate — if your hands or feet tingle, slow down. There's some concern that hyperventilation can decrease oxygen supply to the baby. If moaning or making other noises helps, go ahead. Keep your eyes open and focused and your muscles relaxed.

Breathing to prevent pushing
If you feel the urge to push but your health care provider says your cervix isn't fully dilated and you must hold back, blow out tiny puffs with your cheeks — as if you're blowing out birthday candles — until the urge to push passes.

Breathing for pushing
When your cervix is fully dilated and your health care provider tells you to go ahead and push, take a couple of deep breaths and bear down when you feel the urge. Push for about 10 seconds. Exhale. Then take in another breath and push again. Contractions at this stage will last for a minute or more, so it's important that you inhale at regular intervals and don't hold your breath.

Your personal preferences and the nature of your contractions will guide you in deciding when to use breathing exercises in your labor. You can choose breathing techniques or even invent one on your own. Even if you plan on having pain medication during labor, it's still important to learn breathing and relaxation techniques.

Changing positions

Moving about freely during labor allows you to find the most comfortable positions. So, if possible, change positions frequently, experimenting to find the ones most comfortable for you.

Changing positions during labor is actually a natural method of pain relief. Moving helps improve your circulation. It can also help distract you from the pain. It may even help a slow labor progress.

Try a new position whenever you feel like it, and if it's possible, throughout your labor. For example, you may want to try standing and leaning on your labor coach or getting on all fours while your labor coach massages your back. You may find it helpful to lean on a chair, bed or pillows for support. If you need help finding a comfortable position, ask your health care team to suggest positions for you to try.

Some women find that rhythmic movements, such as rocking in a rocking chair or rocking back and forth on their hands and knees, can be soothing and a distraction from pain.

Heat and cold

Applying heat or cold, or both, can be a soothing, natural pain reliever in labor. The goal of applying heat or cold is to make you more comfortable so that you can better relax.

Heat relieves muscle tension. It can be applied through a heating pad, a warm towel, a hot compress, a hot water bottle or a heated rice-filled pack or sock. You can apply heat to your shoulders, lower abdomen or back to relieve pain. As you near the time to push, you may find it comforting to place a warm blanket over your body if you're trembling, or a hot compress on the area between your vagina and anus (perineum).

Cold can be applied with a cold pack, a chilled soda can or a baggie filled with ice. Some women like a cold pack on their lower back to help relieve back pain. You may find that a cool, moistened washcloth on your face helps ease tension and cools you during labor. Sucking on ice chips also can help to cool you and create a distracting sensation in your mouth.

You may want to use a combination of heat and cold to relieve pain naturally during labor. For example, a hot water bottle alternated with a washcloth soaked in cold water can reduce backache or cramping.

If you apply heat or cold to your skin, don't overdo it. You don't want to burn or freeze your skin.

Shower or bath

Many hospitals and birthing centers have showers in their labor rooms. Some even have bathtubs or whirlpool baths to help ease the discomforts of labor, particularly those of active labor when your contractions are intensifying. The soothing, warm water helps relieve pain naturally by blocking pain impulses to your brain. Warm water is also relaxing. This is a method of pain relief you can try at home, too, before heading to the hospital or birthing center.

If you use a shower, you can sit in a chair and direct water onto your back or abdomen with a hand-held showerhead. Ask your labor coach to bring a bathing suit and join you.

Aromatherapy

To trigger relaxation and ease pain naturally during labor, try using comforting smells. When you're home, light a scented candle or burn incense. When you're at the hospital or birthing center, bring along a pillow scented with your favorite fragrance. Or have your labor coach use a lightly scented oil or lotion when massaging you. Aromatherapy may relax you and reduce stress and tension. However, being in labor can make you sensitive to certain smells, so don't go overboard with fragrances. Simple scents, such as lavender, are probably best.

Music

Music can be a natural pain reliever. It can focus your attention on something other than your pain and help you relax during childbirth. If you've been practicing relaxation techniques or breathing methods to music at home, bring the same cassette tapes or compact discs with you to the hospital or birthing center, or use them during a home birth. Many women use a portable music player to listen to their favorite music during labor and to tune out other distractions.

Birthing ball

A birthing ball is a large rubber ball and tool of natural childbirth. Leaning or sitting on the ball can decrease the discomfort of your contractions, relieve the pain of back labor and aid in the descent of your baby into the birth canal. Your hospital or birthing center may provide one for you. Or you may need to purchase one and bring it with you. Have someone on your health care team show you how to get the most out of a birthing ball. Its use can be combined with massage and touch relaxation.

Other natural pain relief methods

Research continues to find other methods of pain relief that don't involve medication and are safe for both you and your baby. Some examples include hypnosis, acupuncture, reflexology and a procedure called transcutaneous electrical nerve stimulation (TENS), which uses electrical impulses to try to control pain.

If you're considering using any of the following more nontraditional methods of natural pain relief, you may need to arrange for a qualified practitioner to be with you throughout your labor to ensure everything is done correctly. These all may help relax you and reduce pain, or they may distract you from pain during labor. However, the effects may vary. A common feature of nontraditional techniques is the lack of scientific evidence of their effectiveness. With the help of an expert, you may choose to try:

Hypnosis
This works by suggestion — if you believe that you can control the pain, you may be less disturbed by it. Through self-hypnosis, some women are able to achieve deep relaxation during labor and delivery. Self-hypnosis is

taught privately or in specialized childbirth classes. Often, you use audio-tapes for practice and in labor. With this method, you begin self-hypnosis in early labor and continue it for as long as it helps.

Acupuncture

In this method of natural pain relief, an acupuncturist inserts small needles into specific body points to relieve pain. If you're considering acupuncture for pain relief during labor, look for an acupuncturist experienced in using the method on women who are going through labor and delivery.

Reflexology

This method involves applying pressure to specific points on your feet to relieve pain and muscular problems in other parts of your body. Again, look for a therapist — in this case, a reflexologist — who is experienced in using this method on women who are going through labor and delivery. If reflex-ology interests you, you may want to research it on your own. Your labor coach may be able to learn and apply the techniques, to go beyond simply massaging your feet during labor and delivery.

TENS

TENS is performed with the aid of a hand-held, battery-operated device with wires that attach to your body by adhesive pads. The small pads are usually placed on your lower back. When you feel a contraction starting, you press a button on the device's handset. The machine then delivers mild electrical impulses through the wires and pads and through your skin. By electrically stimulating nerves in your lower back, the device helps block the transmission of pain impulses to your brain. The electrical impulses aren't painful. You'll feel a mild tingling sensation, which you may find comforting.

Most hospitals and birthing centers don't have a TENS machine on hand. If you decide to try it, you'll likely have to rent your own set from a hospital supply company and take it with you when you first go into labor. Because TENS is used to treat chronic pain, you may be able to borrow or rent a device from the physical therapy department of a hospital.

The choice is yours

The decision of whether to have pain relief medications during labor is largely up to you. Discuss the topic of pain relief with your health care provider long before your labor begins. Become familiar with natural pain relief methods and consider using them first, if possible, or use them in con-junction with medication.

If during your labor you feel the need for medication, don't insist on it immediately. Try holding out for 15 minutes or longer and putting that time to good use, concentrating hard on your relaxation and breathing techniques and taking in all the comfort your labor coach can give you. You may find that with a little support, you can handle the pain. If not, you know you have pain relief options available to you.

Remember, too, that once your baby is born and you're holding him or her, the experience will have all been worth it!

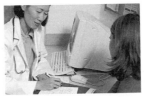

considering vaginal birth after Caesarean birth

In your last pregnancy, your baby was delivered by Caesarean. Can you have a vaginal birth this time?

Maybe. It used to be that once you had a Caesarean birth, all your subsequent deliveries would be by Caesarean as well. Now, vaginal birth after Caesarean birth (VBAC) is possible in many cases.

But it's not without risk. Several factors must be considered before you and your health care provider decide to try VBAC or to arrange a repeat Caesarean.

Women who choose VBAC go through labor. It's the same process that any woman having her child vaginally goes through. You wait for the first signs of labor and then head to the hospital. A home delivery should not be attempted with VBAC.

At the hospital, it's important that you have a doctor and hospital staff closely monitor your active labor. They can be ready to perform a Caesarean birth if necessary. Between 60 percent and 80 percent of women who start through labor have a successful vaginal birth. If the labor isn't successful, a Caesarean birth is performed.

Potential benefits of having a vaginal birth after a Caesarean birth
One advantage to having a vaginal birth is that it's generally safer than a Caesarean because it doesn't involve major surgery. Other advantages of a vaginal birth include:

- Fewer blood transfusions
- Lower risk of infection
- Shorter hospital stay — one to two days instead of three or more days
- More energy after childbirth
- A faster return to normal activities

In addition, you may feel more involved in the delivery process during a vaginal birth because of your efforts to push the baby out. Your labor coach and others may be able to play a larger role in a vaginal delivery.

Potential risks of having a vaginal birth after a Caesarean birth
The possible risks of having a VBAC include:

- Failure to deliver vaginally. This may increase the risk of infection for you and your baby. You may also feel emotionally and physically drained after going through labor and being unable to deliver the child vaginally. A small number of women feel that they have failed, even though events were beyond their control.
- Tearing of the scar from your previous Caesarean birth, called a uterine rupture. The risk of this is typically low in women who choose VBAC. It's largely dependent on the type of uterine incision you received during your first Caesarean birth. But a uterine rupture can cause excessive bleeding and may be life-threatening to you and your baby. Your baby's nervous system may be damaged. In addition, you may need to undergo a hysterectomy if you have a uterine rupture. If you're at high risk of a uterine rupture, your health care provider will probably recommend that you have a repeat Caesarean delivery.

Issues to consider

Are you a good candidate for a vaginal birth after a Caesarean birth (VBAC)? It depends mainly on the type of uterine incision used during your initial Caesarean birth and the reasons you had a Caesarean birth.

Type of incision

During a Caesarean birth, your health care provider creates two incisions. One is in your abdomen, and one is in your uterus. The incision in your abdomen goes through skin, fat and muscles. From this opening, your surgeon makes the incision in your uterus. The incision in your uterus is different from the incision in your abdomen. You can't tell what kind of uterine incision you've had just by looking at your belly. Instead, to find out which type you had, check with your health care provider or look at your medical records.

The three types of uterine incisions are as follows:

- **A low transverse incision** is the most common type. It's made horizontally across the lower portion of the uterus. It usually bleeds less than an incision made higher on the uterus. It also tends to form a stronger scar and presents less danger of rupture during subsequent labors — between a 0.2 percent and 1.5 percent chance. If you have had one or even two of these incisions, you may be a candidate for VBAC.
- **A low vertical incision** is made low on the uterus, where the uterine wall is thinner. It may be used to deliver a baby in an awkward position

or when the doctor thinks that the incision may need to be extended. A low vertical incision presents a slightly higher risk of uterine rupture — 1 percent to 7 percent. But if you've had this type of incision, you may still be a candidate for VBAC.

- **A classical incision,** also called a high vertical incision, is made higher up on the uterus, on the rounded portion. This type of incision was once used for all Caesarean births but is now rare. Because a classical incision is associated with the highest risk of bleeding and of subsequent rupture of the uterus — 4 percent to 9 percent — it's used only in emergency situations. VBAC is not recommended for women who have had a classical uterine incision.

Reasons for a previous Caesarean birth

The causes behind your first Caesarean birth tend to have an influence over a trial of labor afterward:

- If your first Caesarean was performed for a reason that may not necessarily recur, your chance of having a successful vaginal delivery is the same as that of a woman who has never had a Caesarean birth. Examples include an infection, pregnancy-induced high blood pressure (preeclampsia), placental problems and fetal distress.
- If you've had at least one vaginal delivery either before or after your Caesarean birth, you're more likely to have a successful VBAC than is someone who hasn't had a vaginal delivery.
- If you've previously had a difficult labor because of the size of your child or the small size of your pelvis (dystocia), you may still have a successful VBAC. But the chances are somewhat lower than if you had a Caesarean birth for a nonrecurring condition.
- If you have a chronic medical condition where problems may arise again during labor and delivery, you and your health care provider may decide on a repeat Caesarean.

Who might not be a candidate for a VBAC?

In some cases, a repeat Caesarean birth is a better option than VBAC. According to the American College of Obstetricians and Gynecologists, labor should not be attempted in the following situations:

- You have a prior classical or T-shaped incision or another simular type of uterine surgery
- Your pelvic opening is too narrow to allow a baby's head to pass through
- You have a medical or obstetric problem that precludes vaginal delivery
- You're at a facility that can't perform emergency Caesarean birth

Medical experts disagree on whether to attempt labor in these circumstances:
- You've had more than two previous Caesarean births
- You have an unknown uterine scar
- You're carrying more than one baby
- You're more than two weeks past your due date
- Your health care provider suspects that your baby is larger than normal

In these situations, your best bet is to discuss with your health care provider the potential risks and benefits associated with your particular case.

Tips for planning a vaginal birth after a Caesarean birth

Most women who've undergone a previous Caesarean are candidates for a vaginal birth after a Caesarean birth (VBAC). Yet in 2000, only about 20 percent of eligible women went through with it. Given that the success rate is 60 percent to 80 percent, why don't more women choose VBAC?

Part of the reason may be women's fears of the possibility of a long, protracted delivery that ends in surgery. Another possible reason is that not all women have access to facilities that are prepared to handle VBACs.

If you and your health care provider think that VBAC is right for you, don't be afraid to try it. Although it's impossible to predict if a VBAC will be successful, you can increase your chances of a positive experience. Try these ideas:

- Discuss your fears and expectations of an attempt at VBAC with your health care provider. He or she can help you better understand the process and how you may be affected. If you have doubts about your health care provider, you may wish to find another whom you find easier to trust and rely on. Make sure your current health care provider has your complete medical history, including records of your initial Caesarean birth.
- Take a class on VBAC, with your labor coach, if possible. These classes often help you work through concerns you may have about VBAC.
- Plan to have your VBAC at a well-equipped hospital. Look for one that has continuous fetal monitoring, a surgical team that can be assembled quickly and the ability to administer anesthetics and blood transfusions 24 hours a day.
- Try to avoid the use of drugs to induce labor, especially if the cervix is tightly closed and not ready for labor. These drugs can make contractions stronger and more frequent and may contribute to the risk of uterine rupture.
- Make sure your health care provider will be available to you throughout labor. Constant monitoring by your health care provider can decrease the risk of complications.

- Think of yourself as an athlete preparing for an event. Positive thinking, a healthy diet, regular exercise and plenty of rest will help you give your best shot at labor and delivery.
- Keep your ultimate goal in mind. You want a healthy baby and mom, regardless of how you get there.

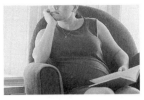

DECISION GUIDE

exploring
elective Caesarean birth

For reasons ranging from safety to convenience, some women choose to have a planned Caesarean birth rather than to deliver vaginally. This is called an elective Caesarean birth.

In an elective Caesarean birth, the baby is surgically removed from the abdomen, usually before the woman goes into labor. This procedure is done according to the woman's choice and not necessarily for medical reasons.

Issues to consider

Elective Caesarean birth is a controversial topic. Those in favor of it say that a woman has a right to choose how she wants to deliver her child. Those against it say that the risks of Caesarean birth outweigh any potential benefits. A verdict based on medical evidence hasn't been reached because the procedure hasn't been studied enough.

Because the procedure is controversial, you might find that health care providers' opinions on this subject are quite varied. Some may be willing to consider it. Others may not, believing that an elective Caesarean birth may be harmful and therefore against their pledge to do no harm.

You may wish to talk to your health care provider about an elective Caesarean birth if you've had difficulty with labor and delivery in the past. Be sure to discuss all of the risks and benefits with your health care provider. He or she can assess your medical history, the state of your pregnancy and the most current medical information.

The best way to make a decision — especially on a controversial issue — is to be as informed as possible about both sides of the issue. Learn the advantages and disadvantages of elective Caesarean birth. If possible, talk to other women who have had Caesarean births. Find someone who has had an elective Caesarean birth because a woman's experience of an emergency

Caesarean birth may not be similar to that of a woman who has had an elective procedure. Also talk to women who have had vaginal births. Then work with your health care provider to make the best decision for you and your child.

Potential risks of elective Caesarean birth

Some say that with advances in surgical techniques, elective Caesarean births are virtually as safe as vaginal deliveries. Others argue that they still carry the risk of more complications than do vaginal births.

Some of the possible risks of elective Caesarean birth for you include:

- **Maternal death.** Death as a result of pregnancy or labor is rare, whether you have a vaginal or Caesarean birth. But Caesarean birth may carry more than twice the risk of vaginal birth, although the rate of Caesarean-related maternal death has been decreasing over the last decade. Some studies now call even this rate into question, suggesting that it may be equal to or lower than the risk associated with vaginal birth. In addition, a planned Caesarean birth has a lower death rate than an emergency Caesarean.
- **Long-term risks.** Women who have had a previous Caesarean birth are at an increased risk of placental problems in subsequent pregnancies. This may complicate later pregnancies. It may lead to removal of your uterus (hysterectomy) and even death. A previous Caesarean birth may also increase your risk of uterine rupture, especially if you decide to try a vaginal birth after Caesarean birth (VBAC). Multiple pregnancies tend to increase the risk of complications with each successive pregnancy. Multiple Caesarean births increase your risk even more.
- **Operative risks.** Because Caesarean birth is a major surgery, it carries higher risks of infection, blood loss and injury. Blood loss during a Caesarean birth can be twice that associated with a vaginal birth. About 3 percent of the time, the mother needs a blood transfusion after a Caesarean birth.

  The medications used during surgery, including those used for anesthesia, can sometimes cause unexpected responses, such as breathing problems. Most planned Caesareans are done with spinal or epidural anesthesia, which numbs your body from the chest down. Another option is general anesthesia, which causes you to be unconscious. Use of general anesthesia can sometimes lead to pneumonia, and it poses a small risk of you vomiting and breathing the vomit into your lungs. However, general anesthesia is usually used only in emergency situations, when the baby needs to be delivered as quickly as possible.

  After delivery, women who had a Caesarean birth are more likely to have an infection of the mucous membrane lining the uterus (endometritis) or a blood clot. Some studies suggest that women who undergo Caesarean birth may be more likely to end up back in the hospital after childbirth.

- **Decreased ability to breast-feed after delivery.** Within the first few hours after delivery, you may not be able to breast-feed or do much with your child. But this is temporary. You'll have plenty of time to feed and bond with your child when you've recovered.

In addition to the risks listed here, Caesarean birth has the added drawback of being generally more expensive than a vaginal delivery. You may wish to check with your insurance company to see if it covers elective Caesarean births.

Some of the possible risks of a Caesarean birth for your baby include:

- **Premature birth.** If the gestational age of your baby hasn't been estimated correctly, your baby may be delivered a week or two prematurely. This can lead to breathing difficulties, low birth weight and other problems.
- **Transient tachypnea.** One of the more common risks to a baby after a Caesarean birth is a mild respiratory difficulty called transient tachypnea. This condition occurs when the baby's lungs are too wet. While your baby is in the uterus, his or her lungs are normally filled with fluid. During a vaginal birth, movement through the birth canal naturally squeezes the baby's chest and pushes the fluid out of the lungs. During a Caesarean birth, the squeezing effect isn't present, so your baby's lungs may still contain fluid after birth. This results in rapid breathing and usually requires additional oxygen delivered under pressure to get the fluid out. The condition usually goes away within a few hours or days.
- **Effects of anesthesia.** Occasionally, anesthesia-induced low blood pressure (hypotension) in the mother may cause decreased oxygen delivery to the baby, resulting in increased acidity in the baby's blood. This condition is usually temporary. With general anesthesia, some of the medication reaches the baby, which can result in depression in the baby's breathing. If necessary, the baby can be given medications to counteract the effects of the anesthesia.
- **Cuts.** Rarely, a baby may be cut during a Caesarean birth.
- **Future risk of stillbirth.**

Potential benefits of elective Caesarean birth

Some of the possible benefits for you that may come with an elective Caesarean birth include:

- **Potential protection of your pelvic muscles.** During a vaginal birth, the effort of pushing your baby out may weaken or damage pelvic muscles or cause injury to pelvic nerves. The resulting damage can lead to urinary or fecal incontinence. Less commonly, it may lead to pelvic organ prolapse, a condition where organs such as your bladder protrude into the vaginal canal.

    Usually, urinary incontinence caused by pregnancy and labor goes away within three months. But some women have permanent damage.

At times, signs and symptoms of weakened pelvic muscles may not show up until years after childbirth. Factors that may increase your risk of pelvic muscle injury include a surgical incision to widen the vaginal opening for birth (episiotomy), large tears during labor and a forceps or vacuum-assisted delivery.

Having a Caesarean birth doesn't guarantee that you won't have incontinence problems. The weight of the baby during pregnancy also may weaken your pelvic muscles. Even women who have never had babies sometimes develop incontinence problems.

A 2003 study of more than 15,000 women found that 10 percent of women who had never had children reported signs and symptoms of incontinence during their lives. This rate increased to 16 percent of women who had all Caesarean deliveries and 21 percent of women who had all vaginal deliveries. Results for women with elective and nonelective Caesarean births were similar. When looking at women age 50 to 64, there was no difference in the rate of incontinence between women who had vaginal deliveries and those women who had Caesarean deliveries.

Women may use Kegel exercises during and after pregnancy to try to strengthen their pelvic muscles and prevent incontinence problems.

- **Avoidance of emergency Caesarean birth.** An emergency Caesarean birth, which is often conducted after a difficult labor that hasn't progressed, has higher risks than both an elective Caesarean and a vaginal birth.
- **Avoidance of difficult labor.** A difficult labor may lead to forceps or vacuum-assisted delivery. These methods usually don't pose a problem. But instrument-assisted deliveries that fail are associated with a higher risk of infant injuries.
- **Greater ease in scheduling.** Scheduling a Caesarean birth may allow you to be better prepared for childbirth. Scheduling may also ease demands on your medical caregiving team, helping to prevent fatigue and inadequate staff levels.

Some of the reduced risks to your baby may include:

- **Fewer childbirth problems.** A planned Caesarean birth may reduce certain rare childbirth problems. It may reduce labor-related infant death, shoulder dystocia, birth injury, which is a particular concern for high-risk women who have large babies, and breathing in of meconium, which occurs when a baby inhales fecal waste during childbirth. The events of labor also carry a very small risk of cerebral palsy.
- **Reduced risk of infectious disease transmission.** With elective Caesarean birth, there may be a reduction in mother-to-child transmission of infectious diseases such as the AIDS virus, hepatitis B, hepatitis C, herpes and human papillomavirus.

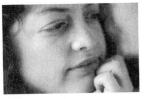

considering circumcision for your son

If you have a baby boy, one of the decisions you may face soon after birth is whether to have him circumcised. Circumcision is a surgical procedure performed to remove the skin covering the tip of the penis. Knowing about the procedure's potential health benefits and risks can help you make an informed decision.

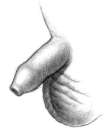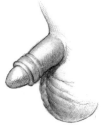

Before circumcision (left), the foreskin of the penis extends over the end of the penis (glans). After the brief operation, the glans is exposed (right).

Issues to consider

Although circumcision is fairly common in the United States, it's still controversial. There's some evidence that circumcision may have medical benefits. But the procedure also has risks. The American Academy of Pediatrics doesn't currently recommend routine circumcision of all male newborns, saying there isn't enough evidence of benefit.

Consider your own cultural, religious and social values in making this decision. For some people, such as those of the Jewish or Islamic faith, circumcision is a religious ritual. For others, it's a matter of personal hygiene or preventive health care. Some parents may not want their son to look different from his family members or peers.

Some people feel strongly that circumcision is disfiguring to the baby's normal appearance. Some feel it's wrong to circumcise a boy when he's too young to consent. Still others feel that circumcision is unnecessary.

As you decide what's best for you and your son, consider these potential health benefits and risks.

Potential benefits of circumcision

Some research suggests that circumcision has health benefits, including:

- **Decreased risk of urinary tract infections (UTIs).** Although the risk of UTIs in the first year is low, various studies suggest that UTIs may be as much as 10 times more common in uncircumcised baby boys than in those who are circumcised. Uncircumcised boys are also more likely to be admitted to the hospital for a severe UTI during the first three months of life. Severe UTIs early in life can lead to kidney problems later on.
- **Decreased risk of cancer of the penis.** Although this type of cancer is very rare, circumcised men show a lower incidence of cancer of the penis than do uncircumcised men.
- **Slightly decreased risk of sexually transmitted diseases (STDs).** Some studies have shown a lower risk of human immunodeficiency virus (HIV) and human papillomavirus (HPV) infections in circumcised men. Still, safe sexual practices are much more important in the prevention of STDs than is circumcision.
- **Prevention of penile problems.** Occasionally, the foreskin on an uncircumcised penis may narrow to the point where it's difficult or impossible to retract, a condition called phimosis. Circumcision may then be

How is circumcision done?

If you decide to have your son circumcised, ask your son's health care provider for advice on whether circumcision is permissible or advisable. Your son's doctor can also answer questions about the procedure and help you make arrangements at your hospital or clinic.

Usually, circumcision is done before you and your son leave the hospital. At times, circumcision is done in an outpatient setting. The procedure itself takes about 15 minutes. It's generally done before the morning feeding.

Typically, the baby lies on a tray with his arms and legs restrained. After the penis and surrounding area are cleansed, an anesthetic is injected into the base of the penis. A special clamp or plastic ring is attached to the penis, and the foreskin is cut away. An ointment, such as petroleum jelly, is applied. The penis is then wrapped loosely with gauze.

After circumcision, it's OK to wash the penis while it's healing. In the first week, there may be a yellowish mucus on the skin, but this is normal. Apply petroleum jelly to the tip of the penis to keep it from sticking to the diaper. It takes about seven to 10 days for the penis to heal.

Problems after circumcision are very rare. But call your baby's doctor immediately if your baby isn't urinating normally, if there's persistent bleeding or if you suspect an infection.

needed to treat the problem. A narrowed foreskin can also lead to inflammation of the head of the penis (balanitis).

- **Ease of hygiene.** Circumcision makes it easy to wash the penis. But even if the foreskin is intact, it's easy to keep clean. Normally the foreskin adheres to the end of the penis in a newborn, then gradually stretches back during early childhood. Simply wash your baby's genital area gently with soap and water. Later, when the foreskin fully retracts, your son can learn to wash it properly by gently pulling the foreskin back and cleansing the tip of the penis with soap and water.

Potential risks of circumcision

In general, circumcision is considered to be a safe procedure, and the risks related to it are minor. Several studies found the overall complication rate of circumcision to be around 0.2 percent. Circumcision does have some risks and possible drawbacks, including:

- **Risks of minor surgery.** All surgical procedures, including circumcision, carry certain risks, such as excessive bleeding and infection. There's also the possibility that the foreskin may be cut too short or too long, or that it doesn't heal properly. If the remaining foreskin reattaches on the end of the penis, a minor surgery may be needed to correct it. These occurrences are uncommon.
- **Pain during the procedure.** Circumcision does cause pain. Typically a local anesthesia is used to block the nerve sensations. Talk to your doctor about what type of anesthesia might be used.
- **Difficult to undo.** Following most circumcisions, it would be difficult to recreate the appearance to look uncircumcised.
- **Cost.** Some insurance companies don't cover the cost of circumcision. If you're considering circumcision, you may wish to check whether your insurance company will cover it.
- **Complicating factors.** Sometimes, circumcision may need to be postponed, such as if your baby is born prematurely. In some situations, circumcision shouldn't be done. That may be the case when the baby's urethral opening is in an abnormal position on the side or base of the penis (hypospadias). This condition is treated surgically and may require the foreskin for repair. Other conditions that may prevent circumcision include an illness with high fever, ambiguous genitalia, or a family history of hemophilia.

Circumcision doesn't affect fertility or prevent masturbation. Whether it enhances or detracts from sexual pleasure for men or their partners hasn't been proved. Research on circumcision is ongoing. More studies are needed to verify some of the claims made about the procedure. The good news is that whatever your choice, negative outcomes are rare and mostly minor.

Circumcision care

If your newborn boy was circumcised, the tip of his penis may seem raw for the first week after the procedure. Or a yellowish mucus or crust may form around the area. This is a normal part of healing. A small amount of bleeding is also common the first day or two.

Clean the diaper area gently and apply a dab of petroleum jelly to the end of the penis with each diaper change. This will keep the diaper from sticking while the penis heals. If there's a bandage, change it with each diapering. Sometimes a plastic ring is used instead of a bandage. The ring will remain on the end of the penis until the edge of the circumcision has healed, usually within a week. The ring will drop off on its own. It's OK to wash the penis as it's healing.

Problems after a circumcision are rare. But call your baby's health care provider in the following situations:

- Your baby doesn't urinate normally within six to eight hours after the circumcision.
- Bleeding or redness around the tip of the penis is persistent.
- The penis tip is swollen.
- A foul-smelling drainage comes from the penis tip or there are crusted sores that contain fluid.

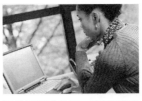

DECISION GUIDE

choosing your baby's health care provider

While you're shopping for cribs, baby blankets and booties, don't forget to shop around for one other essential item — your baby's health care provider.

It's a good idea to choose your baby's health care provider before your child is born. Often, the provider you choose will come to the hospital to check on your baby.

With the provider in place, you'll know in advance where and when to bring your baby in for his or her first checkup. You'll have someone you can call with any questions regarding newborn care — and most first-time parents have lots of questions. Plus, it gives you one less thing to worry about after the baby is born.

Where to start

If you don't already have a health care provider in mind, ask for recommendations from friends or family members who have children. Find out why they like their health care provider and how that may apply to your situation. Your pregnancy health care provider may also be an excellent referral source.

If you've just moved to the area or you want to do some research on your own, the following resources may be helpful:

- Nearby general or pediatric hospitals
- Local medical societies
- Medical directories at your local library
- The local yellow pages
- The Internet. The following Web sites may help you find a medical care provider near you:
  - American Academy of Pediatrics, "Pediatrician Referral Service" *www.aap.org/referral*

- American Academy of Family Physicians, "Find a Family Doctor" *www.familydoctor.org*
- National Nurse Practitioner Directory, "Search for a Nurse Practitioner" *www.nurse.net/cgi-fin/start.cgi/referral/search.html*

Types of providers

Basically, three types of health care providers are qualified to care for children: family physicians, pediatricians and pediatric nurse practitioners.

Family physicians

Family physicians provide health care for people of all ages, including children. They are trained in various areas of medicine, including pediatrics. After going through medical school, they complete a three-year residency program. There, they gain experience in hospital and outpatient medical care. Family physicians take care of most medical problems. They can also refer your child for specialized care if the need arises.

A family physician can see your child from babyhood all the way through adulthood. Also, if the rest of your family sees the same physician, your doctor will gain an overall perspective of your family. That picture may be missed in other health care provider arrangements.

If you already have a family doctor you trust, ask whether he or she will see infants. Some don't see many infants. Others see children only after they have reached a certain age. If your family doctor isn't available for your baby, he or she may be able to suggest a suitable health care provider.

Pediatricians

Pediatricians specialize in the care of children from infancy through adolescence. After medical school, they go through a three-year residency program. There, they focus on preventive health care for children and other aspects of pediatrics. Some pediatricians receive further training in subspecialties such as allergies, infectious disease, cardiology and psychiatry.

Many parents choose pediatricians to care for their children's health because caring for children is what they are trained to do. A pediatrician can be particularly helpful if your child has a health condition or needs special medical attention.

Pediatric nurse practitioners

Nurse practitioners are registered nurses with advanced training in a specialized area of medicine, such as pediatrics or family health. After nursing school, a nurse practitioner must go through a formal education program in his or her specialty field. Most have at least a master's degree. A typical program combines instruction in nursing theory with intense clinical experience under the supervision of a physician or experienced nurse practitioner. A pediatric nurse practitioner focuses on caring for infants, children and teens.

A pediatric nurse practitioner's main goal is to provide your child with primary care, such as maintaining your child's health, preventing disease and helping you and your child learn how to care for yourselves. Most pediatric nurse practitioners can prescribe medications and order medical tests. They work closely with physicians and medical specialists in hospitals, clinics or family practices and can call on them if a more complex health issue arises.

Some parents may feel uncomfortable choosing a pediatric nurse practitioner as a health care provider for their child because of what they see as a lack of training or expertise. But a pediatric nurse practitioner can be a good choice for primary care. In fact, a large study published in 2000 in the *Journal of the American Medical Association* found no significant differences in health outcomes or overall satisfaction rates between people cared for by nurse practitioners and people cared for by physicians. In addition, parents may find that nurse practitioners place a greater emphasis on answering questions and addressing any potential concerns. Their fees also tend to be less than those of physicians.

Issues to consider

No matter what type of provider you choose, it's important that you feel comfortable with that person. He or she will play an important role in your family. With that in mind, you may want to choose a provider who shares some of the same philosophies about parenting, including such topics as breast-feeding, immunizations and general health care.

You may wish to meet with several health care providers before having your baby. Most don't charge a fee for a preliminary interview, but some may. Some factors you may wish to explore include:

- What are the health care provider's professional qualifications?
- How do you rate his or her bedside manner?
- How accessible is your health care provider, either by phone or by appointment? For example, how far in advance will you need to schedule appointments?
- Who will respond to your calls both during and after office hours?
- How likely is it that you can see the health care provider for an emergency? Is there a contingency plan when your provider isn't available?
- If your baby required admission to the hospital, which hospital would

the health care provider use? Would that person care for your child in the hospital, or refer you to others for inpatient pediatric care?
- Is the office staff courteous and helpful?
- Is the office clean and inviting for children?
- What are the costs to you and your insurance company? Will the health care provider's office file insurance claims? If you're in a managed health care plan, check with your insurance company to see if your preferred provider is a participant in the plan's network.

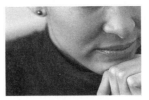

the breast or the bottle?

Do you plan to feed your baby with breast milk or formula?

A great deal of scientific evidence supports the idea that breast milk is best for babies. And many new moms hear the message. According to the Department of Health and Human Services, 65 percent of new mothers in the United States initiate breast-feeding. At six months, almost one-third are still breast-feeding their babies.

For a variety of reasons, other women choose to feed their babies with formula. Today's commercial formulas ensure that babies can be well nourished with bottle-feeding.

No matter whether you choose the breast or bottle, the first few weeks with your newborn are likely to be demanding and exhausting. Both you and your baby are adapting to an entirely new reality, and that takes time.

Throughout this adjustment, remember that feeding your newborn is about more than the nourishment. It's a time of cuddling and closeness that helps build the connection between you and your baby. Whether you feed by breast or bottle, make every feeding a time to bond with your baby. Stroke his or her skin while maintaining eye contact. Find a quiet place to feed the child, where you're both less likely to be distracted. Cherish the time before your baby is old enough to start feeding himself or herself. That time will come soon enough.

Issues to consider

If you're undecided about whether to breast-feed or bottle-feed, consider these questions:

- Does your or your baby's health care provider suggest one or the other? If you or your baby has health problems, discuss how that may affect your decision about how to feed your baby.
- Do you have a solid understanding of both methods? Learn as much as you can about feeding your baby. Seek out a perinatal educator, a lactation consultant or other health care provider.

- Do you plan to return to work? If so, how does that affect your decision? What accommodations are available or can be made for you to express milk at work, if that's your plan?
- How does your partner feel about the decision?
- How have other mothers you trust and respect made their decisions? If they had it to do over again, would they make the same choices?

The facts on breast-feeding

Breast milk has many known benefits. The longer you breast-feed, the greater these benefits are to you and your baby and, in many cases, the longer they last.

Breast milk provides babies with:

- **Ideal nutrition.** Breast milk has just the right nutrients, in just the right amounts, to nourish your baby completely. It contains the fats, proteins, carbohydrates, vitamins and minerals that a baby needs for growth, digestion and brain development. Breast milk is also individualized; the composition of your breast milk changes as your baby grows.
- **Protection against disease.** Research shows that breast milk may help keep your baby from getting sick. It provides antibodies that help your baby's immune system fight off common childhood illnesses. Breast-fed babies tend to have fewer colds, ear infections and urinary tract infections than do babies who aren't breast-fed. Breast-fed babies may also have less asthma, food allergies and skin conditions, such as eczema. They may be less likely to experience a reduction in the number of red blood cells (anemia). Breast-feeding may offer a slight reduction in the risk of childhood leukemia.

  Breast milk may even protect against disease long term. As adults, people who were breast-fed may have a lowered risk of heart attack and stroke — due to lower cholesterol levels — and may be less likely to be obese and to develop diabetes. Breast-feeding, research suggests, might also help to protect against sudden infant death syndrome (SIDS), also known as crib death.
- **Easy digestion.** In addition to its health benefits, breast milk is easier for babies to digest than formula or cow's milk. Because breast milk doesn't remain in the stomach as long as formula, breast-fed babies spit up less. They have less gas and less constipation. They also have less diarrhea, because breast milk appears to kill some diarrhea-causing germs and helps the baby's digestive system grow and function.
- **Other benefits.** Nursing at the breast also helps promote normal development of your baby's jaw and facial muscles. It may even help your baby have fewer cavities later in childhood.

For mothers, breast-feeding:

- **Shrinks the uterus more quickly.** The baby's suckling triggers your body to release oxytocin, a hormone that causes your uterus to contract. This means that the uterus returns to its pre-pregnant size more quickly after delivery than it would if you bottle-feed.
- **Suppresses ovulation.** Breast-feeding delays the return of ovulation and therefore your period, which may help extend the time between pregnancies.
- **May protect long-term health.** Breast-feeding may reduce your risk of getting breast cancer before menopause. Breast-feeding also appears to provide some protection from uterine and ovarian cancers.

What parents say about breast-feeding

Mothers who have breast-fed their children list these advantages:

- **Convenience.** Many mothers find breast-feeding to be more convenient than bottle-feeding. It can be done anywhere, at any time, whenever your baby shows signs of being hungry. No equipment is necessary. Breast milk is always available — and at the right temperature. Because you don't need to prepare a bottle and you can nurse lying down, nighttime feedings may be easier.
- **Cost savings.** Breast-feeding can also save money because you don't need to buy bottles or formula.
- **Bonding.** Breast-feeding can promote intimacy and closeness between mom and baby. It can be extremely rewarding and fulfilling for you both.
- **Rest time for mom.** Breast-feeding also encourages you to rest every few hours while you feed your baby.

Breast-feeding can present challenges, such as:

- **Exclusive feeding by mom at first.** If you breast-feed exclusively, you must be with your baby for all feedings. In the early weeks, it can be physically demanding and tiring for the mother because newborns nurse every two to three hours — day and night — at first. Eventually, you can express milk with a breast pump, which will enable your partner or others to take over some feedings. But it will likely take a month or more before your milk production is well established enough to enable you to collect and store a supply for feedings by someone else.
- **Restrictions for mom.** Drinking alcohol isn't recommended for mothers who are breast-feeding, because alcohol can pass through breast milk to a baby. In addition, you may not be able to take certain medications while nursing.

- **Sore nipples.** Some women may experience sore nipples and, at times, breast infections. These can be remedied with the help of a lactation consultant or your health care provider.
- **Other physical side effects for mom.** When you're lactating, your body's hormones may keep your vagina relatively dry. This may not be conducive to your sex life, although using a water-based lubricating jelly can moderate the problem.

When breast-feeding may not be an option

Almost any woman is physically capable of breast-feeding her baby. The ability to do so has nothing to do with the size of your breasts; small breasts don't produce less milk than large breasts. Women who have had breast reduction surgery or breast implants may still be able to breast-feed.

However, some women may be encouraged to bottle-feed and not to use their breast milk. Discuss this option with your health care provider if:

- You're infected with tuberculosis, HIV, human T cell lymphotropic virus or hepatitis B. These infections can be transmitted to your baby through breast milk.
- You develop a herpes simplex infection, especially shingles (herpes zoster) on your chest.
- You develop West Nile virus or chickenpox (varicella). Using breast milk from a woman with these infections could pose a risk to the baby. Recommendations for women with these infections depend on their individual circumstances.
- You drink heavily or use drugs. Breast milk can pass alcohol and other drugs to your baby.
- You're taking certain cancer treatments.
- You're taking a medication that can pass into your breast milk and might be harmful to the baby, such as anti-thyroid medications, some blood pressure drugs and most sedatives. Before you begin breast-feeding, ask your health care provider, your baby's provider or a lactation consultant about whether you need to discontinue or change any prescription or nonprescription medications you're taking.
- You have a serious illness and aren't ready for the demands of breast-feeding.
- Your baby has a mouth deformity, such as a cleft lip or cleft palate. If so, he or she may have difficulty breast-feeding, necessitating that you use a bottle to feed. However, you do have the option of expressing breast milk and putting it in a bottle for your baby.
- Your newborn has certain health conditions. Some rare metabolic conditions, such as phenylketonuria (PKU) or galactosemia, may require using specially adapted formulas. The rare newborn condition lymphangiectasis may require a special formula.
- Your newborn doesn't grow well. Some infants with poor growth may need to have measured amounts of milk and nutritional supplements. Breast milk may be possible, but you may need to give it by bottle, tube or cup until growth improves.

The facts on bottle-feeding with formula

If you can't breast-feed or choose not to, you can be assured that your baby's need for nutrition can be met.

A wide variety of baby (infant) formulas are on the market. The majority of them are based on cow's milk. Never use regular cow's milk as a substitute for formula. Although cow's milk is used as the foundation for formula, the milk has been changed dramatically to make it safe for babies. It's treated by heat to make the protein in it more digestible. More milk sugar (lactose) is added to make the concentration similar to that of breast milk, and the fat (butterfat) is removed and replaced with vegetable oils and animal fats that are more easily digested by infants.

Infant formulas contain the right amount of carbohydrates and the right percentages of fats and protein. The Food and Drug Administration monitors the safety of commercially prepared infant formula. Each manufacturer must test each batch of formula to make sure it has the required nutrients and is free of contaminants.

Infant formula is designed to be an energy-dense food. More than half its calories are from fat. Many different types of fatty acids make up that fat. Those that go into infant formula are specifically selected because they're similar to those found in breast milk. These fatty acids help in the development of your baby's brain and nervous system, as well as in meeting his or her energy needs.

What parents say about bottle-feeding with formula

Parents who bottle-feed report these advantages:
- **Flexibility.** Using a bottle with formula allows more than one person to feed the baby. For that reason, some mothers feel that they have more freedom when they're bottle-feeding. Fathers may like bottle-feeding because it allows them to share more easily in the feeding responsibilities.

Bottle-feeding can present challenges, such as:
- **Time-consuming preparation.** You have to prepare the bottle for each feeding. You've got to keep a supply of formula at hand. Bottles and nipples always need to be washed. If you go out, you need to take a supply of formula with you.
- **Cost of formula.** Formula is costly, which is a concern for some parents.
- **Baby's tolerance to formula.** It may take time to find a formula that works well for some infants.
- **Breast discomfort.** If you choose not to breast-feed after your baby is born, your breasts may be swollen and somewhat tender for a while and eventually will stop producing milk.

A third option: Combining breast and bottle

You don't have to opt exclusively for either the breast or the bottle. Once breast-feeding is well established, many parents find that a combination of both breast and bottle works well and lets them enjoy the advantages of each.

The basics of breast-feeding

Breast-feeding is quite amazing. Under normal circumstances, the mother's body is able to produce all the food her newborn needs. How does it work?

Early in your pregnancy, your milk-producing (mammary) glands prepare for nursing. By about your sixth month of pregnancy, your breasts are ready to produce milk. In some women, tiny droplets of yellowish fluid appear on the nipples at this time. This fluid is called colostrum. It's the protein-rich fluid that a breast-fed baby gets the first few days after birth. Colostrum is very good for the baby because it contains infection-fighting antibodies from your body. It doesn't yet contain milk sugar (lactose). It's actually the delivery of the placenta that signals your body to start milk production. It clears the way for a hormone called prolactin to start up the mammary glands.

Your milk supply gradually increases, or is said to come in, between the third and fifth days after delivery. What you experience is full and sometimes tender breasts. They may feel lumpy or hard as the glands fill with milk. When a baby nurses, breast milk is released from tiny sacs of the milk-producing glands. The milk travels down milk ducts, which are located just behind the dark circle of tissue that surrounds the nipple (areola). The sucking action of the baby compresses the areola, forcing milk out through tiny openings in the nipple.

Your baby's sucking stimulates nerve endings in your areola and nipple, sending a message to your brain to tell your body to release the hormone oxytocin. Oxytocin acts on the milk-producing glands in your breast, causing the release of milk to your nursing baby. This release is called the let-down (milk ejection) reflex, which may be accompanied by a tingling sensation. Soon you learn to use the let-down reflex as a cue to sit back, relax and enjoy precious moments feeding your baby.

The stimulation of frequent nursing builds up your milk supply. The let-down reflex makes your milk available to your baby. Although your baby's sucking is the main stimulus for milk let-down, other stimuli may have the same effect. For example, your baby's cry — or even thoughts of your baby or the sounds of rippling water — may set things in motion.

Your body produces milk after you have a baby, regardless of whether you plan on breast-feeding. If you don't breast-feed, your milk supply eventually dries up. If you do breast-feed, your body's milk production is based on supply and demand. The more frequently your baby nurses, the more milk your breasts produce.

Getting started

Starting to breast-feed requires patience and practice. It's a natural process, but that doesn't mean it comes easily to all mothers. It's a new skill for both you and your baby. It may take a few attempts — even a few weeks — before you and your baby get the hang of it. Breast-feeding may go smoothly with one baby but not so with your next child.

For many reasons, it's a good idea to take a class on breast-feeding. Often, information on breast-feeding is offered as part of childbirth classes. Or you may need to sign up for an extra class. Most hospitals and birthing centers offer classes on feeding a newborn, which are open to both mothers and fathers.

The time to begin breast-feeding is right after the baby is born. If feasible, put the baby to your breast in the delivery room. After that, you can arrange for your baby to room with you at the hospital or birthing center to facilitate nursing. To help your baby learn how to breast-feed, request that, if possible, he or she not be given any supplementary bottles of water or formula, and preferably no pacifier, until breast-feeding is well established.

As you begin to breast-feed, it's a good idea to seek out expert help and advice. Ask your midwife, nurse or lactation consultant to assist you during your first days of feedings. These experts can provide hands-on instruction and helpful hints. After you leave the hospital or birthing center, you may arrange for a public health nurse who is knowledgeable about infant feeding to visit you at home for additional one-on-one instruction. You can always call a lactation consultant, your health care provider or the baby's provider for advice.

You can also find support and information by calling a chapter of La Leche League, a national organization that promotes breast-feeding. In addition, many books, other literature and Web sites on the subject are available. For example, the La Leche League International can be found at *www.lalecheleague.org,* and the National Women's Health Information Center has information on breast-feeding at *www.4women.gov/breastfeeding.*

Of course, women such as your mother, sister or a well-intentioned friend may offer lots of advice. It's also a good idea to have an expert observe your technique and redirect you if you and your baby aren't yet in sync.

The best advice is to stick with it. If it goes easily for you right from the first feeding, that's wonderful. If not, be patient with yourself. With time, and the support of a lactation consultant or nurse or your health care provider, you may soon be the one giving advice on breast-feeding.

Preparing to breast-feed

Before you bring your baby to your breast, find a quiet location. Have a drink of water, milk or juice at hand for yourself because it's common to feel thirsty when your milk lets down. Put the phone nearby or turn it off. Place a book, magazine or the TV remote control within reach, if you wish.

Next, get into a position to nurse that's comfortable for you and your baby. Whether in your hospital bed or a chair, sit up straight. Put a pillow behind the small of your back for support. If you opt for a chair, choose one with low arm rests or place a pillow under your arms for support. Put your feet up, too, if possible.

When you're comfortable, move your baby across your body so that he or she faces your breast, with his or her mouth near your nipple. Make sure your baby's whole body is facing you — tummy to tummy — with ear, shoulder and hip in a straight line. You don't want your baby's head turned to the side; rather, it should be straight in line with his or her body. Your baby's arms should be on either side of the nursing breast.

Bring your free hand up under your breast to support it for breast-feeding. Place the palm of that hand under your breast with the thumb on top of the breast, behind the areola. All fingers should be well behind the areola. Support the weight of your breast in your hand while squeezing lightly to point the nipple straight forward.

If your baby's mouth doesn't open immediately to accept your breast, touch the nipple to your baby's mouth or cheek. If your baby is hungry and interested in nursing, his or her mouth should open. As soon as your baby's mouth is opened wide — like a yawn — move his or her mouth onto your breast. You want your baby to receive as much nipple and areola as possible.

Let your baby take the initiative; don't push the nipple in an unwilling mouth. It might take a couple of attempts before your baby opens his or her mouth wide enough to latch on properly. You can also express some milk, which may encourage the baby to latch on.

As your baby starts suckling and your nipple is being stretched in your baby's mouth, you may feel some surging sensations. After a few suckles, those sensations should relax a bit. If they don't, sandwich the breast more and draw the baby's head in more closely. If that doesn't produce comfort, gently remove the baby from your breast, taking care to release the suction first. To break the suction, gently insert the tip of your finger into the corner of your baby's mouth. Push your finger slowly between your baby's gums until you feel the release. Repeat this procedure until your baby has latched on properly.

You want your baby to latch on well and create a firm bond of suction. You'll know that milk is flowing and your baby is swallowing if there's a

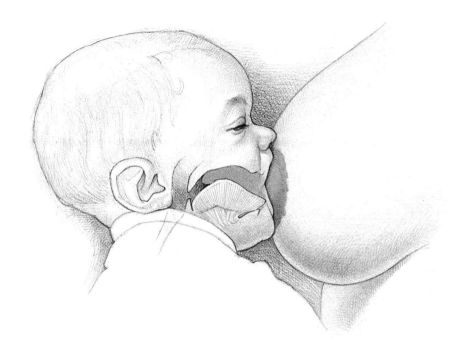

strong, steady, rhythmic motion visible in your baby's cheek. If your breast is blocking your baby's nose, lightly depress the breast with your thumb. Elevating your baby slightly or angling the baby's head back and in also may help provide a little breathing room.

Once nursing begins, you can relax the supporting arm and pull your baby's lower body closer to you. If your baby can comfortably remain attached, you may be able to stop supporting your breast with the other hand.

Offer your baby both breasts at each feeding. Allow your baby to end the feeding on the first side. Then, after burping your baby, offer the other side. Alternate starting sides to equalize the stimulation each breast receives.

Some babies have no trouble figuring out what they're supposed to be doing at the breast. Simply bringing the baby up to your breast and allowing him or her to nuzzle into it may be sufficient, especially after your baby has had some practice.

If your baby attaches and sucks correctly — even if the arrangement feels awkward at first — the position is correct. Your baby's mouth must be comfortably near your nipple. Don't bend over to link the baby with the breast. Instead, bring the baby to the breast.

In general, let your baby nurse as long as he or she wants. The length of feedings may vary considerably. However, on average, most babies nurse for about half an hour, usually divided between both breasts. Ideally, you want the baby to finish one breast at each feeding before switching to the other side. Why? The milk that comes first from your breast, called the foremilk, is rich in protein for growth. But the longer your baby sucks, the more he or she gets the hindmilk, which is rich in calories and fat and therefore helps your baby gain weight and grow. So wait until your baby seems ready to quit before offering him or her your other breast.

Because breast milk is easily digested, breast-fed babies usually are hungry every few hours at first. During those early days, it may seem to you that all you do is breast-feed! But a baby's need for frequent feeding isn't a sign that the baby isn't getting enough; it reflects the easy digestibility of breast milk. If your baby is satisfied after feeding and is growing well, you can be confident that you're doing well.

Positioning the baby at the breast

Different women find different positions comfortable. Here's a sampling of breast-feeding positions to try:

The cross-cradle hold
Bring your baby across the front of your body, tummy to tummy. Hold your baby with the arm opposite to the breast you're feeding with. Support the

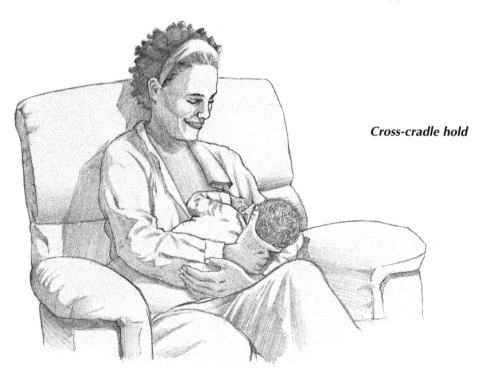

Cross-cradle hold

back of the baby's head with your open hand. This hold allows you especially good control as you position your baby to latch on.

The cradle hold

Cradle your baby in an arm, with your baby's head resting comfortably in the crook of the elbow on the same side as the breast you're feeding with. Your forearm supports your baby's back. Your open hand supports your baby's bottom.

The football (clutch) hold

In this position you hold your baby in much the same way a running back tucks a football under the arm. Hold your baby at your side on one arm, with your elbow bent and your open hand firmly supporting your baby's head faceup at the level of your breast. Your baby's torso will rest on your forearm. Put a pillow at your side to support your arm. A chair with broad, low arms works best.

With your free hand, gently squeeze your breast to align your nipple horizontally. Move your baby to your breast until the nipple meets the lips. When your baby's mouth opens, pull her or him in close to latch on snugly.

Because the baby isn't positioned near the abdomen, the football hold is popular among mothers recovering from Caesarean births. It's also a frequent choice of women who have large breasts or who are nursing premature or small babies.

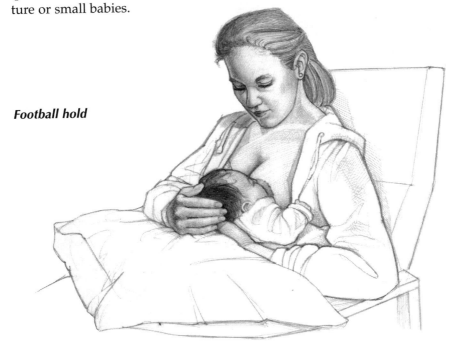

Football hold

Side-lying hold

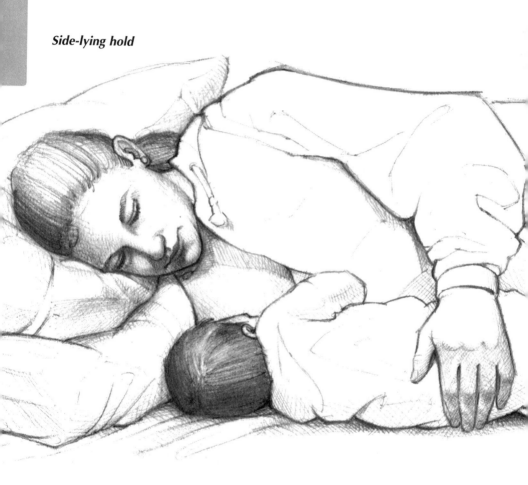

Side-lying hold
Although most new mothers learn to breast-feed in a sitting position, at times you may prefer to nurse while lying down. For example, lying down might be the best position if your baby prefers to snack and doze at the breast. A lying position may help you in getting your baby correctly connected in the early days of breast-feeding, or when you both may simply be tired. Use the hand of your lower arm to help keep your baby's head positioned at your breast.

With your upper arm and hand, reach across your body and grasp your breast, touching your nipple to your baby's lips. After your baby latches on firmly, you can use your lower arm to support your own head and your upper hand and arm to help support your baby.

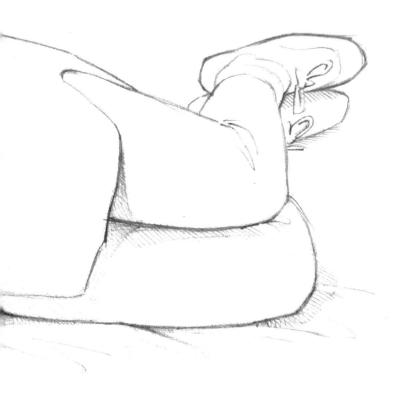

Your needs while you're breast-feeding

If you're like most mothers, your attention will be focused intently on the needs of your baby. Although this commitment is completely reasonable, don't forget about your needs. If your baby is to thrive, he or she needs a healthy mother. Consider:

Nutrition
The specific amounts of foods, fluids and calories you need to support breast-feeding aren't universally agreed on, but you may need fewer calories than was previously thought. The best approach to nutrition while breast-feeding isn't unlike the best approach at other times in your life: Eat foods at

regular intervals from various food groups — a balanced diet. In addition, drink six to eight cups of fluids each day. Water, milk and juice are good choices. *Small* amounts of coffee, tea and soft drinks are fine.

There are no special foods to avoid when you're breast-feeding. However, if you know that certain foods bother you or appear to cause a reaction such as fussiness or gas in your baby, then simply don't eat them. Rarely, a breast-fed baby is allergic to a component of your diet, such as cow's milk. To determine whether your baby is having trouble with your breast milk, cut out all dairy products from your diet for two weeks. Then slowly reintroduce dairy into your diet, one food item at a time, while observing your baby for any negative reactions.

Because many demands are made on your time as a new mother, it can be hard to prepare three healthy meals a day. You may find it easier to snack on healthy foods throughout the day. Partners can help support a breast-feeding mother by bringing her refreshments while she's nursing.

Rest

Try to get rest as a new mother, as hard as that may seem at times. You'll feel more energetic, you'll eat better, and you'll enjoy your new baby best when you're rested. Rest promotes the production of breast milk by enhancing the production of milk-producing hormones.

The tranquilizing effect of breast-feeding can make you feel sleepy. Many mothers nurse their babies while lying down or even take their babies to their bed. Nursing's soothing effect may make you both sleep, and lying down may be just what you need. Remember that some adult beds, such as waterbeds or pull-out sofas, can be hazardous for infants.

Ask others to take over daily chores so that you can rest. Younger children may appreciate being able to help out mother and baby by pitching in around the house.

A nursing bra and nursing pads

If you're going to breast-feed, invest in a couple of nursing bras. They provide important support for milk-laden breasts. They help prevent backaches and reduce leakage of milk. What distinguishes nursing bras from regular bras is that both cups open, usually with a simple maneuver that you can manage unobtrusively while you hold your baby.

Nursing pads are handy to absorb excess milk that leaks from your breasts. Slim and disposable, they can be slipped between breast and bra. They soak up milk leakage while allowing air to circulate to the skin. Nursing pads can be worn continuously or on occasion. Some women don't bother with them. You can purchase nursing pads at most baby supply stores and general retail stores. They're often shelved near the disposable diapers.

Care of your breasts

As you start to breast-feed, you may experience a few problems with your breasts, such as:

Engorgement
A few days after your baby is born, your breasts may become full, firm and tender, making it challenging for your baby to grasp your nipple. This swelling, called engorgement, also causes congestion within your breasts, which makes your milk flow slower. So even if your baby can latch on, he or she may be less than satisfied with the results.

To manage engorgement, express some milk by hand before trying to breast-feed. Support with one hand the breast you intend to express. With your other hand, gently stroke your breast inward toward your areola. Then place your thumb and forefinger at the top and bottom of the breast just behind the areola. As you gently compress the breast between your fingers, milk should flow or squirt out the nipple. You can also use a breast pump to express some milk.

As you release your milk, you'll begin to feel your areola and nipple soften. Once enough milk is released, your baby can comfortably latch on and nurse. As you nurse your baby, gently massage your breast to further relieve the fullness and promote milk flow.

Frequent, lengthy nursing sessions are the best means to avoid engorgement. Nurse your baby regularly and try not to a miss a feeding. Wearing a nursing bra both day and night will help support engorged breasts and may make you feel more comfortable.

If your breasts are sore after nursing, apply an ice pack to reduce swelling. Some women find that a warm shower relieves breast tenderness. Fortunately, the period of engorgement is usually brief, lasting no more than a few days following delivery.

Sore nipples
Sore, tender or cracked nipples can make breast-feeding painful and, frankly, frustrating. Fortunately, most women don't get sore nipples, and if they do, the soreness doesn't last for long. Sore nipples are usually caused by incorrect positioning. At each feeding, you want to make sure that the baby has the areola and not just the nipple in his or her mouth. You also want to be certain that the baby's head isn't turned to the side, out of line with his or her body. This position causes pulling at the nipple.

To care for your nipples, let them air-dry after each feeding. Some women wave a blow-dryer, on a cool setting, across their nipples for a few minutes to dry them.

You don't need to wash your nipples after nursing. There are built-in lubricants around the areola that provide a natural salve. Soap removes these protective substances and promotes dryness, which may cause or aggravate sore nipples. When you bathe, simply splash water on your breasts. Afterward, let your nipples air-dry once again. Don't dry them with a towel.

Some mothers place regular tea bags soaked in cool water on sore nipples to soothe them. Some women find that expressing a little milk after each feeding keeps their nipples supple. You can purchase and apply 100 percent pure lanolin to your nipples after feedings, as long as you're not allergic to wool.

Do your best to relax while breast-feeding, which will enhance the let-down of milk and in turn help prevent your baby from vigorous sucking as he or she waits for the flow of milk.

Blocked milk ducts

Sometimes, milk ducts in the breast become clogged, causing milk to back up. Blocked ducts can be felt through the skin as small, tender lumps or larger areas of hardness. Because blocked ducts can lead to an infection, you should treat the problem right away. The best way to open up blocked ducts is to let your baby empty the affected breast, offering that breast first at each feeding. If your baby doesn't empty the affected breast, express milk from it by hand or by breast pump. It may also help to apply a warm compress before nursing and to massage the affected breast. If the problem doesn't go away with self-treatment, call your lactation consultant or health care provider for advice.

Breast infection (mastitis)

This is a more serious complication of breast-feeding. Infection can be caused by a failure to empty your breasts at feedings. Germs may gain entry into your milk ducts from cracked nipples and from your baby's mouth. These germs are not harmful to your baby; everyone has them. They just don't belong in your breast tissues.

Mastitis causes swelling, burning, redness and pain in one or both breasts, along with flu-like signs such as a fever and chills. If you develop such signs and symptoms, call your health care provider. You may need antibiotics, in addition to rest and more fluids. If you develop mastitis, keep nursing. Mastitis typically doesn't affect your baby. Emptying your breasts during feedings will help to prevent clogged milk ducts, another possible source of the condition. If your breasts are really painful, hand express some milk from them as you soak your breasts in a bath of warm water. (See "Mastitis," page 581.)

Inverted nipples

Although inverted nipples aren't very common, a few women do have them. It's a condition in which the nipples are drawn inward. A baby has a harder time latching onto a nipple that's not pointing outward.

The problem may clear up on its own, as your breasts get larger when your milk comes in. If this doesn't happen, you can wear breast shells between feedings to help your nipples protrude. You can also try a breast pump to draw out your nipples and start the milk flowing. If your nipples are severely inverted or flat, talk with your lactation consultant or health care provider.

Expressing breast milk

You may want to remove (express) your breast milk for feeding your baby by bottle when you're unable to breast-feed. You can express your milk either with a breast pump or by hand. To help with let-down, find a quiet place to express. Relax for a few minutes before starting to express.

Expressing milk with a breast pump

Most breast-feeding mothers find using a breast pump is easier than expressing milk manually. There are many pumps to choose from: hand, battery-operated or electric ones. The type of pump you select will depend on your particular needs. The most effective pumps are those that automatically pulsate. Electric pumps stimulate the breast more effectively than hand pumps, but they're more expensive.

You may want to consider a breast pump that expresses both breasts at the same time. Double breast pumps cut pumping time in half and are the best selection for building a milk supply or maintaining a supply when pumping regularly. Be sure to read the instructions that accompany the breast pump.

You can purchase breast pumps from medical supply stores and most drug and baby stores. You may be able to rent a breast pump. Ask your health care provider or lactation consultant where to rent a breast pump. Some employers provide breast pumps for their employees to use.

Whichever type of pump you choose, make sure you can remove and wash with soap and water all the parts that come in contact with your skin or milk. Some breast pump parts are dishwasher safe. Without proper cleaning, bacteria could grow, and your milk wouldn't be safe for your baby.

Expressing milk by hand

Use these steps to express milk by hand:

- Support your breast in one hand.

- Using your other hand, position your thumb and index finger about 1½ inches behind your nipple (behind the areola).
- Push your thumb and finger back toward the chest wall and then compress them together to squeeze milk from the sinuses. Be careful not to slide them forward and pinch the nipple.
- Rotate the position like hands on a clock to better remove the milk.

Storing breast milk

Store expressed breast milk in bottles or plastic milk-storage bags. Label each container with the date and time of each pumping. Breast milk may be used after it has been stored:

- For no more than 10 hours at room temperature
- In the refrigerator for up to eight days
- In the freezer compartment of the refrigerator for up to two weeks
- In a freezer compartment with a separate door for up to three to four months
- In a separate deep freezer for six months or longer

Thaw milk in the refrigerator or in a container of warm water. Don't thaw it at room temperature.

You can give breast milk straight from the refrigerator if your baby doesn't object. If your baby prefers warm milk, warm the bottle by setting it in a pan of warm water for a few minutes. Then shake the bottle and test it by putting a few drops on the top of your hand. Don't microwave breast milk because extreme heat can destroy some of the natural antibodies that breast milk carries and can cause hot spots that could burn your baby's mouth.

One other note: You may look at expressed breast milk and wonder, "How could this possibly be rich enough for my baby to grow on, when it looks so watery?" Breast milk is normally watery looking. It also has a blue cast, making it look somewhat like skim milk. But don't let looks deceive you. Breast milk is rich in exactly what your baby needs for growth.

Introducing a bottle to a breast-fed baby

During the first several weeks of your child's life, it's best to nurse exclusively to help you and your baby learn how to breast-feed and to be sure your milk supply is being established. Once your milk supply is established and you feel confident that you and your baby are doing well with breast-feeding, you may give your baby an occasional bottle of breast milk. This allows others, such as your partner or a grandparent, an opportunity to feed the baby. If your baby receives a bottle of milk, you may want to pump your breasts for your comfort and to maintain your milk supply.

BREAST-FEEDING TWINS AND TRIPLETS

A mother can certainly breast-feed more than one baby.

If you have twins, you can breast-feed one baby at a time. Or you can nurse them simultaneously, once breast-feeding is established. To accomplish this feat, you can position both babies in the football (clutch) hold. Or you can cradle them both in front of you with their bodies crossing each other. Use pillows to support the babies' heads and your arms.

With triplets, it's possible to breast-feed. One option is to supplement feedings with expressed milk or formula in a bottle. Nurse two babies at the same time and give a bottle to the third. At the next feeding, use the bottle for a different baby. The goal is to have all three babies have a chance to feed at the breast.

If you're the parent of multiples, you may want to discuss a breast-feeding plan with your health care provider or a lactation consultant before you leave the hospital. Ask them to suggest a mother who has successfully breast-fed her twins or triplets — it's nice to have a source of supportive, practical advice.

The feel of a bottle nipple in a baby's mouth is different from that of the breast. The way a baby sucks from a bottle nipple also is different. It may take practice for your baby to be comfortable with a bottle nipple. A baby may initially be reluctant to take a bottle from mom because he or she associates mother's voice and scent with breast-feeding.

When you give your baby a supplementary bottle, follow your baby's cues as to the amount to give. There's no set amount that's right. Your baby may be satisfied at a few ounces.

Working and breast-feeding

With a little planning and preparation, you can combine breast-feeding and employment.

Some mothers work at home or can take their babies with them to work. Some arrange to have their babies brought to them for feedings, or they go to the babies. The mothers can continue to do most of the feedings with only occasional bottle feedings.

If these aren't options for you, you may choose to have your child-care provider give your baby bottled breast milk or infant formula. For a few weeks before your return to work, give your baby a bottle once or twice a week at the times he or she will receive them while you're at work.

You can provide your baby with bottled breast milk by expressing milk during your maternity leave and freezing it, or by pumping while you're at work and saving the milk for the next day. Using a double breast pump is the most effective — it takes about 15 minutes every three to four hours. If you need to increase your milk supply, nurse and pump more often. On your days off from work, nurse your baby as usual.

If you choose not to express your milk while at work, you may pump milk at other times to provide breast milk for the next day. For example, pump after the morning feeding and after the feeding when you return home. As long as all of your milk produced in 24 hours is removed either by your baby or from pumping, you'll maintain a good supply.

You may decide to have your child care provider give your baby infant formula. This will decrease your milk supply but allow enough to remain for nursing at home. To prevent overly full breasts at work, some mothers find they need to give thawed breast milk or formula on days off from work at the same times the child-care provider feeds the baby.

Once in a while, your baby may take a bottle, then later reject the breast. If this happens, give your baby extra cuddling and attention before feeding.

Bottle-feeding: The basics

Infant formulas

The first time you purchase infant formula, you may be surprised by just how many different types are available. Consult your baby's health care provider for advice about choosing the right formula. For most babies, an iron-fortified, cow's-milk-based formula is the best choice.

Several special formulas also are available, such as those containing soy protein and protein hydrolysates. These formulas are made for specific digestive problems and should be used only under a health care provider's direction.

Iron-fortified formula is important for preventing anemia and iron deficiency, which can cause slow development. In general, iron deficiency isn't a risk in the first few months of a baby's life. However, it can occur later in the first year. Iron deficiency in six- to 10-month-old infants was common before iron supplementation became routine.

Infant formulas come in three forms: powder, liquid concentrate and ready-to-feed liquid. Both the powder and concentrate liquid formulas must have a specific amount of water added to them. Dry powder formulas generally are the least expensive. Ready-to-feed brands offer great convenience.

If you decide to bottle-feed your baby with infant formula, instead of breast-feeding, you need to purchase the right supplies to get started. You'll need formula, bottles and nipples on hand when you bring the baby home from the hospital or birthing center where you delivered.

Let the medical staff assisting your birth know of your plans to bottle-feed. The staff at the hospital or birthing center can provide bottle-feeding equipment and formula during your postpartum recovery and show you how to bottle-feed your newborn. But you should stock up on your own supplies.

BREAST OR BOTTLE: TIPS FOR FEEDING YOUR BABY

At first, it may seem that all you do is feed your baby. How often you feed your baby depends on how often your baby is hungry. One feeding may seem to blur into the next. Breast-fed babies likely will want to be fed between eight and 12 times in 24 hours — about every two to three hours. And formula-fed babies probably will want to be fed between six and nine times in 24 hours — about every three to four hours — for the first few months of life.

Your baby won't always feed this often. As your baby matures, he or she will gradually need fewer daily feedings and eat more at each feeding. A feeding pattern and routine will begin to emerge after the first month or two. Expect that a newborn will wake routinely at night for feeding one or more times and that your baby may demand more milk during growth spurts.

Tips for feeding your baby include feeding on demand and letting your baby set the pace:

Feeding on demand

Feeding your baby on demand is suited to your baby's development. Your baby is awake for short periods. His or her nervous system isn't fully developed, so he or she can't distinguish one sensation from another. The size of your infant's stomach is very small, about the size of his or her fist, and the time it takes to become empty varies from one to three hours.

Feeding on demand requires you to be flexible and to read your baby's cues. Watch for these clues that a baby is ready to eat: your baby makes sucking movements with his or her mouth or tongue (rooting), sucks on his or her fist or making small sounds, and, of course, cries. The sensation that hunger produces often makes babies cry. You will soon be able to distinguish between cries for food and those for other reasons — pain, fatigue, illness. It's important to feed your baby promptly when he or she signals hunger. This helps your baby learn which kinds of discomfort mean hunger and that hunger can be satisfied by sucking, which brings food. If you don't respond promptly, your baby may become so upset that trying to feed at this point may prove more frustrating than satisfying.

Letting the baby set the pace

Try not to rush your baby during a feeding. He or she will determine how much and how fast to eat. Many babies, like adults, prefer to eat in a relaxed manner. In fact, it's normal for an infant to suck, pause, rest, socialize a bit and then return to feeding. Some newborns are speedy, efficient eaters, consistently whizzing through feedings in minutes on each breast. Other babies are grazers, preferring snack-sized feedings at frequent intervals. Still others, especially newborns, are snoozers. These babies may take a few vigorous sucks and blissfully doze off, then wake, feed and doze again intermittently throughout a typical nursing session.

Your baby will also let you know when he or she has had enough to eat. When your baby is satisfied, he or she will stop sucking, close his or her mouth or turn away from the nipple. Your baby may push the nipple out of his or her mouth with his or her tongue, or your baby may arch his or her back if you try to continue feeding your baby. If, however, your baby needs burping or is in the middle of a bowel movement, his or her mind may not be on eating. Try offering the breast or bottle again after waiting.

Sometimes, a baby will contentedly suck away at an empty bottle or breast. If you want your baby to let go of the nipple, gently slide your little finger between his or her gums.

Don't expect your baby to eat the same amount every day. Babies vary how much they eat, especially if they're experiencing a growth spurt. At these times, your baby will need and demand more milk and more frequent feedings. It may seem like your baby can't get full. During these times, you may need to put your baby to breast or offer a bottle more often.

Most babies don't eat at precise intervals throughout the day, as you might first expect. Most babies bunch (cluster) their feedings at various times of the day and night. It's common for a baby to eat several times within a few hours and then sleep for a few hours.

If your baby is very sleepy or was born prematurely, he or she may not always give clear signals of hunger. You may need to wake or stimulate the baby to feed him or her. To accomplish this, try gently tickling the top of the baby's head or rubbing his or her foot gently. Removing a few layers of blanket or clothing may arouse him or her to feed. Softly talking to a sleepy baby may be enough to capture his or her attention. Know the signs that your baby is getting enough to eat.

Most babies eat frequently and well enough to support their rapid growth. There are many ways to tell if your baby is getting enough to eat. If you're breast-feeding, you can't precisely measure the amount of milk your baby is getting. But there are signs that reveal how your baby is breast-feeding and whether he or she is getting enough milk. For example, you'll know if your breasts are firm and full before feedings and softer and emptier after nursing. You'll hear and see your baby swallow milk, and you'll see your baby turn away from your breast when he or she has had enough.

Whether on breast milk or formula, your baby's weight gain is the most reliable sign that he or she is getting enough to eat. Most babies lose a few ounces soon after birth, then regain the weight — and then some — by two weeks. If you're unsure about whether your baby is gaining or losing weight, have the baby weighed at the office of your baby's health care provider. Your baby's provider may encourage a return visit within a few days after birth, or you can initiate the visit. Trust your instinct if you believe your baby isn't eating well.

Another trustworthy sign of normal growth is your baby's pattern of diapers. Babies should have six to eight wet diapers and one to three or more bowel movements a day in the first few weeks. Normally, a breast-fed infant will have bowel movements more frequently than a formula-fed infant. The consistency of stools also differs — the breast-fed infant tends to have golden-yellow-colored, looser stools, and the formula-fed infant tends to have tan-colored, soft or formed bowel movements. Contact your baby's health care provider if your baby is urinating or having bowel movements less often than expected.

Equipment for bottle-feeding includes:
- Four 4-ounce bottles (optional, but useful at the beginning).
- Eight 8-ounce bottles.
- Eight to 10 nipples, nipple rings and nipple caps.
- A measuring cup.
- A bottle brush.
- Infant formula. After your baby's born, talk with his or her health care provider about which specific type of formula to use.

In addition to buying the right equipment for bottle-feeding, consider taking a class on newborn care before your baby is born. Often, information on feeding a newborn is offered as part of childbirth classes. If you've never bottle-fed a baby before, it's a good idea to get comfortable with the method by taking a class on it or reading up on the subject before your baby arrives.

Getting started

The bottles for feeding your baby can be glass, plastic or plastic with a soft plastic liner. When your baby is old enough to hold a bottle, you may want to use plastic bottles for safety reasons. Some bottles are shaped to better fit a baby's hands.

Bottles generally come in two sizes: 4 ounces and 8 ounces. The amount the bottle holds isn't an indication of how much your baby needs to drink in a feeding. Your baby may need less or more for any given feeding.

Many types of nipples are on the market. For many babies, it makes little difference which nipples you use. But for a full-term baby, don't select overly soft nipples designed for use by a premature baby. A full-term baby should use a regular nipple. Use only one or two different types of nipples for your baby's bottles. Using too many different types may be confusing to your baby.

It's important that milk flows from the nipple at the correct speed. Milk flow that's either too fast or too slow can cause your baby to swallow too much air, leading to stomach discomfort and the need for frequent burping. Test the flow of the nipple by turning the bottle upside down and timing the drops. One drop per second is about right. Nipples now come in sizes for the newborn, three-month-old, six-month-old, and so on, making the flow out of the nipple appropriate for the child's age.

Preparing formula

Whatever type and form of formula you choose, proper preparation and refrigeration are essential, both to ensure the appropriate amount of nutrition and to safeguard the health of your baby.

Newborns have few defenses against germs. It takes a while for your baby to build up immunity — especially if he or she isn't getting breast milk, which contains antibodies. Formula doesn't have them. That's why it's important to minimize the danger of bacteria contaminating your baby's formula by preparing and storing it safely.

Wash your hands before handling formula or the equipment used to prepare it. All equipment that you use to measure, mix and store formula should be washed with hot, soapy water and then rinsed and dried before every use. Sterilizing bottles and nipples isn't necessary as long as you wash and rinse them well. After use, clean bottles, nipples and preparation equipment with hot, soapy water. Use a bottle brush to wash bottles. Brush or rub the nipples thoroughly to remove any traces of formula. Rinse well. You can also clean bottles and nipples in the dishwasher.

Wash or wipe the tops of formula cans with a clean towel before you open them. You may keep unused liquid concentrate formula in the can after you open it. Cover it tightly and refrigerate. Generally, you can store all prepared formula or liquid concentrate in the refrigerator for up to 48 hours. After that, throw away all unused formula.

Whether using powder formula or liquid concentrate formula, always add the exact amount of water specified on the label. Measurements on bottles may be inaccurate, so pre-measure the water before adding it to the formula. Using too much or too little water can be harmful to your baby. If formula is too diluted, your baby won't get enough nutrition for growth needs or to satisfy hunger. Formula that's too concentrated puts strain on the baby's digestive system and kidneys and could dehydrate your baby.

Warming formula isn't necessary for nutritional purposes, but your baby may prefer it warm. To warm formula, set the bottle in a pan of warm water for a few minutes. Shake the bottle and test the temperature of the milk by dropping a few drops of formula on the top of your hand. Don't microwave formula because this can cause hot spots that can burn your baby's mouth. Once you warm formula, don't refrigerate the leftovers. Discard the unused portions of formula.

In general, it's best to make up formula when you need it, not in advance. However, you may prefer to make up a bottle or two and store them in the refrigerator for use that night. This may make nighttime feedings easier.

Water concerns

If your water comes from a safe municipal water supply, it's acceptable to use for preparing your baby's formula. If your home is supplied by well water, you can have the water checked by your local public health department to make sure it doesn't contain contaminants, such as nitrates, or heavy metals, such as lead. Use bottled water to prepare formula if you have any concerns about your water supply.

When preparing formula, use cold water or water warmed to room temperature. Don't boil water because this concentrates minerals naturally found in water, as well as impurities.

Positioning baby and bottle

The first step to bottle-feeding is to make you and your baby comfortable. Find a quiet place where you and your baby won't be distracted. Cradle your baby in one arm, hold the bottle with the other and settle into a comfortable chair, preferably one with broad, low armrests. You may want to put a pillow on your lap under the baby for support. Pull your baby in toward you snugly but not too tightly, cradled in your arm with his or her head raised slightly and resting in the bend of your elbow. This semi-upright position makes swallowing much easier.

Now that you're ready to start feeding, help your newborn get ready. Using the nipple of the bottle or a finger of the hand holding it, gently stroke your baby's cheek near the mouth, on the side nearest you. The touch will cause your baby to turn toward you, often with an opened mouth. Then touch the nipple to your baby's lips or the corner of the mouth. Your baby will open his or her mouth and gradually begin sucking.

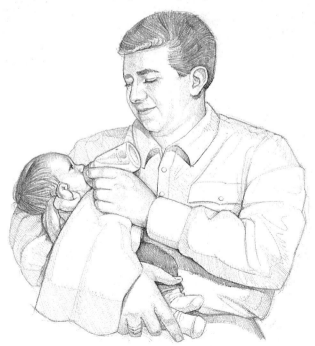

When feeding your baby, position the bottle at about a 45-degree angle. This angle keeps the nipple full of milk. Hold the bottle steady as your baby feeds. If your baby falls asleep while bottle-feeding, it may be because he or she has had enough milk or gas has made your baby full. Take the bottle away, burp your baby, then start to feed again.

Always hold your baby while feeding. Never prop up a bottle against your infant. Propping may cause your baby to vomit and may lead to overeating. In addition, never give a bottle to your baby when he or she is lying on his or her back. This may cause ear infections in your baby.

Although your baby doesn't have teeth yet, they're forming beneath the gums. Don't develop a habit of putting your baby to bed with a bottle. Formula lingers in the mouth of a baby who falls asleep while sucking a bottle. The prolonged contact of sugar in milk can cause tooth decay.

WHY NOT JUST COW'S MILK?

During the first year, the best milk for babies is either breast milk or formula. Cow's milk — the kind that comes in a jug or carton from a grocery store — is a fine food for children, but not before age one. Here's why:

- Cow's milk is not optimal for the intestines and kidneys of human infants. It has about three times as much sodium and three times as much protein as your baby needs. In fact, babies shouldn't drink cow's milk because it can make them sick.
- Cow's milk can cause an allergic response. Your baby can't digest it easily.
- Cow's milk doesn't contain the proper fats to meet infants' needs.

In fact, breast milk or infant formula is the only food your baby needs for about the first six months of life. Don't give your baby cereal in his or her bottle. Don't offer bottles of water or juice until your baby is six months or older, unless your health care provider recommends that you do.

If you have any questions about bottle-feeding your baby, don't hesitate to ask your baby's health care provider.

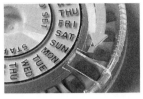

contraceptive choices after delivery

In the blur of sleepless nights and diaper changes, it's easy to forget about birth control. But the fact is, even before your first postpartum menstrual period, there may be a chance that you could become pregnant again if you have unprotected sex. Conceiving again within six months of your delivery carries certain health risks for you and your baby, not to mention the stress of being pregnant while caring for a newborn. For these reasons, it's important to consider your birth control options after your baby is born.

For those who choose to use birth control, there are many different choices. Some may be a better fit for you than others. Some factors to consider include:

- Your ability to stick to a regimen
- Your level of comfort with your body
- Whether you want to have more children
- Whether you have a steady partner
- Your overall health
- Whether you smoke

Following is a brief description of contraceptives currently available that may be appropriate after delivery. Keep in mind that correct use increases a method's effectiveness. Refraining from having sexual intercourse at all (abstinence) is the only 100 percent effective way to prevent pregnancy and sexually transmitted diseases (STDs), including HIV/AIDS. Talk with your health care provider for more information on which choice may be best for you.

Temporary methods of birth control

Birth control pills

Oral contraceptive pills contain synthetic hormones that prevent ovulation and impair fertilization. The two types of birth control pills are those that combine estrogen and progestin and those that contain only progestin (the minipill).

Availability
Prescription

How they're used
You take the pills on a daily basis. It usually takes about a week for the pills to start working, so you may need to use another form of birth control if you have sex in the meantime.

Effectiveness
Combination pills are about 97 percent effective, meaning up to three out of 100 women who use this method as birth control for a year will become pregnant.

Progestin-only pills are 95 percent effective, meaning up to five out of 100 women who use this method as birth control for a year will become pregnant.

Issues to consider
Some health care providers may wait three or more weeks after your delivery to start you on birth control pills. If you're breast-feeding, your health care provider may recommend progestin-only pills because they don't noticeably affect your breast milk. Combination pills may reduce your milk supply slightly. Some women may have side effects such as nausea, dizziness or changes in menstruation, mood and weight.

If you're a smoker over 35 years of age, don't use the combination pill because it can increase your risk of blood clots. In addition, birth control pills aren't recommended for women who have a history of strokes, blood clots or liver disease. Birth control pills don't increase your risk of breast cancer. This method of birth control doesn't protect you from STDs, including HIV/AIDS.

Birth control patch

The patch (Ortho Evra) is a square skin patch worn on your lower abdomen, buttocks or upper body, but not on your breasts. The patch releases a continuous dose of estrogen and progestin hormones into your bloodstream to prevent pregnancy.

Availability
Prescription

How it's used
You wear patches continuously for three weeks, applying a new patch each week and discarding the used one. On the fourth week, you forego the patch so that you can have your period.

Effectiveness
The birth control patch is 99 percent effective, meaning one out of 100 women who use this method as birth control for a year will become pregnant. It's less effective if you weigh more than 198 pounds.

Issues to consider
The patch is convenient, and many women find it easier to keep up with this regimen than a pill regimen. Side effects and risks of the patch are similar to those of birth control pills. It carries an increased risk of blood clots, heart attack and stroke. Like other forms of hormonal birth control, the patch isn't recommended for smokers over age 35 or for women who have liver disease, uncontrolled diabetes, or a history of blood clots, heart attack or stroke. Talk to your health care provider about when to start using it.

Birth control shots

Birth control shots are similar to birth control pills in that both methods use hormones to prevent ovulation and impair fertilization. These injections are given in your arm or buttocks. The shots are available in the form of a progestin-only injection (Depo-Provera).

Availability
Prescription

How they're used
With Depo-Provera, you get an injection every three months.

Effectiveness
Birth control shots are more than 99 percent effective, meaning fewer than one out of 100 women who use this method as birth control for a year will become pregnant.

Issues to consider
Birth control shots are safe immediately after pregnancy and while you're breast-feeding. Your periods may become irregular, or you may stop having them altogether. Return to fertility after you stop using them may be delayed for up to a year. If you weigh more than 160 pounds, you may have a slightly higher chance of becoming pregnant, but your health care provider can adjust your dosage accordingly.
Studies have shown that Depo-Provera decreases bone density, although the loss is largely reversible if you stop receiving the injections. Talk to your health care provider about your risk of osteoporosis, a condition marked by

abnormal loss of bone density as you age. If your risk is high, your health care provider may recommend another form of birth control or a shorter course of Depo-Provera. Birth control shots don't protect you from STDs, including HIV/AIDS.

Diaphragm with spermicide

A diaphragm is a dome-shaped rubber cap with a flexible rim that fits over your cervix. It's used along with spermicidal foam, cream or jelly to block sperm from reaching the egg. Diaphragms come in different sizes, so you need to be fitted by your health care provider in order to use one.

The cervical cap is a similar method of birth control, but it's more difficult to insert and isn't recommended for women who've had children.

Availability
The diaphragm is available by prescription, as is the cervical cap. Spermicide is available over the counter.

How it's used
You insert the diaphragm into your vagina one to two hours before intercourse. Before insertion, you must apply spermicide to the rim and center of the diaphragm. After intercourse, you must leave the diaphragm in place for at least six hours but not more than 24 hours. If you have sex again within those 24 hours, first insert more spermicide into your vagina without removing the diaphragm.

Effectiveness
Diaphragms with spermicide are 84 percent effective, meaning 16 out of 100 women who use this method as birth control for a year will become pregnant. For women who haven't had children, cervical caps are 82 percent to 94 percent effective. Cervical caps have decreased effectiveness (60 percent to 80 percent) when used by women who've had children.

Issues to consider
If you used a diaphragm before you were pregnant, you may need to be refitted after your child is born because your vaginal size may have changed. Diaphragms with spermicide don't protect you against STDs. Previously, spermicide with the ingredient nonoxynol-9 was believed to offer some protection against gonorrhea and chlamydia, but recent studies show that this isn't the case and that it may in fact increase the risk of HIV transmission. Spermicide may also cause vaginal irritation in some women.

Female condom

The female condom (vaginal pouch) is a polyurethane tube-like sheath you insert into the vagina. It's lubricated and can be inserted up to 24 hours before intercourse. Only one brand (FC Female Condom) is currently on the market.

Availability
Nonprescription

How it's used
The female condom comes with a flexible ring on each end. The closed end is inserted into the vagina close to the cervix so that the condom lines the vaginal wall. The penis enters through the open end, which remains outside the vagina. Use once only and then discard.

Effectiveness
Female condoms are 79 percent to 95 percent effective, meaning up to 21 out of 100 women who use this birth control method for a year will become pregnant.

Issues to consider
A female condom gives the woman more control over contraceptive use. Like the male condom, it's inexpensive. However, it may be a little trickier to use. Make sure to use plenty of lubricant so that the condom doesn't get pushed in or pulled out. You may need to add lubricant — use a water-based one. Don't use a male and female condom at the same time, as the friction between them can cause one or the other to come off. Female condoms offer some protection against STDs, including HIV/AIDS, but not as much as the male latex condom.

Hormonal vaginal ring

The hormonal vaginal ring is available under the brand name NuvaRing. This method consists of wearing a flexible ring around your cervix. The ring releases a continuous low dose of the hormones estrogen and progestin. The hormones keep you from getting pregnant.

Availability
Prescription

How it's used
You insert a new ring into your vagina each month and keep it in place for three weeks. During this time, if the ring is out of your vagina for more than

three hours, use an additional method of birth control, such as a male condom, until the ring has been back in place for seven days. You remove the ring after three weeks and then put in a new one. Don't remove the ring during intercourse.

Effectiveness
Hormonal vaginal rings are 98 percent to 99 percent effective, meaning up to two out of 100 women who use this method as birth control for a year will become pregnant.

Issues to consider
Like birth control pills, NuvaRing is a highly effective form of birth control. The advantage is that you don't have to take a pill every day. It's also easily reversible. Talk to your health care provider about when you can start using it after delivery. It may produce some of the same side effects as birth control pills, such as nausea, dizziness, and weight or mood changes.

It's not recommended for smokers over age 35 or for women who have liver disease, uncontrolled diabetes, or a history of blood clots, heart attack or stroke. NuvaRing may also cause increased vaginal discharge and irritation or infection. It doesn't protect against STDs, including HIV/AIDS.

Intrauterine devices

An intrauterine device (IUD) is a small, T-shaped object that's placed inside your uterus. It prevents sperm from reaching the egg and may hinder implantation. Two types are currently available: the Copper T IUD, which can stay in place for up to 10 years, and the intrauterine system (Mirena), which can stay in your uterus for up to five years.

Availability
Procedure performed by your health care provider

How they're used
Your health care provider inserts the IUD through your cervix into your uterus. Many health care providers recommend having it done during your period. Small strings allow you to check that the device is in place. You check the strings about once a month.

Effectiveness
IUDs are 98 percent to 99.9 percent effective, meaning up to two out of 100 women who use this method as birth control for a year will become pregnant.

Issues to consider
This is a very effective long-term form of birth control that's also reversible. It can be inserted soon after delivery and is safe to use while breast-feeding. It can also be used as an emergency contraceptive if placed within seven days after unprotected sex. But it's not for everyone. Most health care providers recommend it for women who have had children, are in a mutually monogamous relationship and have no history of pelvic inflammatory disease. It's not recommended for women with STDs or a history of STDs. Some IUDs may cause increased cramping during your period and can sometimes be expelled spontaneously. They don't protect against STDs, including HIV/AIDS.

Male condom

A male condom is a thin rubber sheath that's used to cover a man's penis when it's erect. It blocks ejaculation fluid from entering the vagina. Condoms made of latex are most common, but they're also available in lambskin or polyurethane materials, for those who are allergic to latex.

Availability
Nonprescription

How it's used
Before intercourse, unroll the condom all the way down the shaft of the penis, leaving a half-inch space at the head of the penis to allow semen to collect. Use once only and then discard.

Effectiveness
Male condoms are 86 percent to 98 percent effective, meaning up to 14 out of 100 women who use this method as birth control for a year will become pregnant.

Issues to consider
Of all birth control methods, male latex and polyurethane condoms are the most effective at protecting against STDs, including HIV/AIDS. Lambskin condoms have tiny pores that may allow viruses to pass through. Condoms are inexpensive and easy to use. Don't use latex condoms with oil-based lubricants, such as petroleum jelly or hand lotion, as they can weaken or damage the condom.

Natural family planning methods

Natural family planning methods, which are also called rhythm methods, involve determining the days during your monthly cycle that you're fertile (ovulating) and avoiding intercourse during those days. No devices or medications are required.

Availability
Nonprescription

How they're used
The following ways can be used to assess when you're most fertile:

- **Calendar method.** Using certain calculations, you determine the first and last days during which you can become pregnant in your cycle.
- **Cervical position and dilation.** Your cervix opens and changes position at the time of ovulation. When using the cervical position and dilation method, you check your cervical position using your finger. During ovulation, your cervix is slightly higher, softer and more open than it is normally. You may be able to determine your fertile time by recording and tracking your positions.
- **Mucus inspection method.** This involves tracking changes in your cervical mucus to determine when ovulation occurs.
- **Temperature method.** Most women have a slight change in body temperature related to ovulation. Their temperature drops during ovulation, then rises slightly after ovulation.
- **Mucothermal method.** This is a combination of the temperature and mucus inspection methods.
- **Symptothermal method.** This is a combination of four methods — calendar, cervical position and dilation, mucus inspection and temperature. Using all methods provides a more accurate picture of your fertile phase because signs noted with one method can confirm those noted with another method.

If you plan on using a rhythm method, it's best to take a class or receive training from a qualified teacher.

Effectiveness
The effectiveness of natural family planning methods depends on your diligence. Used perfectly, effectiveness ratings could reach 90 percent, which means that 10 out of 100 women who use natural family planning as birth control for a year will become pregnant. Few couples use natural family planning perfectly, so they experience slightly lower effectiveness rates.

Issues to consider
These methods are approved by most religious practices, but they require motivation and extended periods of abstinence. Usually, your periods must be very regular in order for this approach to be effective. Plus, you must carefully chart

your cycles and observe physical signs of ovulation. Some research has shown that the timing of a woman's fertility window can be highly unpredictable, even if her cycles are regular. That means you may have the potential for becoming pregnant even when calculations suggest you're not ovulating.

Withdrawal, which involves a man pulling out his penis before orgasm, isn't considered a reliable method of birth control because a man may leak some sperm even before ejaculation. Rhythm methods of birth control don't protect against STDs, including HIV/AIDS.

Spermicide

Spermicide contains a chemical that destroys sperm cells before they can fertilize the egg. It comes in different forms, including gel, foam, cream, film, suppository and tablet. Spermicides are often used in conjunction with diaphragms or male condoms.

Availability
Nonprescription

How it's used
You apply the spermicide inside your vagina near the cervix.

Effectiveness
Spermicides are 69 percent to 85 percent effective, meaning up to 31 out of 100 women who use this method as birth control for a year will become pregnant.

Issues to consider
Spermicides may cause vaginal irritation and urinary tract infection. Some spermicides contain an ingredient called nonoxynol-9, which was previously thought to protect against certain STDs, such as gonorrhea and chlamydia. But recent studies have shown that it doesn't protect against STDs and may even increase the risk of HIV transmission. Researchers are working to find a more effective form of vaginal microbicide, a substance that kills microorganisms such as viruses and bacteria.

Permanent methods of birth control

Nonsurgical sterilization

In November 2002, the Food and Drug Administration approved the first nonsurgical method of sterilization for women (Essure System). It consists of placing a small, metallic device within each fallopian tube. These devices cause scar tissue to form, effectively blocking the fallopian tube and preventing fertilization of the egg.

Availability
Procedure performed by your doctor

How it's done
Your doctor inserts a device into each of your fallopian tubes using a thin, flexible tube (catheter) that's threaded through the vagina into the uterus and on into the fallopian tube. For the following three months, you must use an alternate form of birth control. After this time, you undergo an X-ray to ensure that the scar tissue has grown into place. If the X-ray shows that your tubes are fully blocked, you can discontinue other forms of birth control.

Effectiveness
Within the studies conducted so far, the devices have been 100 percent effective when successfully implanted.

Issues to consider
The advantage of the Essure system is that it doesn't require an incision or general anesthesia. But it's irreversible, so be sure that you don't wish to have any more children. Even in women who have been sterilized, there's a small possibility of pregnancy occurring, and sterilization may increase your risk of an ectopic pregnancy.

Surgical sterilization

Either you or your partner may wish to undergo surgery to permanently prevent pregnancy. A woman may have tubal ligation, a procedure in which her "tubes are tied." A man may have a vasectomy, which keeps sperm from being ejaculated.

Availability
Surgical procedure

How it's done
During tubal ligation, a woman's fallopian tubes are cut and tied. She is usually under general anesthesia during this procedure, and a hospital stay may or may not be required. A tubal ligation can be done immediately after delivery, about six weeks after delivery or at any time after that.

A vasectomy may be done in a doctor's office with a local anesthetic. In this procedure, a man's vas deferentia — ducts through which the sperm travel — are cut and sealed.

Effectiveness for tubal ligation
In the first year following a tubal ligation, the chance of your becoming pregnant is less than 1 percent, meaning fewer than one woman out of 100 will become pregnant in the first year after a tubal ligation. Over time, it's possible that the tubes could fuse together and make it possible to become pregnant. After 10 years, failure rates as high as 5 percent have been reported in women who had the surgery early in their reproductive years. Failure rates are lower in women who are older when they have the procedure.

Effectiveness for vasectomy
The failure rate is less than 1 percent for vasectomy, meaning fewer than one woman out of 100 will become pregnant in the first year after her partner has had a vasectomy. However, vasectomy doesn't provide immediate protection against pregnancy. Most men become free of sperm after eight to 10 ejaculations. Until your doctor determines that the ejaculate doesn't contain sperm, another form of birth control needs to be used.

Issues to consider
Surgical sterilization isn't easily reversed. When a tubal ligation is reversed, it may carry an increased risk of an ectopic pregnancy. Before undergoing sterilization, be sure that you don't wish to have any more children. If you are a woman and have a medical condition that makes surgery risky, talk to your doctor about your options. All surgeries carry certain risks, such as bleeding and infection.

Emergency methods of birth control

If you had unprotected sex or a method of birth control failed during vaginal intercourse, you can use an emergency form of contraception to prevent pregnancy. Two types of pills are dedicated to emergency contraception: Preven, which contains a combination of estrogen and progestin, and Plan B, which contains progestin only. An IUD also may be used as an emergency contraceptive.

These emergency contraceptives prevent pregnancy by preventing ovulation, by preventing the egg from being fertilized or by preventing a fertilized egg from being implanted in your uterus.

Availability
Prescription

How they're used
Timing is important in the use of emergency contraceptives. Emergency contraceptive pills are most effective when taken within 72 hours of intercourse. You take them in two doses, 12 hours apart. In some cases, specific regimens of standard oral contraceptives can be used under a health care provider's advice. Emergency IUDs may be placed within seven days of intercourse.

Effectiveness
Estrogen-progestin combination pills are around 75 percent effective, meaning pregnancy is prevented for 75 out of 100 women using this method. Progestin-only pills are 85 percent effective, meaning pregnancy is prevented for 85 out of 100 women using this method.

The IUD is over 99 percent effective, meaning pregnancy is prevented for more than 99 out of 100 women using this method.

Issues to consider
Emergency contraceptives are generally very safe and have few side effects, but they're not intended for frequent use and aren't recommended as a routine form of birth control. Common side effects are nausea and vomiting, although they may occur more frequently with combination regimens. If you're breast-feeding, your health care provider may recommend a progestin-only regimen. After use of emergency contraceptive pills, your first period may be irregular.

Restrictions and side effects for emergency placement of an IUD are the same as for standard use of an IUD.

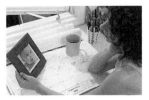

returning to work

"Should I return to work?"

That question weighs on the minds of many women — and, increasingly, men — after the birth of their babies.

Many American women juggle motherhood and a career. In 2001, around 64 percent of mothers with children under 6 years of age were part of the U.S. work force. And although mothers are still the predominant primary caregivers, more and more fathers are taking on that role. In families where mothers worked outside the home, one out of every five fathers provided the majority of child care for their preschoolers. In addition, nearly 200,000 fathers in two-parent homes in the United States were not in the work force primarily so that they could care for the family while their wives worked, according to a survey conducted by the U.S. Census Bureau in 2002. That compares to 11 million children with stay-at-home mothers in the United States.

Advice about parenting abounds. Before the '60s and '70s, it was generally expected that women were the primary caregivers of their children. But as more women began to work outside of the home, the desirability and, indeed, the practicality of the stay-at-home-mom arrangement came into question for many.

These days, there are advocates on both sides of the spectrum — and plenty of people somewhere in the middle. Some insist that to be a good parent, you must be at home to care for your children. Others don't want to give up a hard-won career to stay home full time. Still others try part-time work, home-based work, job sharing, flextime and a host of other arrangements.

Issues to consider

Consider the following points as you decide how to balance work and family matters.

Your concern about the possible effects on your child

Researchers have attempted to evaluate the effect of a working mother on her child. But measuring such a complex factor is difficult, if not impossible.

Results of studies vary. Some studies have found a slightly negative effect on child behavior and mother-child bonding for children whose mothers work during early childhood years. Other child experts assert that participation in high-quality group child care offers children a social setting where they can learn to interact with their peers and other adults.

One thing that research — and common sense — supports is the positive effect of a loving, nurturing relationship between parent and child. The most influential factor in parenting is probably not the sheer quantity of time you spend with your child. Stay-at-home parents don't spend all of their time interacting with their children. They have errands to run, dishes to wash, clothes to fold and various other duties that come with running a household.

One study from the *Journal of Marriage and Family* noted that stay-at-home moms averaged 38 hours a week caring for and socially interacting with their children. Working moms averaged 26 hours a week. In addition, the study said that there were no differences in the quality of mother-child interaction between the working mothers and stay-at-home mothers. What's important is that when you're with your child, you're all there — physically, mentally and emotionally.

Whatever your choice, if you feel happy and fulfilled, it will affect your child. If you resent your current arrangement or feel cheated by it, you'll likely pass on these feelings to your child. The old saying, "Take care of yourself first so that you can care for others," is still true.

Your financial needs

Sometimes you must work in order to make ends meet. You simply may not have the option of staying at home. Although money isn't everything, it is necessary to provide basic care for your family. If you need the income, spending some time away from your child is probably preferable to enduring chronic stress over money issues.

If you or your partner makes enough income to sustain both of you, you may not feel the need to have both of you split your time between work and home. If the loss of income is more stressful than you imagined, however, you might consider taking on a part-time job or a job that you can do from home.

If you're somewhere in the middle, carefully review your finances before making a decision. Consider not only salaries but also the cost of having two people working. Review costs such as commuting, parking, clothing and child care.

Your desire to maintain a career

Women and men who have worked hard to attain a certain position or whose occupation is meaningful to them often feel reluctant to give it up. You may desire and enjoy the intellectual challenges and adult interaction that comes from working outside the home. Because these needs are being met at work, you may feel more prepared to function fully at home.

Your desire to be a full-time parent

Perhaps your job is just a job to you. Or perhaps you value your job, but being your child's primary caregiver is more important to you than keeping your job.

Your ability to manage stress

It takes energy to handle the juggling act of parenting and working outside the home. Some people manage the stress that comes with these dual roles just fine. Others struggle with it.

Consider how well you can handle multiple roles and responsibilities. If you work, can you provide your children with the sort of attention you'd like them to have? Will your performance at work and at home decline? Will you have the support of friends and family to help you through some of the more difficult days?

There is no social right or wrong in this decision, but there's probably a choice that's best for you. Think carefully about your options. Talk it over with your partner and friends and family who have made different choices. Then make the best decision for you and your family. In this case, there's no wrong decision.

Sources of child care

If you decide you'll go back to work after your leave, it's important to find appropriate care for your child. Several options may be available to you, including an in-home caregiver, family child care and a child-care center.

In-home caregiver

Under this arrangement, someone comes to your home to provide child care. The person may live with you, depending on your agreement. Some examples of in-home caregivers are relatives, nannies and au pairs. Au pairs typically come to the United States on a student exchange visa and provide child care in exchange for room and board and usually a small salary. The advantage of hiring an in-home caregiver is that your child can stay at home, you set your own standards, and you have more flexibility with your work hours. But you also have certain legal and financial obligations as an employer.

Family child care

Some people provide care in their homes for small groups of children. The home usually has to meet state or local safety and cleanliness standards. Family child care allows your child to be in a home setting with other children, often at a lower cost than that of an in-home caregiver or a child-care center. Quality varies widely though, so before you leave your child there be sure to visit the home and get references from current or previous clients.

Child-care centers

Child-care centers are organized facilities with staff members who are trained to care for groups of children. Such centers are typically required to meet state or local standards. Some of the advantages of child-care centers include socialization with other children, a large selection of toys and activities and they're fully staffed, which can relieve worries about finding backup care. Child-care centers may not let you bring your child if he or she is mildly ill, and they usually require you to be fairly punctual. When considering a center, check the ratio of children to caregiver. If one adult has too many children to care for, your child may not get as much individual attention. The American Academy of Pediatrics recommends three children to one staff member, for infants up to 12 months.

If you don't already have a child-care arrangement in mind, a good place to start your search for high-quality care in your area is through Child Care Aware, a program of the Nation's Network of Child Care Resource and Referral. You can call the program at (800) 424-2246 or use its online search tool at *www.childcareaware.org*. It also has advice on what to look for and what questions to ask when evaluating a provider.

Once you've found child care you feel comfortable with, you can return to work with confidence knowing that your child is in good hands. Often, when mothers first return to work after their baby is born, they feel guilty for leaving the child. Or they're anxious that the child may bond more with the caregiver than with them. But don't worry, you'll still have time to spend with your child. The bond between mother and child, and father and child, is unique and can't be replaced.

Transitioning back to work

An important step in going back to work can be accomplished while you're still pregnant. Find out what family-leave benefits your company provides. See if other types of time off, such as vacation days or sick leave, can lengthen your leave.

Talk to your employer about your situation well ahead of your leave. If you're interested, ask if you can work flextime, part time or from home for a few months to help ease the transition. Don't expect special considerations, but be ready to be proactive when discussing opportunities with your boss. Offer potential solutions instead of ultimatums.

When's the best time to return to work? Although there's no perfect time frame, experts suggest spending three to four months at home with your baby if you can. That may give you time to settle into a schedule, bond emotionally and learn to care for your child. Fatigue is a big factor for both parents during those first few months. You'll benefit from plenty of time to rest and recover.

If possible, set your start date for a Wednesday, Thursday or Friday. This will give you a shorter workweek and a weekend to regain some energy.

THE FATHER AS PRIMARY CAREGIVER

Some research suggests that stay-at-home dads develop a stronger bond with their children than do traditional fathers who work outside the home. Two studies undertaken during the mid-1990s found that kids who have an at-home dad feel equally comfortable going to either parent when they are hurt or wake up in the middle of the night.

And although the father may occupy a position traditionally held by the mother, this doesn't necessarily mean there's a role reversal. At-home fathers still tend to clean the gutters and fix the dishwashers. But they also get their kids dressed, give them their meals and play with them. When mothers come home from work, they tend to resume the traditional mother role by helping with dinner, bathing the children and putting them to bed. As a result, fathers get to participate more in parenting, and children receive a strong influence from both mother and father.

Fathers cited two main reasons for staying at home. They didn't want to place their children in child care, and the working parent made more money.

Just as the decision for the mother to stay at home is unique to each couple, so, too, is the decision for the father to stay at home. The good news is, this type of arrangement is becoming increasingly acceptable. More and more fathers are discovering the joy and fulfillment that comes from caring for their children.

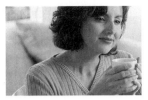

DECISION GUIDE

thinking about when to have another child

You think you want another child. But when might be the best time?

Only you and your partner can answer that question. If you wait for circumstances to be just right, you might never have any more children. The truth is that any child who is received with love and attention will probably do well, regardless of when he or she arrives.

The following information can help you examine and prioritize your goals as you plan for any future children.

Issues to consider

A few key factors need to be considered when thinking about the birth of your next little one. To begin, here are some general questions:

- Are you ready for the responsibility of raising another child? Caring for a growing family can be physically, mentally and emotionally taxing, despite its many rewards.
- How will another child affect your career? Is it important for you to reach another level in your field before you take on pregnancy, childbirth and caring for an infant again?
- What are your financial priorities? Will you or your partner need to stay home to care for your children? Are you willing to sacrifice certain things in order to cover baby costs? Do you wish to save for your children's college tuition?

Spacing

Is there an ideal amount of time you should wait between children? In some ways yes; in other ways, not really. Below are some of the advantages and disadvantages of the various ways you might space your children.

1 to 2 years

Having children one to two years apart can be the ultimate test of your endurance. In addition, it may carry some health risks. But that doesn't mean it can't work.

Advantages

- Your children will be close in age as they grow up. They may share many of the same interests and activities, making it easier to juggle family schedules. Parents often hope that siblings close in age will also be close companions.
- You get through the phase of carrying, feeding, diaper changing, sleep deprivation and toilet teaching all at once. Also, you may not need to baby-proof your home as many times as you would if you had your children further apart.
- Your first child may have an easier time adjusting to a sibling and may barely remember what life was like without him or her.

Disadvantages

- Caring for two in diapers is likely to leave you exhausted much of the time and with little personal space for a few years.
- Stress and fatigue can take their toll on your marriage. You and your partner will need to work as a team to meet the challenges ahead. And you'll need to set aside some quality time for each other.
- Supplies for two infants can be costly.
- Sibling rivalry may be an issue as your children grow up.
- Several studies have indicated that conceiving less than 18 months after the birth of your last child can increase the risk of low birth weight and premature birth. This may be because your body hasn't had a chance to recover from childbirth. It may still be depleted of necessary nutrients.
- Short gaps between pregnancies may affect the mother's health. Some studies suggest that becoming pregnant again in less than six months may increase the risk of certain maternal complications, such as anemia and third-trimester bleeding. Again, this may be due to your body not having fully recovered from the first pregnancy.
- If you had a Caesarean birth and allow for less than an 18-month interval before your next child is born, you may increase your risk of uterine rupture if you decide to try a vaginal birth.
- If you choose to breast-feed, you're less likely to conceive while doing so, but it can happen. If you do get pregnant while breast-feeding and decide not to wean your baby, you'll need to take extra care with your diet. You may want to meet with a dietitian to be sure you're meeting your nutritional needs.

2 to 5 years

A spacing of two to five years is what most experts recommend. Your first child is a little more independent, and you and your partner have had some time to regain much-needed strength and energy.

Advantages
- During the interval between pregnancies, you'll have time to bond with your first child and give him or her your undivided attention.
- Your first child will have the opportunity to be the baby of the family without any competition.
- When the new baby arrives, the older sibling will be more likely to play on his or her own at times, giving you some one-on-one time with the baby.
- Your children will still be close enough in age to bond easily.
- You're only paying for diapers for one. Some baby supplies, such as a crib or stroller, can be recycled.
- There's no rush to breast-feeding, and your body has time to restore its nutritional supply for the next pregnancy.
- Some research suggests an optimum pregnancy interval — the time between birth and subsequent conception — to be between 18 and 23 months, which poses the least risk of complications to mother and child.
- If you've had a Caesarean birth, waiting two to five years before giving birth again gives you a reduced risk of uterine rupture if you try a vaginal birth.

Disadvantages
- Your first child may feel jealous of the new baby. It's not uncommon for 3- and 4-year-olds to revert to baby-like behavior when faced with having to compete for a parent's attention. This usually goes away with time, though.
- Rivalry issues regarding toys and activities may occur as the baby gets older and starts getting around on his or her own.
- The further apart your children are, the more different each child's activities are. Coordinating the various schedules in your household may require considerable organization and planning. It can be quite stressful for the parents.

5 years or more

Having your kids as far apart as five years or more has both benefits and challenges. It also presents some possible health risks for you and your baby.

Advantages

- You get a big break between babies. This may give you some time to go back to doing things you enjoyed before having an infant, such as going out for dinner or a movie or taking adventurous vacations. It may also give you a chance to refocus on your career or your marriage.
- Each child gets plenty of individual attention during infancy.
- Because of the difference in age, sibling rivalry tends to be less intense.

GETTING YOUR CHILD READY FOR A NEW BABY

Your older children may beg you to "bring home a new baby" for the family. Yet children often react quite differently when the new little brother or sister actually arrives.

The reaction may not be what you expect. It's not abnormal for children to feel some jealousy or resentment when a new sibling is born. These feelings may stem from possible fears that they're no longer loved or that they aren't good enough for their parents anymore. Often, children aren't able to articulate these fears and may express them by regressing to earlier behaviors, such as using a pacifier or reverting to baby talk, whining or clinging to you.

A new baby's arrival can be a stressful time for the whole family. But with a little forethought and planning, you may be able to ease some of the tension surrounding it and increase your other children's sense of security. Following are some suggestions for preparing your children for the new baby.

Before birth

You don't have to rush to tell your children you're pregnant. You might even wait until the later stages of your pregnancy when the changes are obvious and they can see what's happening. Other things you might do with your children while you're pregnant:

- Help your children create their own baby books so that they can understand what it was like when they were babies and see how far they've come. Explain to them that the new baby will have many of the same experiences.
- Look at picture books that depict the baby's stages of development in the uterus. Try to use correct anatomical terms whenever possible.
- Spend time with families who have infants. Explain to your children that they may have special duties when the new baby comes, such as singing quiet songs or smiling and laughing with the baby.
- Have your children make big brother or big sister birth announcements to give to friends and classmates.
- Introduce your children well ahead of time to any changes that are necessary before the baby is born, such as changing rooms. Celebrate the changes as something special because they're growing up.
- Begin to adjust your routines. Perhaps you'll want to cut back on how often you pick up and carry your children.
- Make child-care arrangements before you go to the hospital, preferably with someone your children enjoy being with.

Instead, your younger child may regard his or her older sibling as more of a hero, while the older child may assume a more protective or guardian-like role.

- Waiting five years or more can also give you a financial break and allow you to save money for the next baby.
- Depending on the age of your first child, you may even have a built-in baby sitter.

- Take your children to a sibling class at your local hospital or read them stories about the arrival of a new baby.

In the hospital

Make the time in the hospital special for your children as well as the baby:

- Many hospitals now allow siblings to join their parents in the birthing suite. This can promote the sense that they are participating in the process of childbirth.
- Reconnect with your older children and give them each some undivided attention before you introduce them to the new baby.
- Have your children and baby exchange gifts from one another.
- Have a small family birthday party for the baby with a cupcake and a zero candle.

At home

When you get home, let the answering machine get the phone and spend some time with just your immediate family. Also, you may:

- Make use of the birth announcements your children have made. Emphasize the big brother or big sister aspect of having a new family member.
- Give your children age-appropriate responsibilities if they wish. However, don't force them to assist. Examples include bringing fresh diapers at changing time or talking or singing to the baby, especially when the baby's fussy.
- Reserve certain spaces for your children that are exclusively theirs, such as a bedroom or toy area, and respect that space.
- Try to spend time one-on-one with your other children on a regular basis. It doesn't have to be every day, but make it a priority when you do schedule it. Try reading, taking a short walk or coloring a picture with your older children.
- If your child expresses regressive behavior, don't criticize him or her. Rather, praise any positive behavior and downplay the negative. Try to stick to your normal daily routine, including school or child care for your child, if possible. Include your child in family activities and spend time alone with your child. This will reassure him or her that although some things have changed, your love is still the same, and his or her needs are still important.

Disadvantages

- After several years of being out of baby mode, you may have a hard time getting back into it. You tend to forget how much work caring for an infant can be and how exhausted you become.
- Your body may not be as flexible as it once was. It may be a challenge to keep up with your grade schoolers or teenagers while caring for a baby.
- Schedules in your household will probably vary widely. It may be stressful to keep them all coordinated.
- Some parents liken having two far-apart children to having two only children. Due to the age difference, your children may not share many of the same interests. They may not be as close as children who are more similar in age.
- Long gaps between pregnancies may increase the risk of certain complications for both you and your baby. Some studies suggest that women who conceive five years or more after the birth of a previous child have a higher risk of developing high blood pressure during pregnancy (preeclampsia), which can lead to a life-threatening condition characterized by seizures (eclampsia). Newborns arriving after a long pregnancy interval may be at a higher risk of premature birth and low birth weight. Researchers speculate that women who wait five years or more to have another baby may lose some of the protective effects generated by the first pregnancy.

PART 3

pregnancy reference guide

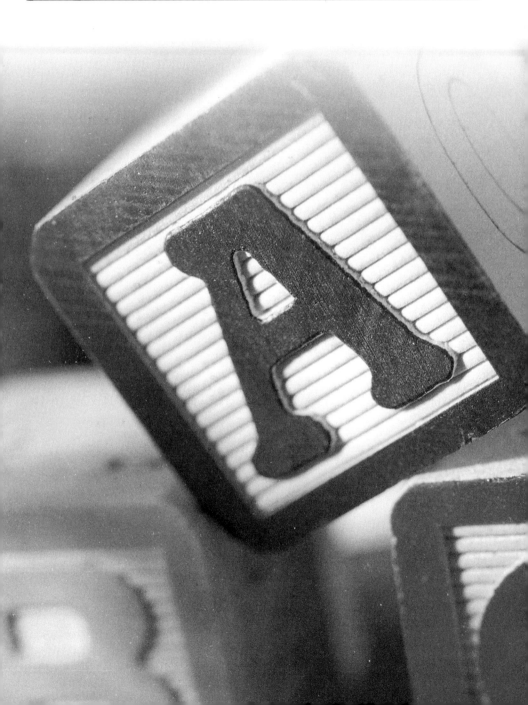

Pregnancy can bring with it a host of concerns, everything from acne to morning sickness, fatigue to heartburn. The Pregnancy Reference Guide offers self-care tips and insights on when to seek medical care for many pregnancy concerns.

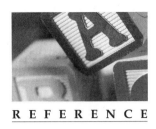

pregnancy reference guide

Abdomen, pressure in the lower

▤ *1st, 2nd, 3rd trimesters*

When not accompanied by other symptoms, a feeling of pressure in the lower abdomen is probably nothing to worry about. In the first trimester, this sensation is common. Most likely, you're feeling your uterus starting to grow. You may also be feeling increased blood flow. In the second or third trimester, the pressure likely has to do with the weight of the growing uterus. In all of these cases, the bladder and rectum are compressed by the growing uterus, which provokes feelings of pressure.

▤ *When to seek medical help for pressure in the lower abdomen*

If the pressure is accompanied by pain, cramping or bleeding early in your pregnancy, these might be signs and symptoms of miscarriage or ectopic pregnancy. An ectopic pregnancy occurs when the embryo implants outside the uterus, usually in a fallopian tube. Later in your pregnancy, pressure in the lower abdomen could indicate preterm (before the 37th week) labor.

Contact your health care provider if the abdominal pressure lasts for four to six hours or longer or is accompanied by any of the following:

- Pain
- Vaginal bleeding
- A low, dull backache that lasts four hours or longer
- Abdominal cramps
- Regular contractions or uterine tightening
- Watery vaginal discharge
- Ruptured membranes (your "water breaks")

Abdominal discomfort or cramping

▤ *1st, 2nd trimesters*

Pain in the lower abdomen during the first and second trimesters often stems from normal pregnancy changes. As the uterus expands, the ligaments and muscles that support it stretch. This stretching may cause twinges, cramps or pulling sensations on one or both sides of your lower abdomen. You may notice the pain more when you cough, sneeze or change position.

Another fairly common cause of abdominal or groin discomfort in midpregnancy is stretching of the round ligament, a cord-like muscle that supports the uterus. The discomfort usually lasts for several minutes and then goes away. (See also **Round ligament pain.**)

If you've had abdominal surgery, you may have pain from stretching or pulling of adhesions, the bands of scar tissue that adhere to the walls of the abdomen or other structures. The increasing size of your abdomen can cause these bands of tissue to stretch or even pull apart, which can be painful.

Lower abdominal discomfort that's relatively minor and comes and goes irregularly is probably nothing to worry about. If it's regular and predictable, consider whether you might be entering labor, even if you are still far from your due date.

Prevention and self-care for abdominal discomfort or cramping
It may help to sit or lie down if abdominal pain is bothering you. You may also find relief by soaking in a warm bath or doing relaxation exercises.

When to seek medical help for abdominal discomfort or cramping
Pain that's severe and unrelenting may be a sign of a problem, such as ectopic pregnancy or preterm labor. The first sign of an ectopic pregnancy usually is pain in the abdomen or pelvis. This pain is usually described as sharp and stabbing. Your abdomen may feel tender. You may have bleeding, nausea and low back pain.

In midpregnancy and beyond, lower abdominal pain accompanied by continuous low back pain or contractions may signal preterm labor. Call your health care provider right away if:
- Pain is severe, persistent or accompanied by fever
- You experience vaginal bleeding, vaginal discharge, gastrointestinal symptoms, dizziness or lightheadedness
- You have pain in the shoulder and neck
- You have contractions, which may feel like a tightening in the abdomen and a sensation similar to menstrual cramps

Abdominal tenderness due to muscle separation
2nd, 3rd trimesters
During pregnancy, your growing uterus stretches the muscles in your abdomen. This may cause the two large parallel bands of muscles that

meet in the middle of the abdomen to separate. This separation, called diastasis, can also cause a bulge where the two muscles separate.

For most women, the condition is painless. Others experience some tenderness around the bellybutton. The muscle separation can also contribute to back pain.

The condition may first appear during the second trimester. It may become more noticeable in the third trimester. In subsequent pregnancies, it's likely to be worse. But the problem generally goes away after delivery.

■ *Prevention and self-care for abdominal muscle separation*
If abdominal muscle separation is causing a backache or back pain, a number of simple strategies can help make your back more comfortable (see also **Backaches and back pain**).

■ *Medical care for abdominal muscle separation*
Usually no medical care is needed for abdominal muscle separation. Your health care provider can evaluate whether the amount of muscle separation is more than usual. He or she may suggest ways to remedy the separation after your baby is born.

Absent-mindedness
See **Forgetfulness**

Acne
■ *1st, 2nd, 3rd trimesters*
Because pregnancy hormones increase oil secretion from skin glands, you may develop acne early in your pregnancy. These skin changes are temporary and will likely disappear after you give birth.

■ *Prevention and self-care for acne*
Most acne can be prevented or controlled with good basic skin care. Try the following techniques:
- Wash your face as you normally would. Avoid facial scrubs, astringents and masks because they tend to irritate skin and can make acne worse. Excessive washing and scrubbing can also irritate skin.
- Avoid irritants such as oily cosmetics, hair-styling products or acne concealers. Use products labeled water-based or noncomedogenic,

which are less likely to clog pores. If the sun makes your acne worse, protect yourself from direct sunlight.

- Watch what touches your face. Keep your hair clean and off your face. Avoid resting your hands or objects on your face. Tight clothing or hats also can pose a problem, especially if you're sweating. Sweat, dirt and oils can contribute to acne.

Medical care for acne

Don't take any medications for acne without your health care provider's advice. Some drugs used to treat acne can harm a fetus. These include:

- *Isotretinoin (Accutane)*. This acne medication, taken orally, is known to cause birth defects such as hydrocephalus, cardiac abnormalities and ear defects. Women who take Accutane must wait at least three months after stopping use of the drug before becoming pregnant.
- *Hormonal therapy*. Hormones, including estrogen and the anti-androgens spironolactone and flutamide, are sometimes used to treat acne. They shouldn't be taken during pregnancy.
- *Tetracyclines*. These antibiotic medications are often used to treat acne. They may cause slowed bone growth and discolored teeth in the fetus as well as severe liver disease in expectant mothers. They shouldn't be used during pregnancy.

If you're concerned about acne or skin breakouts, talk to your health care provider.

Alcohol, use of

1st, 2nd, 3rd trimesters

Don't drink alcohol during your pregnancy. No level of alcohol has been proved safe during pregnancy. Drinking alcohol during pregnancy can cause fetal alcohol syndrome, which can result in both physical and mental birth defects.

If you have a drink or two before you realize you're pregnant, don't panic. It's unlikely that drinking a small amount of alcohol early in the pregnancy will do harm. However, stop drinking alcohol as soon as you suspect you're pregnant — better still, quit before you try to become pregnant.

When to seek medical help for use of alcohol

If you find it hard to stop drinking, get help. Talk with your health care provider about your options.

Allergies

1st, 2nd, 3rd trimesters

Many women have allergies, either seasonal or year-round, before getting pregnant. Others develop a stuffy nose during pregnancy, even if they haven't had that problem before.

During pregnancy, elevated levels of estrogen appear to increase mucus production and swelling in the nose, causing congestion. In addition to a runny or stuffed nose, you may experience sneezing and itchy, watery eyes.

Many of the usual remedies for these signs and symptoms should be avoided in pregnancy:

- *Antihistamines.* Use caution when considering the use of antihistamines, which are commonly used to relieve cold and allergy signs and symptoms such as itching, sneezing and a runny nose. Talk with your health care provider to see if antihistamines would help and for direction on which product to use.
- *Decongestants.* There is reason for concern regarding pregnant women's use of decongestants, which come in either nasal or oral form and work by shrinking blood vessels to relieve nasal congestion. Decongestants are sold under many brand names, including Afrin, Dristan, Drixoral, Naphcon Forte, Neo-Synephrine, Otrivin, Sudafed, and Vicks Sinex. Use decongestants only on a health care provider's advice.
- *Combination antihistamines and decongestants.* Many prescription and nonprescription products combine antihistamines and decongestants. Some over-the-counter medications of this type include Allerest, Benadryl Allergy & Sinus, Claritin-D, Contac Day & Night Allergy/Sinus, Sudafed Severe Cold Formula and Vicks DayQuil. Avoid all medications of this type while pregnant because combination drugs may have combined effects on the fetus.

Preferred medications for problems in pregnancy include:

- *Nasal sprays.* Steroid nasal sprays reduce inflammation and mucus production and may improve night sleep and daytime alertness. Nasal sprays include beclomethasone (Beconase, Vancenase), budesonide (Rhinocort), flunisolide (Aerobid), fluticasone (Flonase), mometasone furoate (Nasonex) and triamcinolone (Nasacort). Steroid nasal sprays are thought to be safe during pregnancy, but discuss your options carefully with your health care provider before taking them.
- *Cromolyn.* Cromolyn (NasalCrom) also is a nasal spray that reduces inflammation, but it's not a steroid. It's not as effective as the steroid sprays, but it's effective for treating mild allergies. It's often a good treatment option for pregnant women with mild allergies.
- *Allergy shots.* Allergy shots (immunotherapy) are safe for pregnant women who are already receiving them. If you haven't been getting

shots, don't start them during pregnancy unless you've talked about this option with your health care provider.

Prevention and self-care for allergies

As a first step, try to determine what you're allergic to. Try to avoid exposing yourself to those things. Common irritants or allergens include pollen, dust mites, animal dander and hair, molds, fungi and cockroaches. Keep in mind that smoking or being in a smoke-filled room can make your allergies worse. Air filters and air conditioning can help control pollen allergies.

Here are some other tips to help you deal with allergy signs and symptoms:

- Use a nasal wash to clear a congested nose. Dissolve ¼ teaspoon of salt in 1 cup of warm water. Lean over the sink with your head down and to the side. Pour some of the saline solution into the palm of your hand and inhale it through a nostril while holding the other nostril closed with your finger. The solution will move through your nasal passages and into your mouth. Spit the remaining solution out, and gently blow your nose. Tilt your head to the other side and repeat with the other nostril. You can also administer the wash with a large rubber syringe, available at pharmacies. You can do nasal washes several times a day. Make a fresh solution each time.
- You may be able to clear a stuffy nose by breathing steam from a hot shower, a pot of boiling water taken off the stove, a cool mist humidifier or a vaporizer. Be sure to keep humidifiers and vaporizers clean because bacteria and mold can grow in them.
- Place warm, moist towels on your face to clear your nose and chest.
- Use your fingers to massage your sinuses — rub on the bony ridge above and under your eyebrows, under your eyes and down the sides of your nose.

When to seek medical help for allergies

If your signs and symptoms are severe or don't improve with self-care techniques, talk to your health care provider. He or she may suggest an appropriate medication. Don't take any medication for allergies without consulting your health care provider. Studies haven't found any benefit from most alternative therapies, including high-dose vitamins, homeopathic remedies and most herbal remedies. And they aren't any safer than medications.

Baby 'drops'

See **Lightening**

Baby movement, decreased

3rd trimester

Most pregnant women get to know their baby's typical patterns of movement and are attuned to changes in the frequency or intensity of those movements. You may notice a slight decrease in your baby's activity in the last few days before birth. In late pregnancy, the number of fetal movements you perceive often declines gradually. The baby has less room to move around in the uterus, especially after his or her head drops into the pelvis.

Although a baby who isn't very active in the womb may be perfectly healthy, decreased fetal movement can be a sign that something is wrong. A significant drop in fetal activity in the last trimester of pregnancy may indicate that the baby is in jeopardy, possibly because of decreased oxygen. This may be caused by a variety of problems, such as a knotted or compressed umbilical cord. A problem with the placenta also may lead to problems for the baby.

Self-care for decreased baby movement

If you're concerned about the baby's activity, take a break from other activities. Sit down and drink a glass of juice or regular — not diet — soda. Concentrate on your baby's movements. In most cases, you'll find your baby is more active than you realized. Almost all babies will move at least four times each hour.

When to seek medical help for decreased baby movement

Don't hesitate to contact your health care provider if you're worried about a decrease in your baby's movement. Call your health care provider immediately if:

- You feel no fetal movement for more than one hour.
- You notice a significant decrease in your baby's movements — fewer than 10 movements in a two-hour period.

Your health care provider can check the condition of your fetus. Decreased fetal movement is often noted in time to help the baby if he or she is in trouble. When a possible problem is found, the baby may need to be delivered immediately, often by emergency Caesarean birth, during which the baby is removed through an incision in the mother's abdomen. Prompt action may prevent serious problems.

Baby's hiccups

2nd, 3rd trimesters

Starting about midway through your pregnancy, you may occasionally notice a slight twitching or little spasms in your abdomen. Your baby probably has the hiccups. Fetal hiccups develop as early as the 15th week of gestation, even before breathing movements become common. Some fetuses get hiccups several times a day, and others never get them. After they're born, most babies have frequent bouts of hiccups. They're common after a feeding, particularly after burping. No one knows why they occur — in babies or adults — or why babies have them so often.

Fortunately, hiccups pose no danger to babies before or after birth. There's no reliable way to stop hiccups in a baby. They don't cause the same discomfort in babies as they do in adults, though a newborn with hiccups may fuss or cry.

Backaches and back pain

1st, 2nd, 3rd trimesters

Pregnant women are prone to backaches and back pain for a number of reasons. During pregnancy, the joints and ligaments in your pelvic region begin to soften and loosen in preparation for the baby to pass through your pelvis. As your uterus grows, your abdominal organs shift, and your body weight is redistributed, changing your center of gravity. Gradually you begin to adjust your posture and the ways you move. These compensations can lead to backaches and back pain. (See also **Abdominal tenderness due to muscle separation; Sciatica.**)

Prevention and self-care for backaches and back pain

Try these suggestions to help your back feel more comfortable:
- Practice good posture. Tuck your buttocks under, pull your shoulders back and downward, and stand straight and tall. Be aware of how you stand, sit and move.
- Change position often, and avoid standing for long periods of time.
- Avoid lifting heavy objects or children.
- Lift correctly. Don't bend over at the waist. Instead, squat down, bend your knees, and lift with your legs rather than your back.
- Place one foot on a low stool when you have to stand for a long time.
- Wear supportive, low-heeled shoes.
- Exercise (swim, walk or stretch) at least three times a week. Consider joining a prenatal exercise or yoga class.
- Try to avoid sudden reaching movements or stretching your arms high over your head.
- Sit with your feet slightly elevated.
- Sleep on your side with one knee or both knees bent. Place a pillow between your knees and another one under your abdomen. You may also find relief by placing a specially shaped total body pillow under your abdomen.

- Apply heat to your back. Try warm bath soaks, warm wet towels, a hot water bottle or a heating pad. Some people find relief by alternating ice packs with heat.
- Have a back massage or practice relaxation techniques.
- Wear maternity pants with a low, supportive waistband. Or consider using a maternity support belt.
- Do pelvic tilt exercises. Rest comfortably on your hands and knees with your head in line with your back. Pull in your abdomen, arching your back upward. Hold the position for several seconds, then relax your abdomen and back. Repeat three to five times, working gradually up to 10.

When to seek medical help for backaches and back pain

Pain relief medications other than acetaminophen (Tylenol, others) — including aspirin, ibuprofen (Advil, Motrin, others) and "superaspirins" (COX-2 inhibitors such as Celebrex) — cause some concern for your unborn baby. If your back pain is severe, ask your health care provider about appropriate treatment. He or she may suggest a variety of approaches, such as special stretching exercises, to alleviate pain without causing concern about your baby.

Back pain may be a sign of a more serious problem if it's severe and unrelenting or if it's accompanied by other signs and symptoms. A low, dull backache may be a sign of labor or preterm labor.

Contact your health care provider if your back pain lasts four to six hours or longer or if you're also experiencing any of the following:

- Vaginal bleeding, which may come and go
- Cramping or abdominal pain
- Passing of tissue from the vagina
- Fever
- Regular uterine contractions (every 10 minutes or more often), which may feel like a tightening in your abdomen
- A feeling of heaviness or pressure in the pelvis or lower abdomen
- Watery discharge (clear, pink or brownish fluid) leaking from your vagina
- Menstrual-like cramps, which may come and go and may be accompanied by diarrhea
- Ruptured membranes, that is, the breaking of the amniotic sac, a normal part of going into labor (your water breaks)

Birth control pills, safety of, after conception

1st trimester

It rarely happens, but birth control pills can fail. If you get pregnant while you're taking birth control pills, stop taking them immediately. The hormones in the pills should be avoided during pregnancy. The risk is low, but there is a potential for harm.

If you're planning to become pregnant, most health care providers recommend that you stop taking the pill two to three months before conception. For birth control during this time, you may want to use condoms or a diaphragm. Conceiving during the first month after you stop taking the pill doesn't pose a serious risk to fetal development, however.

Bleeding, vaginal
See **Vaginal bleeding**

Bleeding gums
1st, 2nd, 3rd trimesters
Like the rest of your body, your gums are receiving more blood flow during pregnancy. This can cause your gums to swell or become softer. As a result, they may bleed a little when you brush your teeth.

Prevention and self-care for bleeding gums
Don't neglect your dental care during pregnancy. Brushing, flossing and regular dental exams and cleaning are important. Make sure you're getting enough vitamin C from foods or your vitamin supplement because this vitamin helps keep your tissues strong.

When to seek medical help for bleeding gums
If bleeding is heavy or accompanied by pain, redness or inflammation, make an appointment soon with your dentist to check for infection and tell your health care provider about the problem.

Bloating
See **Gas and bloating**

Bloody show
3rd trimester
This dramatic and alarming term refers to the passage of the thick mucus that plugs the cervix during pregnancy. The mucous plug blocks the cervical opening to prevent bacteria and other germs from entering the uterus. As your body prepares for labor, the cervix begins to thin out and relax, and the mucous barrier is dislodged.

You may have a vaginal discharge that's clear, pink or blood-tinged. It may come out as a thick or stringy mass or as a constant or intermittent discharge. Some women don't notice anything at all.

The bloody show or mucous discharge is a sign that the big day is coming, but you probably don't need to rush to pack your bags. The process can start just before labor or up to a week or two before labor.

■ *When to seek medical help for bloody show*
There's no need to report passage of the mucous plug to your health care provider unless your discharge is watery, foul smelling or suddenly becomes bright red, especially if it amounts to more than about two tablespoons. Actual bleeding could indicate premature separation of the placenta or placenta previa. These conditions require prompt medical attention.

Blue lines or veins under skin
■ *2nd, 3rd trimesters*
Veins throughout your body become larger during pregnancy to accommodate increased blood flow to the baby. These enlarged blood vessels show up as fine bluish, reddish or purplish lines under the skin, most often on the legs and ankles. Blood vessels in the skin over your breasts also become more visible and appear as blue or pink lines. These lines usually disappear after pregnancy.

About one in five pregnant women develops varicose veins — protruding, swollen veins, particularly in the legs. Varicose veins may surface for the first time or worsen during late pregnancy, when the uterus exerts greater pressure on the veins to the legs. (See also **Varicose veins.)**

Blurred vision
■ *1st, 2nd, 3rd trimesters*
Changes in your eyes during pregnancy can cause slightly blurred vision. Because your body retains extra fluid, the outer layer of your eye (cornea) becomes about 3 percent thicker.

This change may become apparent by the 10th week of pregnancy and persists until about six weeks after the baby is born. In addition, the pressure of fluid within your eyeball (intraocular pressure) decreases during pregnancy. In combination, these changes can in rare cases cause blurred vision.

If you wear contact lenses, particularly hard lenses, you may find them uncomfortable because of these changes.

■ *Prevention and self-care for blurred vision*
If your contact lenses are uncomfortable, you may want to wear glasses more often instead. But it's not necessary to change your eye lens prescription during pregnancy. Your vision will return to normal after you give birth.

■ *When to seek medical help for blurred vision*
If you experience sudden onset of blurred vision, have it evaluated. That's especially critical if you have diabetes. Talk to your health care provider about establishing good control of your diabetes, monitoring your blood sugar and about any vision problems you experience.

Blurred vision may also be caused by preeclampsia, a disease that produces an increase in blood pressure. Talk to your health care provider if you notice a sudden change in your vision, if your vision is very blurry or if you're seeing spots in front of your eyes. High blood pressure can lead to serious problems with the pregnancy.

Braxton-Hicks contractions
See **Contractions**

Breast discharge
■ *3rd trimester*
In the final weeks of pregnancy, you may notice a thin, yellowish or clear substance leaking from one or both nipples. This discharge is colostrum, the yellowish fluid produced by your breasts until your milk comes in.

Colostrum can range in color and consistency, but such variations are normal. It may be sticky and yellow at first and become more watery as you approach your due date.

The older you are and the more pregnancies you've had, the more likely it is you'll have some breast discharge. But it's no cause for concern if you don't leak colostrum — it doesn't mean you won't be able to produce breast milk.

If you're breast-feeding, you'll notice that you produce colostrum for the first few days after your baby is born.

■ *Prevention and self-care for breast discharge*
If you're leaking colostrum, you might want to wear disposable or washable breast pads. It may also be helpful to allow your breasts to air-dry a few times a day and after showers.

■ *When to seek medical help for breast discharge*
Call your health care provider if your nipple discharge is bloody or contains pus, which could indicate a breast abscess or other problem.

Breast enlargement
■ *1st, 2nd, 3rd trimesters*
One of the first signs of pregnancy is an increase in breast size. As early as two weeks after conception, your breasts start to grow and change in

preparation for producing milk. Stimulated by estrogen and progesterone, the milk-producing glands inside your breasts get bigger, and fatty tissue increases slightly.

By the end of your first trimester, your breasts and nipples will be noticeably larger, and they may keep growing throughout your pregnancy. Breast enlargement accounts for at least a pound of the weight you gain while pregnant. Your breasts may remain enlarged for a while after your baby's birth.

Self-care for breast enlargement

As your breasts grow and become heavier, wear a bra that fits well and provides good support to ease the strain on your breasts and back muscles. If your breasts make you uncomfortable at night, try sleeping in a bra. Over the course of your pregnancy, you may need to replace your bras several times as your breasts change size.

To help prevent premature sagging of your breasts, wear a bra at all times until your breasts return to their pre-pregnancy size.

Breast tenderness

1st trimester

Often the first hint of pregnancy is a change in the way your breasts feel. By a few weeks of gestation, you may notice tingling sensations in your breasts, and they may feel heavy, tender and sore. Your nipples may be more sensitive.

As with breast enlargement, the primary reason for these changes is increased production of the hormones estrogen and progesterone. Breast tenderness normally disappears after the first trimester.

Self-care for breast tenderness

A good support bra that fits well can help alleviate breast soreness. Try a maternity bra or a larger-sized athletic bra — these tend to be breathable and comfortable. At night you may feel more comfortable sleeping in a bra.

Breath, shortness of

2nd, 3rd trimesters

Having trouble catching your breath? Many pregnant women experience mild breathlessness beginning in the second trimester. This is because your expanding uterus pushes up against your diaphragm — the broad, flat muscle that lies under your lungs. The diaphragm rises about $1^{1}/_{2}$ inches from its usual position during pregnancy. That may seem like a small amount, but it's enough to crowd your lungs and alter your lung capacity — the amount of air your lungs are able to take in.

At the same time, your respiratory system makes some adaptations to allow your blood to carry large quantities of oxygen to the placenta and to remove more carbon dioxide than it normally does. Stimulated by the hormone progesterone, the respiratory center in the brain causes you to breathe more deeply and more frequently. Your lungs will inhale and exhale 30 percent to 40 percent more air with each breath than they did before. These changes may give you the feeling that you're breathing hard or short of breath.

The larger your uterus becomes, the harder you may find it to take a deep breath because your diaphragm is pushing against the baby. A few weeks before you give birth, the baby's head may move down in the uterus (drop), taking the pressure off the diaphragm. When the baby drops, you'll find it easier to breathe. But this may not happen until the start of labor, especially if you've had a baby before.

Despite the discomfort of feeling short of breath, you don't have to worry that your baby isn't getting enough oxygen. Thanks to your expanded respiratory and circulatory systems, the oxygen level in your blood increases during pregnancy, ensuring that your growing baby is getting plenty of oxygen.

Prevention and self-care for shortness of breath

If you're short of breath, try these tips:

- Practice good posture. It will help you to breathe better, both during pregnancy and afterward. Sit and stand with your back straight and shoulders back, relaxed and down.
- Do aerobic exercise. It will improve your breathing and lower your pulse rate. But take care not to overexert yourself. Talk to your health care provider about a safe exercise program for late pregnancy.
- Sleep on your side to help lessen the pressure on your diaphragm. Prop yourself up with pillows that support your abdomen and your back or use a total body pillow.

When to seek medical help for shortness of breath

While mild breathlessness is common in pregnancy, severe shortness of breath or breathing problems may indicate a more serious problem, such as a blood clot in a lung.

Call your health care provider immediately or go to an emergency room if you have:

- Severe shortness of breath along with chest pain
- Discomfort while taking a deep breath
- Rapid pulse or rapid breathing
- Lips or fingertips that seem to be turning blue

Burning sensation in hands

See **Carpal tunnel syndrome**

Caffeine

▪ *1st, 2nd, 3rd trimesters*

It's best to avoid caffeine whenever possible during pregnancy. At the very least, don't overindulge. Study results on the subject have been mixed. But overall, studies show that a moderate intake of caffeine — 200 milligrams (mg) or less a day, which is the amount found in about one to two cups of coffee — has no negative effects on pregnant women and their babies. However, high amounts of caffeine — 500 mg or more a day, for example, five or more cups of coffee — may cause a decrease in your baby's birth weight and head circumference. Coffee, tea and carbonated beverages all can contain caffeine. To reduce your intake of caffeine, consider switching to decaffeinated versions of the beverages you like.

Calf pain or tenderness

See **Leg cramps**

Carpal tunnel syndrome

▪ *2nd, 3rd trimesters*

Carpal tunnel syndrome is most often caused by repetitive movements of the hand and wrist, such as typing. You may be surprised to learn that it's also common in pregnant women. That's because hormonal changes, swelling and weight gain can compress the nerve beneath the carpal tunnel ligament in your wrist.

Carpal tunnel ligament

Median nerve

Symptoms of carpal tunnel syndrome include numbness, tingling, weakness, pain or a burning sensation in the hands. In pregnant women carpal tunnel syndrome often occurs in both hands.

The carpal tunnel ligament is a tough membrane that holds the wrist bones together. A nerve called the median nerve enters the hand through the carpal tunnel, a space between the wrist bones and the carpal tunnel ligament. This passageway is rigid, so any swelling in the area can pinch or compress the median nerve, which supplies sensation to the ball of the thumb, the first two fingers and half of the ring finger.

▪ *Self-care for carpal tunnel syndrome*

You may be able to relieve the discomfort by rubbing or shaking your hands. The first line of treatment is to wear a wrist splint at night and during activities that make the symptoms worse, such as typing, driving a car or holding a book. Applying cold compresses or heat to your wrists may help.

Medical care for carpal tunnel syndrome

Carpal tunnel syndrome almost always disappears after delivery. In the rare cases when it doesn't, or when the effects are severe, you may be given steroid injections. Sometimes, minor surgery is needed to correct the problem.

Chickenpox and shingles

1st, 2nd, 3rd trimesters

Most pregnant women are immune to the viral illness chickenpox (varicella) because they had it or were vaccinated as a child. Once you've had the disease, you're immune for life. So if you had chickenpox or have been vaccinated against it, there's no need for concern if you're exposed to it during pregnancy.

If you haven't had chickenpox, it poses risks to you and your fetus if you get the disease while pregnant. That's why during a preconception or prenatal visit your health care provider will likely ask whether you've already had chickenpox. If you haven't or if you don't know, he or she may recommend a blood test to determine whether you're immune. Although a vaccine is available to prevent chickenpox, pregnant women shouldn't be vaccinated.

If you're not immune to chickenpox and haven't been vaccinated, you'll want to take steps to avoid exposure and prevent complications for you and your baby. In rare cases, chickenpox early in pregnancy can result in birth defects. If you develop chickenpox the week before giving birth, your newborn is at risk of developing a severe and potentially fatal chickenpox infection. A chickenpox infection in a baby is rare. Chickenpox in a pregnant woman also is a cause for concern. Pregnant women are much more likely to have severe infections, including varicella pneumonia.

Shingles (herpes zoster) is caused by a limited reactivation of the chickenpox virus, usually years after you were infected. Shingles causes painful clusters of blisters. If you develop shingles while pregnant, there's little cause for concern. There is no risk of birth defects caused by shingles in the mother.

Prevention and self-care for chickenpox

If you're not immune to chickenpox, avoid contact with anyone who has the disease, which is highly infectious. Children are most infectious from two days before the rash appears until three days after the rash appears. Stay away from other susceptible people who've been in recent contact with an infected person.

In rare instances, a child who has recently been vaccinated against chickenpox may pass the virus on to others if he or she develops sores around the injection site. If you're not immune, talk to your health care provider about whether to postpone vaccination of any children at home until after you deliver.

When to seek medical help for chickenpox

Notify your health care provider if you're not immune to chickenpox and you suspect that you've been exposed to it. In pregnancy, you'll likely receive an injection of anti-chickenpox antibodies (varicella-zoster immune globulin, or VZIG). VZIG is safe for both you and your baby. When given within 96 hours after exposure, VZIG helps prevent chickenpox or at least lessens its severity. This can help prevent complications such as pneumonia, which seems to occur more commonly in pregnant women than in other adults with chickenpox. Researchers have not determined whether taking VZIG will help protect your fetus from infection.

If you develop chickenpox the week before giving birth, your newborn is at risk of developing severe chickenpox infection. The severity of the infection can usually be reduced if the baby is treated promptly after birth with VZIG. If serious symptoms develop despite use of VZIG, antiviral drugs can help.

Clumsiness

2nd, 3rd trimesters

During pregnancy, you may feel like you're all thumbs — or all feet or elbows. You find yourself stumbling or tripping, bumping into things, dropping everything you pick up. You may worry that you're going to fall and hurt your baby.

It's perfectly normal to be clumsier than usual at this time. As your uterus grows, your sense of balance is thrown off. Your usual ways of moving, standing and walking change.

In addition, the hormone relaxin, produced by the placenta, relaxes the binding ligaments that hold the three pelvic bones together. This allows the pelvis to open wider so that the baby's head can move through the pelvis. It can also contribute to the feeling of clumsiness.

Other factors that may make you clumsier include water retention, lack of concentration (see also **Forgetfulness)** or lack of dexterity due to carpal tunnel syndrome (see also **Carpal tunnel syndrome).** Late in pregnancy, your large uterus can block your view of stairs or hazards on the floor. All of these effects are temporary, and you'll be back to your old self again after the baby is born.

If you do fall, your baby probably won't be harmed. An injury would normally have to be severe enough to hurt you before it would harm your baby. (See also **Falls.**)

Prevention and self-care for clumsiness
You can't do much about the physical changes that can make you feel like a bull in a china shop. But you can decrease your chances of falling by taking a few precautions:
- Avoid wearing high heels or pumps. Instead, wear stable, flat shoes with soles that provide good traction.
- Avoid situations that require careful balance, such as perching on ladders and stools.
- Take a little extra time with tasks that require many changes of position.
- Use extra caution when going up or down stairs and in other situations that put you at risk of tripping or falling, such as walking on an icy sidewalk.

When to seek medical help for clumsiness
If you fall and strike your abdomen or you're just worried about the welfare of your baby, see your health care provider for reassurance or treatment, if needed. If you fall on your abdomen late in pregnancy, your health care provider will likely monitor the baby to be sure that the placenta's attachment to the uterus wasn't damaged.

Colds

1st, 2nd, 3rd trimesters
Most women catch a cold at least once during pregnancy. Although the signs and symptoms can make you miserable, even a bad cold isn't a hazard to your baby. Colds tend to last longer during pregnancy because of changes in your immune system.

Prevention and self-care for colds
To keep from catching a cold, the best strategy is to eat well, get plenty of rest, exercise regularly and avoid close contact with anyone who has the sniffles or a sore throat. If you're around family members or co-workers with colds, wash your hands often. Cold germs are easily passed from one person to another.

If you do come down with a cold, take care of yourself using minimal medications. Many cold remedies that you may be accustomed to using —

including aspirin, ibuprofen (Advil, Motrin, others), decongestants, cough syrups, antihistamines, nasal sprays, herbal remedies such as echinacea and megadoses of vitamin C and zinc — aren't recommended during pregnancy. Acetaminophen (Tylenol, others) is a good choice for fever, headaches and body aches associated with a cold. If you're miserable with a cold, call your health care provider for advice regarding products that generate the least risk.

To treat your cold, consider these tips:

- Get plenty of rest. Being run down puts a strain on your body.
- Drink extra fluids. Fever, sneezes and a runny nose will cause your body to lose fluids that you and your baby need. In addition to helping your body fight the cold, drinking plenty of fluids can also keep your stuffy nose clearer. Choose citrus juices, water or broth.
- Help clear nasal congestion by using a humidifier in your bedroom at night or by putting a towel over your head and breathing the steam from a pan of boiling water removed from the stove. When you're lying down or sleeping, ease your breathing by keeping your head elevated on a couple of pillows. Nasal strips, which gently pull your nasal passages open, also may help.
- To soothe a sore throat, most health care providers think that topical anesthetic sore throat lozenges are OK. You can also try sucking on ice chips, drinking warm liquids or gargling with very warm salt water (1/4 teaspoon of salt in 8 ounces of water).
- Continue eating well. If you don't have an appetite and can't tolerate large meals, eat smaller amounts more frequently throughout the day. Choose foods that appeal to you. Vitamin-rich fruits and vegetables and soup are good choices when you have a cold.

When to seek medical help for colds

Call your health care provider if:

- Your fever reaches 102 F
- You're coughing up greenish or yellowish mucus
- You have a cough with chest pain or wheezing
- Your signs and symptoms are severe enough to keep you from eating or sleeping
- Your sinuses are throbbing or you have facial pain or painful teeth
- Your signs and symptoms persist for more than a few days with no signs of improvement

It may be possible to treat your signs and symptoms with a cold medication. Your health care provider will recommend one that's considered safe during pregnancy. Although cold medicines can relieve signs and symptoms, they don't affect the severity and duration of a cold. If you have a secondary infection, such as bronchitis or a sinus infection, your health care provider may prescribe an antibiotic.

Don't put off calling the health care provider or refuse to take a prescribed medication because you don't want to take any drug during pregnancy. Many cold treatments aren't harmful for your baby — but your health care provider should make the decision.

Coloring your hair
1st trimester

Studies have not linked hair dyes to birth defects, and the chemicals in the dyes are not readily absorbed through the skin. Still, some experts advise pregnant women to err on the side of caution and avoid any possible risk by switching to a toxin-free hair dye or not getting hair colored during the first trimester. Your colored hair's appearance also may be a concern — hormonal changes can cause your hair to react differently when you're pregnant, leaving you with an unexpected color.

Constipation
1st, 2nd, 3rd trimesters

Constipation is one of the most common side effects of pregnancy, affecting at least half of all pregnant women at some point. It's usually more troublesome in women who were prone to constipation before pregnancy.

When you're pregnant, an increase in the hormone progesterone causes digestion to slow down, so food passes more slowly through the gastrointestinal tract. In the later months, the ever-expanding uterus puts pressure on the lower bowel. In addition, your colon absorbs more water during pregnancy, which tends to make stools harder and bowel movements more difficult.

Other factors that can contribute to the problem include irregular eating habits, stress, changes in environment and added calcium and iron in your diet. Constipation can give rise to hemorrhoids (see **Hemorrhoids).**

Prevention and self-care for constipation

The first step in dealing with the problem is to evaluate your diet. Eating fiber-rich foods and drinking plenty of fluids each day will help prevent or ease constipation. Follow these suggestions:

- Eat high-fiber foods, including fresh and dried fruits, raw and cooked vegetables, bran, beans and whole-grain foods, such as whole-wheat bread, brown rice and oatmeal. The age-old remedy of prunes — now marketed as dried plums — can help, as can fruit juices, especially prune juice.
- Eat small, frequent meals and chew your food thoroughly.

- Drink plenty of fluids, especially water. Aim for eight 8-ounce glasses a day. Drink a glass of water before going to bed.
- Get more exercise. Just adding a little time to your daily walks or other physical activities can be effective.
- Iron supplements can cause constipation. If your health care provider has recommended iron supplements and you have constipation, take the iron pills with prune juice.

Medical care for constipation

If self-care measures don't work, your health care provider may recommend a mild laxative such as milk of magnesia, a bulk-producing agent such as Metamucil or Citrucel, or a stool softener containing docusate. Sometimes, stronger measures are needed, but they should only be used on the advice of your practitioner.

Don't take cod liver oil because it can interfere with the absorption of certain vitamins and nutrients.

Contractions

3rd trimester

When you're about to go into labor, you'll notice an increase in contractions, the tightening and relaxing of the uterine muscles. During labor, the uterus repeatedly contracts, causing the cervix to thin (efface) and open up (dilate) so that you can push your baby out. The contractions gradually dilate the cervix until it's wide enough for the baby to pass through.

During the early phase of labor, contractions can vary greatly from one woman to another. They might last 15 to 30 seconds at the beginning and be irregularly spaced, 15 to 30 minutes apart. Or they might start out fast and then slow down. But they will continue to increase in frequency and duration as the cervix dilates.

Contractions may be relatively painless at first but gradually build in intensity. You may feel like your uterus is knotting up. Or the pain may feel like an aching sensation, pressure, fullness, cramping or a backache.

For more information about contractions and labor, see Chapter 11, "Labor and childbirth."

False labor vs. true labor

If you've never given birth before, you might assume that having contractions is a sure sign that you're starting labor. Not necessarily. Most expectant mothers feel occasional painless contractions before they're actually in labor. Occasionally these can be uncomfortable.

In the last weeks of pregnancy, your uterus might start to cramp. When you put your hands on your abdomen, you can sometimes feel your uterus tighten and relax. These mild contractions are called false labor (Braxton-Hicks contractions). Your uterus is warming up, preparing for the big job ahead.

As you approach your due date, these contractions become stronger and may be uncomfortable or even painful at times. It can be easy to mistake them for the real thing.

The difference between false labor and true labor is that in true labor the contractions cause your cervix to dilate. But you might not be able to tell the difference. And false labor often happens just when you expect to go into labor.

One good way to distinguish true labor from false labor is to time the contractions. Using a watch or clock, measure how long each lasts and how long it is from the start of one to the start of the next. As indicated in the chart below, such timing can reveal a pattern to the contractions if you're truly in labor.

Even after monitoring all these signs, you may not know whether you're truly in labor. Sometimes the only way to know is to see whether the cervix is dilating, which requires a pelvic exam. The start of labor is different for everyone. Some women have painful contractions for days

IS IT FALSE LABOR OR TRUE LABOR?

Contraction characteristic	False labor (Braxton-Hicks contractions)	True labor
Frequency of contractions	• Irregular • Don't get consistently closer together	• Regular pattern • Grow closer together
Length and intensity of contractions	• Vary • Usually weak • Don't get stronger	• At least 30 seconds at onset • Get longer (up to 75 seconds) • Get stronger
How contractions change with activity	• Usually stop if you walk, rest or change positions	• Don't go away no matter what • May grow stronger with activity, such as walking
Location of contractions	• Centered in lower abdomen and groin	• Wrap around from back to abdomen • Radiate throughout your lower back and high on abdomen

with no cervical changes, while others may feel only a little pressure and a backache. You might leave for the hospital with regular contractions that are three minutes apart, and as soon as you arrive they stop. Or you may go in for your regular checkup, only to find that you're dilated enough for your health care provider to send you to the hospital.

It's possible to have contractions for hours before you're actually in labor. Labor begins when the cervix begins to dilate. But if your contractions continue to get longer, stronger and closer together, you're on your way!

Self-care for contractions

If false labor contractions are making you uncomfortable, take a warm bath and drink plenty of fluids.

If you're in true labor, and walking feels comfortable, go ahead and walk, stopping to breathe through contractions, if necessary. Walking may help your labor. It also helps determine if labor is false or real. You might want someone to support you during contractions while you're walking. Some women find that as the pain intensifies, rocking in a rocking chair or taking a warm shower helps them relax between contractions.

If you feel the urge to push, hold back until you've been told you're fully dilated. This helps to prevent your cervix from tearing or becoming swollen.

When to seek medical help for contractions

Monitor your contractions closely to see if they:

- Last at least 30 seconds
- Occur regularly
- Occur more than six times in an hour
- Don't go away when you move around

If you're in doubt about whether you are in labor, call your health care provider. He or she will want to know what other symptoms you're feeling, how far apart your contractions are and whether you can talk during them. If it's not clear that you're in labor, your health care provider may want to do a vaginal exam to check whether your cervix is dilating.

Go to the hospital if:

- Your membranes rupture (your water breaks), even if you're not having contractions. You may not experience contractions even if your water has broken.
- Your contractions come five minutes apart or closer. Frequent contractions may be a sign of a rapid delivery.
- You have constant, severe pain.

If you're having regular contractions or you have a sudden release of fluid from your vagina three weeks or more before your due date, seek medical attention because you may be in preterm labor.

Cramping or continuous pain
1st, 2nd, 3rd trimesters

Abdominal cramping or pain and back pain often go along with the normal processes of pregnancy (see also **Abdominal discomfort or cramping; Backaches and back pain; Pelvic pressure).** However, in early pregnancy, cramping and back pain accompanied by bleeding may be signs and symptoms of miscarriage or an ectopic pregnancy.

In midpregnancy and beyond, cramping and constant back pain could be warning signs of preterm labor. Sudden, constant, severe abdominal pain can be an indication of placental separation. In combination with fever and vaginal discharge, abdominal pain may signal an infection.

Contact your health care provider if cramping or back pain is severe, persistent or accompanied by fever, bleeding, contractions or vaginal discharge.

Dehydration after stomach flu
1st, 2nd, 3rd trimesters

If you've had a stomach flu (gastroenteritis), you've probably lost a lot of fluids as you endured the misery of diarrhea and vomiting. Dehydration is the most common complication of gastroenteritis. Signs and symptoms of dehydration include:

- Excessive thirst
- Dry mouth
- Dark yellow urine or infrequent or no urination
- Severe weakness, dizziness or lightheadedness

After a bout with gastrointestinal illness, it's essential that you take in enough fluids to replace those lost from diarrhea and vomiting.

Although gastroenteritis is often called stomach flu, it's not the same as influenza. Real flu (influenza) affects your respiratory system — your nose, throat and lungs — rather than your intestines. But you may become dehydrated after having the flu because you lose your appetite and stop eating and drinking while sick.

Prevention and self-care for dehydration after stomach flu

A flu shot is your best line of defense against influenza, although it won't prevent gastroenteritis. Health experts at the Centers for Disease Control and Prevention recommend that any woman who will be beyond the first trimester of pregnancy during the flu season get a flu shot. Talk with your health care provider about whether that applies to you.

To keep from catching stomach flu, follow common-sense measures such as washing your hands thoroughly, avoiding close contact with people who are sick, and avoiding sharing eating utensils, glasses and plates. Food preparation problems are the most common cause of gastroenteritis.

If you do get a stomach bug, take steps to replenish lost fluids and prevent dehydration:

- Take frequent sips of water and other clear liquids, such as weak, decaffeinated tea, broth, noncaffeinated sports drinks or orange juice diluted with water. Try to drink at least eight to 16 8-ounce glasses of liquid a day.
- Suck on ice chips or ice cubes.
- Avoid caffeine-containing beverages such as colas, coffee and tea. Caffeine increases the loss of fluids from the body. Milk products may provoke more diarrhea.

When to seek medical help for dehydration after stomach flu
Call your health care provider if you have signs of dehydration, if you're not able to keep liquids down for 24 hours or if you're vomiting for more than two days. If you're dehydrated, your health care provider may recommend a rehydration fluid. For severe dehydration, treatment may involve blood tests and intravenous fluids.

Dizziness
See **Faintness and dizziness**

Dreams, vivid
1st, 2nd, 3rd trimesters
You're being grabbed around the middle by a gorilla ... flying over tall buildings ... talking to your newborn, who is talking back! Vivid dreams and nightmares are common during pregnancy. Dreams may be the mind's way of processing unconscious information. During this time of emotional and physical changes, your dreams may seem more intense and strange. You may find that you're dreaming more frequently or remembering your dreams more clearly when you wake up. Indeed, if you're regularly waking up during the night to urinate or shift to a more comfortable position, you're more likely to interrupt a cycle of dream-filled rapid eye movement (REM) sleep.

You may have anxiety dreams or nightmares. Try not to be disturbed about them. They reflect your apprehension and excitement about this major life change.

One way to enjoy your heightened dream world is to record your dreams in a dream journal. Writing about dreams can be a way to reflect on and come to terms with your experiences.

If disturbing dreams or nightmares are causing you distress, it might be helpful to talk with a therapist or counselor to help discover what's troubling you.

Dyeing your hair
See **Coloring your hair**

Eye changes
▨ *1st, 2nd, 3rd trimesters*
Some of the changes your body undergoes during pregnancy can affect your eyes and your vision. During pregnancy, the outer layer (cornea) of the eyes becomes a little thicker, and the pressure of fluid within your eyeballs (intraocular pressure) decreases by about 10 percent. These changes occasionally result in slightly blurred vision (see also **Blurred vision**).

In addition to blurred vision, you may experience other changes related to your eyes:

- *Vision (refractive) changes.* Changes in hormone levels appear to temporarily alter the strength you need in your eyeglasses or contact lenses.
- *Dry eyes.* Some pregnant women develop dry eyes, which may involve a stinging, burning or scratchy sensation, increased eye irritation or fatigue, and difficulty wearing contact lenses.
- *Puffy eyelids.* Because of water retention during pregnancy, you may have puffiness around the eyes. Puffy eyelids can interfere with peripheral vision.

Monitor your vision closely during pregnancy. Diabetes complications such as diabetic retinopathy — which damages the retina of your eyes — can worsen during pregnancy. It's essential to have your eyes examined during pregnancy if you have diabetes. Women with high blood pressure (hypertension) also are susceptible to vision problems. Hypertension during pregnancy requires close observation. Occasionally, newly blurred vision may be a sign of a serious high blood pressure problem in late pregnancy.

▨ *Prevention and self-care for eye changes*
If you're having trouble with blurred vision or a change in your vision early in pregnancy, there's usually no great cause for worry or a need to change your eyeglass or contact lens prescription. Your vision will return to its normal state after you give birth.

To lessen the discomfort of dry eyes, use lubricating eyedrops, also referred to as artificial tears. Lubricating eyedrops are safe to use during pregnancy. Dry eyes is usually a temporary condition that goes away after delivery.

If your contacts are uncomfortable because of dry, irritated eyes, try cleaning the lenses with an enzymatic cleaner more often. If they remain uncomfortable, don't worry. Your eyes will likely return to normal within a few weeks of delivery.

▨ *When to seek medical help for eye changes*

Contact your health care provider immediately if you have a new onset of blurred vision or blind spots at any time. If you have diabetes or high blood pressure, work with your health care provider to closely monitor your vision. Diabetic retinopathy requires treatment before, during and after pregnancy. To minimize vision complications from retinopathy, see an ophthalmologist regularly. If you're concerned about any changes in your vision, you may want to talk to an eye doctor.

Faintness and dizziness

▨ *1st, 2nd, 3rd trimesters*

Feeling a little faint? It's common for pregnant women to experience light-headedness, faintness or dizziness. These sensations can result from circulatory changes during pregnancy, such as decreased blood flow to your upper body because of the pressure of your uterus on the blood vessels in your back and pelvis. You're particularly susceptible to this early in the second trimester, when your blood vessels have dilated in response to pregnancy hormones but your blood volume hasn't yet expanded to fill them.

Dizziness or faintness may also occur during hot weather or when you're taking a hot bath or shower. When you're overheated, the blood vessels in your skin dilate, temporarily reducing the amount of blood returning to your heart.

Low blood sugar (hypoglycemia), common in early pregnancy, also can cause dizziness, as can having too few red blood cells (anemia). Finally, stress, fatigue and hunger can make you feel dizzy or faint. Less commonly, the flu, diabetes, high blood pressure or a thyroid disorder may contribute to faintness or dizziness.

▨ *Prevention and self-care for faintness and dizziness*

To prevent faintness and dizziness, follow these suggestions:

- Move slowly as you get up from lying or sitting down, and change positions slowly.
- Move or walk at a slower pace. Take frequent rest breaks.
- Avoid standing for long periods of time.
- Avoid lying flat on your back. Instead, lie on your side, with a pillow tucked under your hip.
- Avoid getting overheated. Stay away from warm, crowded areas. Dress in layers. Make sure your bath or shower isn't too hot. Leave the door or window open to keep the room from getting too hot.
- Eat several small meals or snacks each day instead of three large meals. Munch on snacks such as dried or fresh fruits, whole-wheat bread, crackers or low-fat yogurt.

- Stay physically active to help with your lower body circulation. Good activities include walking, water aerobics and prenatal yoga.
- Drink plenty of fluids, particularly early in the day. Sports drinks may be most effective.
- Eat foods that are rich in iron, such as beans, red meat, green leafy vegetables and dried fruits.

When to seek medical help for faintness and dizziness

It's always a good idea to tell your health care provider if you've been feeling faint or dizzy.

If faintness or dizziness is severe and occurs with abdominal pain or vaginal bleeding, it may be a sign of ectopic pregnancy, in which the fertilized egg attaches outside the uterus, or another serious complication. Always report significant vaginal bleeding to your health care provider.

Falls

1st, 2nd, 3rd trimesters

You've taken a tumble and are terrified that you may have hurt your baby. It's easy to panic if you fall during pregnancy. But your body is designed to protect your developing baby. An injury would have to be severe enough to seriously hurt you before it would directly harm your baby.

The walls of your uterus are thick, strong muscles that help keep your baby safe. The amniotic fluid also serves as a cushion. And during the early weeks of pregnancy, the uterus is tucked behind the pelvic bone, so there's even more protection. If you do fall, you can take comfort in knowing that your baby most likely won't be hurt.

In late pregnancy, a direct blow to the abdomen can give rise to placental abruption, in which the placenta separates from the wall of the uterus. This complication is very unlikely unless you've been injured. But if you break a bone, the possibility of this complication means that you must be evaluated.

Prevention and self-care for falls

When you're pregnant, your sense of balance is thrown off as your uterus grows. With this in mind, take a few extra precautions to avoid tripping or falling:

- Wear stable, flat shoes with soles that provide good traction. Put away your heels or pumps for the duration of your pregnancy.
- Avoid situations that require careful balance, such as climbing ladders or standing on stools.
- Take a little extra time when going up and down stairs, during tasks that require several changes of position or in situations that pose a risk of falling, such as walking on an icy sidewalk or wet surface.

When to seek medical help for falls

If you're worried about the welfare of your baby after a fall, see your health care provider for reassurance. Most practitioners want to hear about any spills you take after the 24th week of pregnancy because the possibility of placental abruption must be considered.

Seek medical attention immediately if:

- Your fall results in pain, bleeding or a direct blow to the abdomen
- You're experiencing vaginal bleeding or leaking of amniotic fluid
- You feel severe pain or tenderness in your abdomen, uterus or pelvis
- You have uterine contractions — abdominal tightening that may or may not be painful
- You notice a decrease in fetal movement

In most cases, your baby will be fine. But your health care provider may want to monitor the fetal heart rate or do blood tests to make sure the placenta wasn't injured.

False labor

See **"False labor vs. true labor"** under **Contractions**

Fatigue

1st, 3rd trimesters

"I'm so tired!" This is one of the most common refrains of pregnancy. Most women are more tired than usual in pregnancy. During the early months, your body is working hard — pumping out hormones, producing more blood to carry nutrients to the fetus, speeding your heart rate to accommodate the increased blood flow and changing the way you use water, protein, carbohydrates and fat. High progesterone levels actually make you sleepy in a direct way. During the last couple of months of pregnancy, carrying the extra weight of the baby is tiring.

In addition to physical changes, you're dealing with a range of feelings and concerns that may sap your energy and disturb sleep. It's natural to have conflicting feelings about a pregnancy, whether it's planned or unplanned, your first or your fourth. Even if you're overjoyed, you're probably facing added emotional stresses. You may have fears about whether the baby will be healthy, anxiety about how you will adjust to motherhood and concerns about increased expenses. If your job is demanding, you may worry about being able to stay productive throughout pregnancy.

These concerns are normal and natural. It's important to recognize that emotional issues also play a part in how you feel physically.

Prevention and self-care for fatigue

Remember that it's normal to feel tired during pregnancy. Fatigue is a sign from your body that you need extra rest. Don't push yourself. Here are some ways to keep fatigue from getting the best of you:

- *Rest.* Accept the fact that you need extra rest during these nine months, and plan your daily life accordingly. Take naps when you can during the day. At work, finding time to sit back comfortably with your feet up can renew your energy. If you can't nap during the day, maybe you can take one after work or before dinner or your evening activities. If you need to go to bed at 7 p.m. to feel rested, do it. It may help if you avoid drinking fluids for a few hours before bedtime so that you won't have to get up as often during the night to go to the bathroom.
- *Avoid taking on extra responsibilities.* Cut down on volunteer commitments and social events if they're wearing you out.
- *Ask for the support you need.* Get your partner or other children to help out as much as possible.
- *Exercise regularly.* Regular physical activity will increase your energy level. Moderate exercise, such as walking for 30 minutes a day, can help you feel more energized.
- *Eat well.* Eating a nutritious, balanced diet is more important now than ever. Make sure you're getting enough calories, iron and protein. Fatigue can be aggravated if your diet is short on iron or protein.

Medical care for fatigue
No medications for fatigue are safe or effective during pregnancy. Avoid stimulants such as caffeine, which may be harmful in high doses.

Fears about baby, pregnancy
See **Irrational fears**

Feet, enlarged
2nd, 3rd trimesters
If you like shopping for shoes, you'll appreciate this aspect of pregnancy. Your feet may be spreading, changing your shoe size. Hormonal changes that relax the ligaments and joints in your pelvis in preparation for delivery also relax all the other ligaments and joints in your body, including those in your feet. While these changes are normal and necessary, they can make the arch ligament of the foot (the plantar fascia) stretch under your body's extra weight. As a result, the arch may lose some of its supporting strength, and your feet grow flatter and wider. They may be as much as a full shoe size larger.

On top of these changes, your feet may swell due to the normal fluid retention of pregnancy. And if your weight gain is significant, your feet may carry a little extra fat.

The swelling in your feet should go down shortly after delivery. But it can take up to six months for the other changes in your feet to reverse themselves and your feet to return to their normal size and shape. If the plantar fascia has been stretched excessively, your feet may be permanently larger.

Prevention and self-care for enlarged feet

As your feet expand, it's important to wear shoes that will provide comfort and support for your feet and ankles. Buy a couple of pairs of shoes that fit you well now and will remain comfortable if your feet continue to grow. Avoid narrow-toed or high-heeled shoes. Look for low heels, non-skid soles and plenty of space for your feet to spread out.

Canvas or leather shoes are good choices because they allow your feet to breathe. Good running shoes are a wise choice. You should also be able to find work and dress shoes that meet these criteria. If your feet are aching and tired at the end of the day, try wearing elasticized slippers.

Medical care for enlarged feet

Some shoes and orthotic inserts are specially designed for pregnancy. They're meant to make your feet more comfortable and reduce back and leg pain. Ask your health care provider for a recommendation.

Flu

See **Influenza**

Food aversions

1st trimester

Early in pregnancy, you may find yourself repulsed by certain foods, such as fried foods or coffee. Even the smell of these foods may send a wave of nausea through your stomach. You may have a mildly metallic taste in your mouth that contributes to the problem. Most food aversions disappear or weaken by the fourth month of pregnancy.

Food aversions, like so many other complaints of pregnancy, can be chalked up to hormonal changes. Most pregnant women find that their food tastes change somewhat, especially in the first trimester, when the hormones are having the strongest impact. Food aversions can be accompanied by a heightened sense of smell and, at times, increased salivation, making your distaste even more acute.

Prevention and self-care for food aversions

As long as you continue to eat a healthy diet and get all the nutrients you need, appetite changes aren't a cause for concern. If your aversion is to coffee, tea or alcohol, that works in your favor because you'll find it easier to give up these foods. But if your aversion is to healthy foods such as fruits or vegetables, you'll have to find other sources of the nutrients they provide.

Food cravings

1st trimester

You may not have had the classic pickles-and-ice-cream craving. But chances are you've had a strong desire for certain types of food during your pregnancy. Most expectant mothers do experience food cravings, which are likely caused by pregnancy hormones.

You may wonder if a food craving is a signal from your body that you need the nutrients in that food. But such body signals are unreliable. A craving for ice cream doesn't mean your body needs the saturated fat. And even if you're not in the mood for citrus fruits, it doesn't mean you don't need vitamin C.

Most food cravings disappear or weaken by the fourth month of pregnancy. Cravings that last longer may be a sign of iron deficiency and the anemia that results.

Prevention and self-care for food cravings

As long as you're eating a healthy diet and getting the nutrients you need, you don't have to worry about changes in your food tastes. It's OK to indulge occasionally. However, try not to use your cravings as an excuse for overeating. You can respond to cravings without compromising your own or your baby's nutritional needs.

Try to satisfy your food urges without filling up on empty calories. For example, if you crave chocolate, choose chocolate frozen yogurt rather than ice cream or a frozen chocolate bar, or if you crave sweets, try trail mix instead of candy. If you have a craving for a food that you know isn't the best choice, try diverting your attention by taking a walk, reading a good book or playing a computer game. Usually an exercise-related distraction is most successful.

When to seek medical help for food cravings

Rarely, some pregnant women have a craving for unusual, inedible and possibly harmful substances. These may include items such as clay, laundry starch, dirt, baking soda, ice chips or frost from the freezer, ashes or road salt. Such uncommon cravings result from a disorder known as pica. It can be dangerous and may be caused by an iron deficiency. If you experience a craving to eat something that isn't food, report it to your health care provider.

Forgetfulness

1st, 2nd, 3rd trimesters

You misplace your keys, forget an appointment, can't focus on your work. If you feel like you've turned into a scatterbrain since getting pregnant, you're not alone. Some women become more forgetful or absent-minded during pregnancy. You may have trouble concentrating and feel like you're in a fog. These symptoms, similar to what some women experience premenstrually, are a temporary effect of hormonal changes.

Prevention and self-care for forgetfulness

Consider these tips to feel more in control:

- Accept that being a little absent-minded during pregnancy is normal. Getting uptight about it will just make it worse. Now's the time to have a sense of humor.
- Reduce the stresses in your life as much as possible.
- Keep lists at home and at work to keep from forgetting things you need to do. Some women benefit from using an electronic organizer.

Medical care for forgetfulness

No medical treatment has been shown to improve mental alertness. The herbal remedy ginkgo is touted as a memory booster, but it's not considered safe for use during pregnancy.

Gas and bloating

1st, 2nd, 3rd trimesters

Gas, bloating, flatulence — more fun aspects of being pregnant! Under the influence of pregnancy hormones, your digestive system slows down. Food moves more slowly through your gastrointestinal tract. This slowdown serves an important purpose: It allows nutrients more time to be absorbed into your bloodstream and to reach the fetus. Unfortunately, it can also cause bloating and gas. The problem may be aggravated during the first trimester, when many women have a tendency to swallow air in response to nausea.

Prevention and self-care for gas and bloating

To minimize the amount of gas and bloating you experience during pregnancy, follow these suggestions:

- Keep your bowels moving. Constipation is a common cause of gas and bloating. To avoid it, drink plenty of liquids, eat a variety of high-fiber foods and stay physically active on a regular basis. (See also **Constipation.**)
- Eat small, frequent meals, and don't overfill your stomach.

- Eat slowly. When you eat in a hurry, you're more likely to swallow air, which can contribute to gas. Take a few deep breaths before meals to relax.
- Avoid gas-producing foods. These vary from one person to another, but some common culprits include cabbage, broccoli, cauliflower, brussels sprouts, onions, carbonated beverages, fried foods, greasy or high-fat foods, rich sauces, and, of course, beans.
- Don't lie down immediately after eating.

Medical care for gas and bloating

Don't take an antacid for gas, bloating or indigestion without talking to your health care provider first. Many antacids contain sodium, which can increase swelling and water retention. They may also contain aluminum, which can cause constipation and aggravate the problem. Antacids that contain magnesium can lead to diarrhea.

Gum disease

1st, 2nd, 3rd trimesters

An old saying has it that "a woman loses one tooth with every pregnancy." While that's clearly a tale from the days before professional dental care, you are more susceptible to dental problems when you're pregnant. The oral changes of pregnancy are linked to an increased amount of plaque, the sticky, colorless film of bacteria that coats your teeth. Hormonal changes also make your gums more susceptible to the damaging effects of plaque. If plaque hardens, it turns into tartar.

When plaque and tartar build up along the part of your gums around the base of your teeth (gingiva), they can irritate your gums and create pockets of bacteria between your gums and teeth. This condition is called gingivitis, a form of gum disease. Gingivitis is characterized by red, swollen, tender gums that may easily bleed, especially when you brush your teeth (see also **Bleeding gums).**

Many pregnant women are affected by gingivitis to some extent. It usually starts in the second trimester. If you already have some degree of gum disease, it's likely to worsen during pregnancy.

Left untreated, gingivitis can develop into a more serious form of gum disease called periodontitis. This gum infection can cause teeth to loosen and fall out. And serious gum disease poses even more threats to a pregnant woman. It may increase your risk of having a preterm or low-birth-weight baby and also may increase your risk of developing preeclampsia.

Prevention and self-care for gum disease

Because your teeth are more susceptible to the harmful effects of bacteria while you're pregnant, it's important to keep up good dental hygiene. Follow these preventive dental care steps to keep your gums healthy:

- Brush your teeth with fluoride toothpaste at least twice a day and after each meal when possible. Brush before bedtime and again in the morning. To further reduce bacteria in the mouth, brush your tongue when you brush your teeth.
- If brushing your teeth triggers nausea, rinse your mouth with water or with anti-plaque and fluoride mouthwashes.
- Floss your teeth thoroughly each day. Flossing removes plaque between your teeth and helps massage your gums. Waxed and unwaxed floss are both fine.
- You may need more frequent dental exams when you're pregnant. Even if you're not having problems with your teeth or gums, schedule an appointment to have your teeth checked and cleaned at least once during your nine months. Dental X-rays can be performed without risk to the baby.
- Good nutrition can help keep your teeth and gums healthy and strong. Vitamins C and B-12 are particularly important for oral health.

Medical care for gum disease

If you have severe gum disease, have it treated promptly to avoid problems with your pregnancy. Contact your dentist and your health care provider if you have signs and symptoms of periodontitis:

- Swollen or recessed gums
- An unpleasant taste in your mouth
- Bad breath
- Pain in one of your teeth, especially with hot, cold or sweet foods
- Loose teeth
- A change in your bite
- Drainage of pus around one or more teeth

Treatment for severe gum disease may include special cleaning techniques and antibiotics. In some cases, surgery may be necessary. If you need major dental work while pregnant, you'll want to thoroughly discuss your options with both your dentist and your regular health care provider to ensure safety.

Hair coloring

See **Coloring your hair**

HCG tests

1st trimester

Human chorionic gonadotropin (HCG) is a protein hormone produced in the placenta of a pregnant woman. The test to determine whether you're pregnant detects the presence of HCG in your urine or blood. During the early weeks of pregnancy, HCG is important in the corpus luteum, which is the mass of cells that remains in the ovary after the egg's release from a mature follicle (the sac where the egg develops in your ovary). In a normal pregnancy, production of HCG increases steadily, doubling about every two or three days during the first 10 weeks. Levels then fall slowly during the remainder of the pregnancy.

The HCG test is routinely used to confirm pregnancy, either in a home test of urine or a blood or urine test at a clinic or lab. It takes six to 12 days after fertilization before HCG can be detected in urine.

Abnormal levels of HCG can indicate problems such as ectopic pregnancy, impending miscarriage or development of an abnormal mass of cells in the uterus after fertilization (molar pregnancy). In an ectopic pregnancy or one destined to end in miscarriage, the rate of increase of HCG is much slower than normal. If your health care provider suspects one of these problems, you may be given several blood HCG tests over a number of days to determine whether the hormone is increasing at a normal rate.

A higher-than-usual HCG level may indicate a multiple pregnancy or a molar pregnancy. HCG tests are also used to monitor women after a molar pregnancy, miscarriage or ectopic pregnancy to make sure the pregnancy tissue is gone.

Headaches

1st, 2nd, 3rd trimesters

Many pregnant women are troubled by headaches. Early in pregnancy, increased blood circulation and hormonal changes can cause headaches. Other possible causes include stress or anxiety, fatigue, nasal congestion, eyestrain, and tension. If you suddenly eliminated or cut down on caffeine when you learned you were pregnant, this "withdrawal" also can cause headaches for a few days.

If you suffer from migraines, they may stay the same, improve or worsen when you're pregnant. They might be worse in the first trimester, then improve in the second.

Prevention and self-care for headaches

One way to avoid getting headaches is to determine what triggers them and avoid those things. Triggers may include cigarette smoke, stuffy rooms, eyestrain and certain foods. Here are some other suggestions for minimizing the pain of headaches:

- Get plenty of sleep each night, and rest during the day when possible.

- Drink plenty of liquids.
- Soothe a sinus headache by applying a warm washcloth to the front and sides of your face, around your nose, eyes and temples. If you feel a tension headache coming on, apply an ice pack or cold compress to your forehead and the back of your neck.
- Take a warm shower or bath.
- Massage your neck, shoulders, face and scalp, or ask your partner or a friend to give you a massage.
- Practice relaxation techniques and exercises, such as meditation.
- Get some fresh air. Take a walk outside if possible.
- Minimize the stresses in your life. Although some stresses can't be avoided, you can boost your coping skills. If you're under more stress than you feel you can handle, it might be helpful to talk to a therapist or counselor. Talk to your health care provider about it.

When to seek medical help for headaches

Contact your health care provider right away if you're having headaches that are severe, persistent or frequent, or that are accompanied by blurred vision or other vision changes. If you have high blood pressure, it's important to report any headache.

Talk to your health care provider before taking any pain relievers or headache medications, including aspirin or ibuprofen (Advil, Motrin, others), which could cause problems if they're taken during pregnancy. Acetaminophen (Tylenol, others) is a better choice during pregnancy. It appears to be very safe. It's usually the first choice for pain and fever relief during pregnancy.

If you have migraines, talk to your health care provider about how to manage them during pregnancy. Don't take any migraine medications without checking with your health care provider. He or she may tell you to avoid some medications used to treat migraines, including aspirin, propranolol and especially ergotamine-containing medications.

Heartburn

3rd trimester

More than half of all pregnant women get heartburn — and for many, it's their first experience with it. Heartburn, also called gastroesophageal reflux disease (GERD), actually has nothing to do with your heart. It's caused by the backward flow of stomach contents passing up into the esophagus, the tube that carries food from your mouth to your stomach. When this happens, stomach acids irritate the lining of the esophagus. The resulting burning sensation at about the level of the heart gives the condition its misleading name.

Heartburn is more common during pregnancy for a number of reasons. Pregnancy hormones cause your digestive system to slow down. The wave-like movements of the esophagus that push food down into your stomach become slower. Your stomach also takes longer to empty. These changes give nutrients more time to be absorbed into your bloodstream and to reach the fetus. But they can also cause indigestion and heartburn. The muscle between the stomach and the esophagus also relaxes, which may allow stomach acids to move upward.

In addition, during the later months of pregnancy, your growing uterus continually pushes on your stomach, moving it higher and higher and compressing it. The pressure can force stomach acids upward, causing heartburn.

The typical symptom of heartburn is a burning discomfort behind the breastbone or a burning feeling in your chest. It may feel like indigestion, a sour stomach, pain in the upper abdomen or a feeling of fullness after eating a small amount of food. You may have a burning sensation in your chest when you lie down, bend over or exercise. Some people describe a backing up of sour liquid into their throat or mouth, especially when they're lying down or sleeping. You may belch, feel bloated or have more saliva than usual. Occasionally, GERD will also give the sensation of a lump in the throat.

Prevention and self-care for heartburn

Heartburn is unpleasant, but you can take steps to prevent it or treat it:

- Eat more frequent but smaller meals. For example, have five or six small meals a day rather than three large meals.
- Some foods are more likely to cause irritation than are others. Determine which foods give you heartburn, and avoid them. Stay away from fatty, greasy or fried foods, coffee and tea, chocolate, peppermint, alcohol, carbonated beverages, very sweet foods, acidic foods such as citrus fruits and juices, tomatoes and red peppers and highly spiced foods.
- Drink plenty of fluids, especially water.
- Don't smoke. Cigarette smoking increases stomach acidity — and, of course, it's bad for your baby.
- Sit with good posture when eating. Slouching can put extra pressure on your stomach.
- Wait an hour or longer after eating before you lie down.
- Avoid eating for two to three hours before you go to bed. An empty stomach produces less acid.
- Avoid movements and positions that seem to aggravate the problem. When picking things up, bend at the knees, not the waist.

- Avoid lying flat on your back. When resting or sleeping, prop yourself up on pillows to elevate your head and shoulders, or raise the head of your bed 4 to 6 inches.

Medical care for heartburn

If heartburn is a significant problem, your health care provider may prescribe an antacid to reduce stomach acid. Don't take any antacid or acid blocker without consulting your health care provider, however. Antacids often are high in salt and can increase fluid buildup in body tissues during pregnancy.

Avoid heartburn medications that contain aspirin, such as Alka-Seltzer. Report to your health care provider any history of ulcers, gastrointestinal disturbances or hiatal hernia. Rarely, the problem is severe enough to warrant a procedure called endoscopy to view the inside of your esophagus. When GERD is severe, it can be treated appropriately during pregnancy.

Heart rate — fast heartbeat or rapid pulse

2nd, 3rd trimesters

Throughout pregnancy your heart pumps more blood, faster, than it does normally. This helps meet the fetus's needs for oxygen and nutrients, which are carried in the blood through the placenta.

As the heart pumps 30 percent to 50 percent more blood, your heart rate speeds up as well. Your heart beats progressively faster throughout pregnancy. By the third trimester, your heart rate may be 20 percent faster than it was before you were pregnant.

Medical care for fast heart rate

Because of increases in blood volume, many pregnant women develop heart murmurs. Their occurrence is normal because more blood is flowing through your heart valves. Occasionally, however, the murmur may sound different enough that your health care provider will investigate the cause. Heart murmurs can result from changes in the heart valves, as in mitral valve prolapse, or from damage caused by rheumatic fever.

Hemorrhoids

2nd, 3rd trimesters

Some pregnant women develop hemorrhoids — varicose veins in the rectum. Hemorrhoids are caused by increased blood volume and pressure from the uterus on the veins in your rectum. The veins may enlarge into firm, swollen pouches underneath the mucous membranes inside or outside the rectum. Hemorrhoids may occur for the first time during pregnancy or become more frequent or severe.

Constipation also can contribute to hemorrhoids because straining can enlarge the rectal veins. Constipation is common throughout pregnancy, especially during the later months, when your uterus may push against your large intestine. (See also **Constipation.)**

Hemorrhoids can be painful, and they may bleed, itch or sting, especially during or after a bowel movement. Usually, hemorrhoids recede or disappear after birth.

Prevention and self-care for hemorrhoids

The best way to deal with hemorrhoids is to avoid constipation. This is especially important if you've had them before getting pregnant. To prevent hemorrhoids and ease the discomfort, try the following:

- Avoid becoming constipated by eating high-fiber foods, fruits and vegetables and drinking plenty of fluids.
- Exercise regularly, which can help keep bowel movements regular.
- Avoid straining during bowel movements, as this puts pressure on the veins in your rectum and can aggravate or cause hemorrhoids. Put your feet on a stool to reduce straining, and avoid sitting on the toilet for long periods of time.
- Keep the area around your anus clean. Gently wash the area after each bowel movement. Pads of witch hazel may help relieve pain and itching. You can refrigerate the pads, which may be more soothing when applied cold. You may also want to try a warm sitz bath — a shallow basin that fits over the toilet and allows you to submerge your buttocks and hips.
- Use an ice pack to provide some relief.
- Try warm soaks in a tub or sitz bath to help shrink hemorrhoids and provide relief. Add an oatmeal bath formula or baking soda to the water to combat itching.
- Avoid sitting for long periods, especially on hard chairs.

Medical care for hemorrhoids

Stool softeners or bulk-producing laxatives may help, but consult your health care provider before using any over-the-counter remedy for hemorrhoids. If self-care measures don't work, your health care provider may prescribe a cream or an ointment that can shrink them.

Occasionally a hemorrhoid may become filled with blood clots (thrombosed). If this happens, the swollen vein won't shrink to its normal size. Minor surgery may be needed to remove the hemorrhoid.

Heparin

See "Anticoagulants" under **Medications**

Herbal medications

1st, 2nd, 3rd trimesters

It's best not to take any herbal products while you're pregnant. Because herbals aren't regulated by the Food and Drug Administration, companies that make herbal products don't have to prove the safety or quality of their products. Herbal products can be dangerous to your health and your pregnancy. Popular herbs that could cause problems include echinacea, ginkgo and St. John's wort, among many others. Be sure to talk with your health care provider about any herbal products you're taking or planning to take.

Hiccups

See **Baby's hiccups**

Hip pain

3rd trimester

It's not uncommon to feel some soreness or pain in your hips during pregnancy, especially when you're sleeping on your side at night. In preparation for the birth of your baby, the connective tissues in your body soften and loosen up. The ligaments in your hips stretch, and the joints between the pelvic bones relax. The greater flexibility makes it easier for the baby to pass through the pelvis at birth.

In late pregnancy, your heavier uterus might contribute to changes in your posture, adding to your hip soreness. Hip pain is often stronger on one side because the baby tends to lie more heavily to one side.

Prevention and self-care for hip pain

Exercises to strengthen your lower back and abdominal muscles may ease hip soreness. Warm baths and compresses and massage also may help. Try elevating your hips above the level of your chest for a few minutes at a time.

Hunger

1st, 2nd, 3rd trimesters

Do you feel like raiding the refrigerator constantly since you got pregnant? Feeling hungrier than usual is normal — most women experience an increase in appetite throughout pregnancy. That makes sense because you need about 300 extra calories a day to nurture your baby's growth and development.

Some women have the opposite problem: a lack of appetite due to nausea. Or you may be hungry for a certain type of food, such as fruits, chocolate, mashed potatoes or cereal. Especially during the first trimester, hormonal changes can cause changes in appetite.

As long as you're eating a variety of nutritious foods, you don't have to be too concerned about appetite changes, including increased hunger and cravings. If you're frequently hungry, eat small meals throughout the day. Focus on eating low-fat, healthy foods. If you're frequently nauseated, try eating small amounts of bland foods throughout the day. If nausea or lack of appetite makes you eat less once in a while, don't worry that your baby will be harmed. The fetus gets first dibs on the nutrients you consume. (See also **Nausea throughout the day.**)

Increased perspiration
See **Perspiration**

Indigestion
See **Gas and bloating; Heartburn**

Influenza
1st, 2nd, 3rd trimesters
Influenza affects your respiratory system — your nose, throat and lungs — rather than your intestines.

Prevention and self-care for influenza
The Centers for Disease Control recommends the flu shot for women who will be beyond their first trimester of pregnancy during the flu season (October to April). Talk with your health care provider about whether that applies to you.

In addition, it's important to wash your hands often, especially before touching your eyes or mouth. Use soap and warm water to wash all skin surfaces, rubbing vigorously for 15 to 30 seconds. Encourage those around you to cover their mouths when they cough or sneeze.

If you think you have influenza, talk with your health care provider. Drink plenty of fluids so that you stay hydrated.

Medical care for influenza
Seek medical care if you have signs of dehydration (see also **Dehydration after stomach flu).**

Insomnia
2nd, 3rd trimesters
You go to bed exhausted, sure you'll nod off the minute your head hits the pillow. Instead you find yourself wide awake, watching the minutes tick by. Or you wake up at four in the morning, unable to fall back asleep. Insomnia — a condition in which you have problems falling asleep or

staying asleep — is very common during pregnancy. Considering all the changes you're going through, both physically and emotionally, it's not surprising that your sleep is affected.

Although many women sleep more during the first trimester than before they were pregnant, hormonal changes may make it harder for some women to sleep through the night. As your growing uterus puts pressure on your bladder, the frequent need to urinate can get you out of bed to go to the bathroom several times a night.

As the baby gets larger, you may find it harder to find a comfortable position for sleeping. An active baby also can keep you awake. Heartburn, leg cramps and nasal congestion are other common reasons for disturbed sleep in the later months of pregnancy.

Then there's the natural anticipation, excitement and anxiety you're bound to feel about your baby's arrival. You may have worries about the health of the baby and the changes the baby is going to create in your life. These feelings can make it hard to relax your mind and body. You may have frequent and vivid dreams about birth and the baby, which can also contribute to insomnia.

Although insomnia can be frustrating for you, it won't hurt your baby.

Prevention and self-care for insomnia

Worrying about lack of sleep will only compound the problem. If you have difficulty falling or staying asleep, try these suggestions:

- Start winding down before going to bed. Take a warm bath or do relaxation exercises. Ask your partner for a massage.
- Make sure your bedroom is a comfortable temperature for sleeping and that it's dark and quiet.
- Cut down on your fluids in the evening.
- Exercise regularly, but avoid overexertion.
- The best position for sleeping in late pregnancy is on your left or right side, with your legs and knees bent. Lying on your side takes pressure off the large vein that carries blood from your legs and feet back to your heart. This position also takes pressure off your lower back. Use one pillow to support your abdomen and another to support your upper leg. You can also try placing a bunched-up pillow or rolled-up blanket in the small of your back. This will help relieve pressure on the hip you're lying on.
- Don't lie awake worrying about not sleeping. Get up and read, write a letter, listen to relaxing music, or do needlework or some other calming activity.
- If possible, take short naps during the day to make up for missed sleep at night.

Medical care for insomnia

No medications for insomnia, including herbal remedies, are completely safe to use during pregnancy. If anxiety is keeping you awake at night, ask your health care provider about relaxation exercises that may help, or use the relaxation techniques you learned in childbirth classes.

If you're concerned that you may have a serious sleep disorder, consult your health care provider. If ongoing disturbing dreams or nightmares are causing you distress, it might be helpful to talk with a therapist or counselor.

Irrational fears

1st, 2nd, 3rd trimesters

What if something is wrong with my baby? This is a universal fear among expectant parents. As they head toward the birth experience, all women and men have some fears, especially about the health and condition of the baby. You may also have fears about labor — such as not making it to the hospital in time, having a Caesarean delivery or being exposed in front of strangers.

It's normal to feel a moderate amount of worry that doesn't respond to reassurance. But fears that are all-consuming and interfere with your day-to-day functioning may need attention.

True, some babies are born with problems, and sometimes babies die. But serious problems and death occur in only a small percentage of cases. The numbers are in your favor.

Prevention and self-care for irrational fears

Sit down and make a list of your fears. Share them with your partner or labor companion. Talking about your fears can lighten an unnecessarily heavy emotional load. You might also want to talk with your practitioner and with other expectant mothers, perhaps in a pregnancy class or online chat room. When you voice your fears, they have less power over you.

Childbirth preparation classes offer a unique opportunity to talk with other couples who have the same worries. The instructor also can help address fears about giving birth.

When to seek medical help for irrational fears

If your fears are interfering with your functioning, especially if they're keeping you from eating or sleeping, talk to your health care provider. If you're extremely anxious, particularly if you have a specific reason to fear for your baby's health, your health care provider may do an ultrasound evaluation of the fetus or other prenatal tests. Although the tests can't detect every potential problem, they can tell you a great deal about the health of the fetus. The tests, along with your health care provider's reassurance, can help you let go of some of your fears and get on with caring for yourself and your developing baby.

If nothing seems to reduce your anxiety, your health care provider may recommend professional counseling.

Irritability

See **Mood swings**

Itchiness

2nd, 3rd trimesters

You expected to get bigger, more easily fatigued ... but itchier? It happens to about one-fifth of pregnant women. The itchiness may be on your abdomen or all over your body, and it may cause patches of red, flaky rash. Skin stretching over the abdomen probably accounts for some of the itching and flaking. Generalized itchiness usually goes away shortly after you give birth.

A common skin problem called pruritic urticarial papules and plaques of pregnancy (PUPPP) also can occur during pregnancy. With this condition, you break out with itchy bumps called papules or plaques on your abdomen or possibly on your thighs, buttocks or arms.

Rarely, women have a specific cause for general itchiness called cholestasis of pregnancy. In this condition, bile isn't cleared from the liver as quickly as it should be. It causes components to build up in the skin, triggering severe itching.

Prevention and self-care for itchiness

Scratching isn't the best way to relieve an itch. Try these measures:
- Moisturize your skin with lotion, creams or oils.
- Wear loose clothing made from natural fibers, such as cotton.
- Use an oatmeal bath formula.
- Avoid getting overheated because you'll probably itch more if you're too warm.

When to seek medical help for itchiness

If self-care measures don't provide relief for your itches, your health care provider may prescribe medication or other treatment techniques that can help. PUPPP can be treated with prescription medications.

If severe itching develops late in your pregnancy, your health care provider may order blood tests to check your liver function. Cholestasis of pregnancy can cause severe itching. Very rarely, it can also cause vomiting, loss of appetite and fatigue. This problem goes away after the baby is born.

Labor pains
See **Contractions**

Lactose intolerance
1st, 2nd, 3rd trimesters

Pregnant women are commonly told to drink milk. But this advice doesn't sit well with those who avoid milk and milk products because of lactose intolerance. People with lactose intolerance have trouble digesting lactose, the sugar in milk, because they have low levels of the enzyme lactase.

Lactose intolerance is a common condition, affecting about 15 percent of the adult white population in the United States and 75 percent or more of the adult black, American Indian and Asian-American populations.

Signs and symptoms of lactose intolerance include loose stools, diarrhea, abdominal bloating and pain, gas, nausea, and rumbling or gurgling in the stomach and bowels. The signs and symptoms occur after you consume milk or other dairy products.

For many women, the ability to digest lactose improves during pregnancy, especially as the pregnancy progresses. So even if you're normally lactose intolerant, you may find that while you're pregnant you can consume milk and other dairy products without any bothersome signs and symptoms.

Because people with lactose intolerance often avoid milk products, they may not get enough calcium in their diet. The Institute of Medicine recommends a daily calcium intake of 1,000 milligrams (mg) for women age 19 and older, including pregnant women, and 1,300 mg for pregnant teens under age 19. It can be hard to meet this requirement if you don't consume milk and other dairy products, which are the best sources of calcium.

Prevention and self-care for lactose intolerance

If you have lactose intolerance or dislike milk or other dairy products, it's important to make sure you're getting enough calcium in your diet. Consider the following suggestions:

- Most people who are lactose intolerant can drink up to a cup of milk with meals without causing symptoms. If that amount bothers you, try reducing the portion to half a cup, twice a day.
- Try using lactose-free or lactose-reduced products, including milk, cheese and yogurt.
- Yogurt and fermented products such as cheeses are often better tolerated than regular milk. The lactose in yogurt is already partially digested by the active bacteria cultures in yogurt.
- Try using lactase enzyme tablets such as Lactaid and Lactrase, which help with lactose digestion. They're not effective for everyone.

- Choose a variety of other calcium-rich foods, such as sardines or salmon with bones, tofu, broccoli, spinach and calcium-fortified juices and foods.

Medical care for lactose intolerance
No medical treatment is necessary for lactose intolerance. But if you're concerned about not getting enough calcium in your diet, talk with your health care provider. Many calcium supplements are available to choose from.

Leg cramps
2nd, 3rd trimesters
Cramps in the lower leg muscles are fairly common in the second and third trimesters. They most frequently occur at night and may disrupt your sleep. Although the exact cause of leg cramps is unknown, slow blood return, fatigue or pressure from the uterus on nerves in your legs may cause the problem.

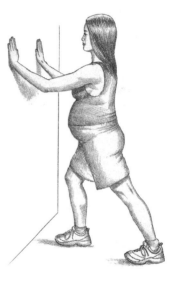

Prevention and self-care for leg cramps
Here are some tips for relieving the discomfort of leg cramps or calf tenderness:

- Stretch the affected muscle. Try straightening your knee and gently flexing your foot upward.
- Walk. You may find it uncomfortable at first, but it helps relieve the cramping.
- Do exercises to stretch your calf muscles, particularly before bed.
- Wear support hose, especially if you stand a lot during the day.
- Take frequent breaks if you sit or stand for long periods.
- Apply local heat.
- Massage your calves.
- Try resting with your legs up on pillows or the arm of a sofa.
- Wear shoes with low heels.

When to seek medical help for leg cramps
If leg cramps persist, talk to your health care provider. They might be caused by a circulation problem. Call him or her if you notice redness, swelling or an increase in pain or if you have a history of a blood-clotting disorder or thrombophlebitis, which is a blood clot and inflammation in a vein.

Lightening

■ *3rd trimester*

As you approach your due date, you may feel that the baby has settled deeper into your pelvis (dropped). The common term for the descent of the baby's head into the pelvis is *lightening.* You may indeed feel lighter, as the position relieves some of the pressure on your diaphragm and stomach. You can breathe again, and digestion is easier. At the same time, you'll probably feel the need to urinate more often because of the increased pressure on your bladder.

If this is your first baby, lightening may occur weeks before the onset of labor. In women who have had children, it usually doesn't happen until labor begins.

When lightening does occur, your abdomen may shift down and forward, or sag lower. The change may be noticeable enough that your friends comment on it. Or you might not be aware of it at all. Some women feel pressure or aches and pains in their pelvic area and groin. You may feel sharp twinges in the vagina or perineal area as the baby's head presses on the pelvic floor.

■ *When to seek medical help for lightening*

Lightening is usually a sign that the baby's head is engaged — that it has moved below the upper part of the pelvis in preparation for birth. Your health care provider can examine you during the last weeks of pregnancy to check whether engagement has occurred. Nothing needs to be done in response to this event except to prepare for your baby's delivery.

If your baby has dropped and you have other signs of labor, such as regular contractions, contact your health care provider. (See also **Contractions.)**

Lightheadedness

See **Faintness and dizziness**

Linea nigra

■ *1st, 2nd, 3rd trimesters*

The barely noticeable pale line that runs from your navel to your pubic bone, called the linea alba ("white line"), often darkens during pregnancy. Then it's referred to as the linea nigra ("black line"). As with so many other changes that occur during pregnancy, skin darkening is the result of hormones that cause the body to produce more pigment. You can't prevent the linea nigra, but it will fade after delivery. (See also **Skin changes.)**

Lower abdominal pain

See **Abdominal discomfort or cramping**

Mask of pregnancy
 1st, 2nd, 3rd trimesters

More than half of all pregnant women develop mild skin darkening on the face. Commonly called the mask of pregnancy, this brownish coloration is also known as chloasma or melasma. It can affect any woman who's pregnant, though women who are dark-haired and fair-skinned are more susceptible. Melasma usually appears on sun-exposed areas of the face, such as the forehead, temples, cheeks, chin, nose and upper lip. It tends to be matching on both sides of the face (symmetrical).

Melasma is often aggravated or intensified by exposure to sunlight or other sources of ultraviolet (UV) light. The condition usually fades after delivery, although it may not fade completely, and it can return with additional pregnancies.

 Prevention and self-care for mask of pregnancy

Because exposure to sunlight often worsens skin darkening, protect yourself from getting too much sun:

- Always wear sunscreen with a sun protection factor (SPF) of 15 or greater when you're outdoors, whether it's sunny or cloudy. The sun's UV rays can reach your skin even when the sky is overcast.
- Avoid the most intense hours of sunlight, during the middle of the day.
- Wear a wide-brimmed hat that shades your face.
- If your mask is extreme, covering makeup may help.

 Medical care for mask of pregnancy

Avoid creams or other agents that bleach the skin. If your skin darkening is extreme, your health care provider or a dermatologist may prescribe a medicated ointment. If melasma persists long after you've delivered your baby, consult a dermatologist. He or she may recommend a medicated cream or ointment or a chemical peel.

Medications
 1st, 2nd, 3rd trimesters

When pregnant, you're still susceptible to all the usual illnesses that the general population faces. And pregnancy itself can give rise to health conditions that require treatment.

But many women have concerns about using medications during pregnancy. Should you avoid all medications? Which medications are safe? What if you're already taking a drug to treat an ongoing health condition? Should you stay on it?

As a general rule, it's best to use caution and avoid use of medications during pregnancy. Some drugs can cause an early miscarriage or harm the developing fetus. Exposure to drugs is thought to account for 2 percent to 3 percent of birth defects. Very few drugs have been proved to be completely safe in pregnancy, but many have been found to be safe enough that their benefits outweigh any tiny, unknown risk. Before you take any medicine — prescription or over-the-counter — check with your health care provider for specific advice based on your health history and the medication in question. A pharmacist also can provide general guidelines.

If you have a health condition that requires regular medication, or were taking a medicine regularly before getting pregnant, your health care provider will evaluate whether it's safest for you to continue taking the medication, discontinue it or switch to a different medication that poses less risk to you and your baby. *A medication that was important for your health before pregnancy most likely will be important during pregnancy, too.* It's always best to outline a plan regarding medications when you anticipate becoming pregnant.

Below is a guide to the risks for pregnant women regarding some commonly used medications.

Acne medications. Don't take any medications for acne without your health care provider's advice. Some drugs used to treat acne can harm a fetus. These include:

- *Isotretinoin (Accutane).* This acne medication, taken orally, is known to cause birth defects such as hydrocephalus, cardiac abnormalities and ear defects. Women who take Accutane must wait at least three months after stopping use of the drug before becoming pregnant.
- *Hormonal therapy.* Hormones, including estrogen and the anti-androgens spironolactone and flutamide, are sometimes used to treat acne, but shouldn't be taken during pregnancy.
- *Tetracyclines.* These antibiotic medications are often used to treat acne. They may cause slowed bone growth and discolored teeth in babies as well as severe liver disease in expectant mothers. They shouldn't be used during pregnancy.

(See also **Acne.**)

Allergy medications. Allergy remedies include antihistamines, decongestants, nasal sprays and allergy shots. During pregnancy, avoid most antihistamines and decongestants unless your health care provider recommends them. Your health care provider can help you select medications that minimize the risk to your baby.

Steroid and nonsteroid nasal sprays are generally safe to use during pregnancy, although if you use them, do so with a health care provider's supervision. Allergy shots are safe for pregnant women who were already receiving them before they got pregnant, although most caregivers don't start them during pregnancy. (See also **Allergies.**)

Antacids and acid blockers. Antacids are generally safe when taken as directed, but their side effects might be bothersome. Sodium, a common ingredient in antacids, can worsen swelling and water retention. Other possible side effects are diarrhea and constipation. Because antacids can reduce your absorption of other medications and vitamins, take them at least an hour apart from other medications or vitamins.

Acid blockers, both histamine (H-2) blockers and proton pump inhibitors, are considered safe to use under a health care provider's supervision. H-2 blockers include cimetidine (Tagamet), famotidine (Pepcid) and ranitidine (Zantac). Proton pump inhibitors include esomeprazole magnesium (Nexium) and omeprazole (Prilosec). (See also **Heartburn.**)

Antibiotics. If you get a bacterial infection, such as a sinus infection or strep throat, your health care provider may prescribe an antibiotic. Most antibiotics, including penicillin, are safe to use during pregnancy, but the exceptions are serious. Always make your health care provider aware of your pregnancy when an antibiotic is to be prescribed.

Anticoagulants. Anticoagulants decrease the clotting ability of blood and help prevent harmful clots from forming in the blood vessels.
- *Heparin.* Heparin is the medication of choice for pregnant women who require an anticoagulant medication. Heparin may be prescribed for women who have a hereditary clotting disorder or who are at risk of developing blood clots while pregnant. Because heparin doesn't cross the placenta, it's safe to use during pregnancy and doesn't harm the fetus.

   Heparin is administered by injection. The treatment must be stopped briefly at the time of delivery to prevent excessive blood loss. Management of heparin treatment is a job for an experienced obstetrician.
- *Low molecular weight heparins.* New, low molecular weight heparins (dalteparin, enoxaparin) also are safe in pregnancy and have some advantages. However, they're extremely expensive.
- *Warfarin.* Warfarin (Coumadin) is another anticlotting drug, but it has been shown to cause birth defects and is not used during pregnancy.

If you've had blood clots or are at risk of developing them, your health care provider will determine what the best course of treatment is for you.

Antidepressants and mood stabilizers. Women who are using medications for depression, anxiety and other mood disorders may need to change their use of these drugs during pregnancy. If you were taking any antidepressant or other psychiatric medication before becoming pregnant, talk to your health care provider about whether you should keep taking it. Medications used for these conditions include the following:

- *Tricyclic antidepressants.* Use of this family of drugs during pregnancy causes concern. More effective medications are now available, so there's rarely a need to consider using this group of drugs during pregnancy.
- *Selective serotonin reuptake inhibitors (SSRIs).* Multiple studies have evaluated use of fluoxetine (Prozac, Sarafem), sertraline (Zoloft) and paroxetine (Paxil) during pregnancy and haven't found evidence of increased risk of birth defects. The effect these medications may have on the unborn child's future behavior is unknown. These drugs usually should be continued if they were prescribed for serious depression.
- *Other antidepressants.* Bupropion (Wellbutrin) hasn't been shown to cause birth defects. However, its future effect on children and adults exposed during their mother's pregnancy is unknown. Bupropion is also sold as a stop-smoking aid under the name Zyban.
- *Mood stabilizers.* Lithium (Lithobid), valproic acid (Depakene) and carbamazepine (Tegretol) are used to treat bipolar disorder. If used during pregnancy, they may harm the developing fetus. If you're using any of these drugs and want to become pregnant, first talk to your health care provider or a perinatal specialist about their risks and benefits. Lithium and valproic acid are strongly linked to birth defects.

Cold medications. A wide variety of medications, including dozens of types of decongestants, cough syrups and nasal sprays, are marketed to treat the symptoms of the common cold. Most of these drugs have at least some concern attached with their use in pregnancy. The medicines may relieve signs and symptoms, but they don't cure or shorten the illness. If you're pregnant, the best treatment plan for a cold includes rest, fluids, increased humidity and time. Often you and your health care provider can find an approach to your cold that minimizes risk to your pregnancy. (See also **Colds.**)

Laxatives. Constipation is a common aggravation of pregnancy. Nonprescription laxatives are generally safe, but check with your health care provider for a recommendation. Overuse of laxatives can cause diarrhea and a degree of dependence. It's best to try to prevent constipation. (See also **Constipation.**)

Pain relievers

- *Acetaminophen.* This nonaspirin medication is sold under various brand names, including Tylenol. In recommended doses, it's considered safe to use during pregnancy. In addition to relieving pain, acetaminophen can lower a fever.
- *Aspirin.* Avoid taking aspirin when you're pregnant, unless your health care provider specifically recommends it. Maternal use of aspirin has been associated with some birth defects and bleeding problems in the mother or infant.
- *Ibuprofen and other nonsteroidal anti-inflammatory drugs (NSAIDs).* Ibuprofen (Advil, Motrin, others), indomethacin (Indocin), katoprofen (Orudis) and other NSAIDs should be used during pregnancy only under a physician's direction, as they could pose risks to the fetus.
- *Narcotics.* Some pain relievers combine acetaminophen with a narcotic medication such as codeine or oxycodone. Brand names include Tylenol with Codeine, Darvocet, Vicodin and Percocet. Oxycodone medications have not been linked with birth defects, but they have high addiction potential and may cause withdrawal or other problems in the infant if used for many days in the last weeks before delivery. These medications are never appropriate for noncancer chronic pain, due to their addictive potential.

For pain relief, you might also consider nonpharmaceutical alternatives. For example, if you have a headache, try resting, avoiding light and using a cool pack on your head. For sore muscles or aches caused by arthritis, try a warm bath or massage.

For more specific information about medications used to treat other conditions, see **Headaches; Herbal medications; Morning sickness.**

Melasma

See **Mask of pregnancy**

Migraines

See **Headaches**

Mood swings

1st, 2nd, 3rd trimesters

One minute you're giddy with happiness. A few minutes later, you feel like crying. Especially in the first trimester and toward the end of the third trimester, mood swings are common. Your emotions may run from exhilaration and joy to exhaustion, irritation, weepiness or depression. If you've typically experienced premenstrual syndrome, you may have more extreme mood swings when you're pregnant.

What causes this moodiness? Some of it may be linked to pregnancy-related discomforts such as nausea, frequent urination, swelling and backache, all of which can interfere with sleep. Fatigue, changing sleep patterns and new bodily sensations can all influence how you feel. You may also be adjusting to a new body image, especially during your first pregnancy. Your fatigue and discomfort are reasons enough to feel stressed emotionally, and in turn, feeling down can affect how you feel physically.

Mood changes may also be caused by the release of hormones and changes in your metabolism. Just as fluctuations in progesterone, estrogen and other hormones are linked to the blues many women feel before their period or after giving birth, these hormonal changes may play a role in the mood changes of pregnancy.

In addition, pregnancy brings a number of new stresses to your life. Adjusting to lifestyle changes and preparing for new responsibilities may leave you feeling up one day and down the next. Added financial responsibilities are another common source of stress, as are worries about the health of the baby and your ability to be a good parent.

Pregnancy has a major impact on your body, your relationships and many other aspects of your life. It's a time when you need extra support from your partner, family, employer and community. Unfortunately, that support isn't always there.

Mood swings are normal during pregnancy and are usually nothing to worry about. But they can make it more difficult to cope with stress. When stress builds up to uncomfortable levels, it can cause fatigue, insomnia, anxiety, poor appetite or overeating, headaches, and backaches. Stress over a long period of time can contribute to potentially serious health problems.

If you're coping well with stress — you're feeling energized rather than drained, and you're functioning well — some added stress won't be a hazard to your health or your baby's health.

Prevention and self-care for mood swings
Simply knowing more about why you're feeling moody — and knowing that these mood swings are temporary — can help you weather the storms, as can the following healthy habits. And practicing these habits may even help you prevent mood swings altogether:

- Keep yourself healthy and fit by eating a nutritious diet, getting plenty of sleep, avoiding alcohol, cigarettes and drugs, and exercising regularly. Exercise is a natural stress reducer and can help prevent backache, fatigue and constipation.
- Boost your support network. This may include your partner, family, friends and a support group. A good support network can provide emotional support and help with tasks around the home.

- Be sure to make time to relax each day. Try relaxation techniques such as meditation, guided mental imagery and progressive muscle relaxation. These kinds of relaxation exercises are often taught in childbirth classes.
- Accept that you may not be able to accomplish everything you did before getting pregnant. Cut back on unnecessary activities that are contributing to your stress or discomfort.

When to seek medical help for mood swings

Moods that interfere with your ability to function may be more than a passing case of fatigue, stress or the blues. Exaggerated mood swings that last more than two weeks may be a sign of depression. Mild depression is quite common in pregnant women. If you're consistently feeling sad, weepy or worthless and you notice that your eating and sleeping are affected, your work is disrupted or you take less pleasure in things you normally enjoy, you may be experiencing depression.

If your mood swings seem to be more than you can handle alone or if you have signs and symptoms of depression, talk to your health care provider about them. Depression is a serious disease that you have no more control over than strep throat. During pregnancy, depression may be treated with counseling, psychotherapy, medications or a combination of those. Be sure to seek help if you have the signs and symptoms of depression.

Morning sickness

1st trimester

Morning sickness is one of the classic signs of early pregnancy. The majority of expectant mothers — up to 70 percent — experience nausea and vomiting.

Although these signs and symptoms are commonly known as morning sickness, the name is misleading because nausea and vomiting can occur at any time of the day. The signs and symptoms typically first start at four to eight weeks of gestation and subside by 13 to 14 weeks. But some women have nausea and vomiting beyond the first trimester. Morning sickness may be more severe in a first pregnancy, in young women and in women carrying multiple fetuses.

The cause of morning sickness isn't completely understood, although the relaxation of the stomach muscle probably plays a part. The stomach empties somewhat more slowly under the influence of pregnancy hormones. Another possible cause is the rapidly rising levels of estrogen produced by the placenta and fetus. Emotional stress, fatigue, traveling and some types of food may aggravate the problem.

Although morning sickness can be quite distressing, it seldom leads to more serious problems such as dehydration or significant weight loss. Morning sickness doesn't affect your baby or mean that your baby is sick. In fact, nausea is generally a sign the pregnancy is progressing well.

Prevention and self-care for morning sickness

Dietary measures. You may be able to alleviate nausea by keeping some food in your stomach — by avoiding having a stomach that's completely empty or completely full. Here are some other dietary suggestions for preventing or relieving nausea:

- Eat smaller meals or snacks frequently throughout the day.
- Before getting out of bed in the morning, eat a couple of soda crackers or a piece of dry toast. Rise slowly, allowing some time for digestion to occur before you get up.
- Have a small snack at bedtime and when you get up to go to the bathroom at night.
- Avoid foods and smells that trigger nausea.
- Drink fewer fluids with your meals.
- Eat more carbohydrates, such as white rice, dry toast or a plain baked potato.
- Try eating low-fat, bland foods or high-protein foods such as peanut butter on apple slices, nuts, cheese and crackers, milk and yogurt. Other good choices are gelatin desserts (Jell-O), popsicles and chicken broth. Some women find it helpful to eat salty and tart foods in combination, such as pretzels and lemonade.
- Avoid foods that are high in fat and salt and low in nutrition. Avoid greasy, rich and spicy foods.
- Suck on hard candy.
- If you're in the habit of drinking ginger ale when you're feeling nauseated, you may have science on your side. Several studies have found a benefit from ginger in reducing nausea and vomiting, with no apparent risks. Some ways to consume the spice include ginger soda or tea, ginger snaps or ginger in capsule form. You can also buy whole ginger root. Cut a slice or grate it and boil it. Let it steep for about five minutes, then sweeten it with honey if you like.

Lifestyle and alternative measures. Some other simple steps that you might find helpful are as follows:

- Keep rooms well ventilated and free of cooking odors and cigarette smoke, which can aggravate nausea.
- Get plenty of fresh air. Take a walk or try sleeping with a window open.

- Rest. The fatigue that's common in early pregnancy can contribute to nausea. Lying down may help.
- Some studies have shown a benefit from acupressure and acupuncture. Acupressure involves stimulating points in the body without use of needles or electricity. Elastic bands worn on the wrists may help counter morning sickness. These bracelets exert a steady pressure over an acupressure point on the inside of the wrist. Because these bands are also used for seasickness, you can usually find them at boating stores or travel agencies.
- The iron in prenatal vitamins may cause nausea. Switching to a children's chewable vitamin with folic acid may help. Talk to your health care provider before changing your vitamins.
- Ask your health care provider about taking a vitamin B-6 supplement. Studies have found that this vitamin reduces nausea and vomiting during pregnancy. The recommended dosage is 25 milligrams three times a day.

When to seek medical help for morning sickness

In rare instances, nausea and vomiting may be so severe that you can't maintain proper nutrition and fluids and gain enough weight. Severe or persistent nausea and vomiting may also be caused by other rare but serious diseases, such as liver disease or thyroid disease.

Call your health care provider if:
- Morning sickness doesn't improve, despite trying self-care remedies
- You're vomiting blood or material that looks like coffee grounds
- You lose more than 2 pounds
- You have prolonged, severe vomiting

Severe cases of nausea and vomiting may require treatment with medications, including antiemetics, which control nausea. Some women find relief with over-the-counter antacids or with motion sickness drugs or antihistamines. Your health care provider will discuss your options with you. (See also **Nausea throughout the day.**)

Mucous discharge

3rd trimester

As you approach your delivery date, you may notice an increase in mucous discharge from your vagina. During pregnancy, the opening of the cervix becomes blocked with a thick plug of mucus that keeps bacteria and other germs from entering the uterus. As you get closer to labor, your cervix begins to thin and relax, and the mucous plug may loosen, causing the discharge to increase and thicken. The plug is sometimes dislodged as thick, stringy or blood-tinged mucus. (See also **Bloody show.)**

■ *Prevention and self-care for mucous discharge*
Mucous discharge is normal toward the end of pregnancy. If you want
something to absorb the flow, use sanitary napkins rather than tampons.
Keep your genital area clean, and wear cotton underwear. Avoid tight or
nylon pants, and don't use perfume or deodorant soap in the genital area.

■ *When to seek medical help for mucous discharge*
Call your health care provider if your discharge is foul smelling, yellow,
green or causes itching or burning. These could be signs of an infection.
Mucous discharge before 35 weeks could be a sign of preterm labor.
Report it to your health care provider.

Mucous plug
See **Bloody show**

Nasal congestion
See **Allergies; Colds; Stuffy nose**

Nausea
See **Morning sickness**

Nausea throughout the day
■ *1st trimester*
What if you don't just have morning sickness — you also have afternoon,
evening and night sickness? Because the nausea and vomiting of pregnancy are commonly referred to as morning sickness, you may wonder if
there's something wrong if you're experiencing these symptoms throughout the day. In fact, morning sickness is a misnomer because nausea can
occur any time of day.

In one study of 160 pregnant women, less than 2 percent had nausea
only in the mornings. For most women, nausea lasted throughout the day.
Other research has found similar results. (See also **Morning sickness;
Vomiting.**)

■ *When to seek medical help for nausea throughout the day*
Nausea and vomiting can become a problem if you can't keep foods or
fluids down and you begin to lose weight. Call your health care provider
if your nausea and vomiting are severe or persistent.

Navel soreness
■ *2nd trimester*
Along with the other aches and pains associated with your expanding

uterus, your navel area may feel tender or sore. This tenderness might be most noticeable as you pass the 20th week of pregnancy and then subside as your belly grows. You may feel most uncomfortable when sitting upright.

The stretching and separation of the two large bands of muscles that run along your abdomen also can cause some soreness around your belly-button. (See also **Abdominal tenderness due to muscle separation.**)

Self-care for navel soreness

To relieve tenderness around your navel, use the pads of your fingers to massage your abdomen in a circular pattern, or ask your partner to do this for you. Apply a cold or warm compress to your bellybutton to soothe it. If pain around your navel is accompanied by severe loss of appetite, this could be a more serious problem. A call to your health care provider is in order.

Nesting instinct

3rd trimester

As your due date nears, you may find yourself cleaning cupboards, washing walls, organizing your closets, cleaning out the garage, sorting the baby's clothes or decorating the nursery. The powerful urge to clean, organize and decorate before the baby arrives is called the nesting instinct. It's usually strongest just before delivery.

Nesting gives you a sense of accomplishment before the birth and allows you to come home afterward to a clean house. The desire to prepare your home can be useful because it'll give you more time later to recover and spend time with your baby. But don't overdo it and wear yourself out. You'll need your energy for the hard work of labor.

Cleaning precautions. No evidence links normal use of household cleaners with birth defects. Always follow safety instructions from the manufacturer, and that goes double when you're pregnant. Never mix ammonia with chlorine-based products, such as bleach, because the combination produces toxic fumes. Wear gloves when cleaning, and don't directly inhale any strong fumes. (See also **Painting.**)

Nipple darkening

2nd trimester

Like other areas of the skin, the skin on or around the nipples often darkens during pregnancy. Skin darkening is the result of pregnancy hormones, which cause the body to produce more pigment. The increased pigment isn't distributed evenly like a smooth tan, but often appears as splotches of color.

Darkening of the nipples and other areas of skin typically fades after delivery. In the meantime, avoid using agents that bleach the skin.

Nipple discharge
See **Breast discharge**

Nosebleeds
1st, 2nd, 3rd trimesters
Some women have nosebleeds during pregnancy, even though they never or rarely did before. With the extra blood flowing throughout your body, the tiny blood vessels lining the nasal passages are more fragile and likely to rupture.

Prevention and self-care for nosebleeds
To stop a nosebleed:
- Sit up and keep your head elevated. Pinch the soft parts of your nose together between your thumb and index finger.
- Press firmly but gently, compressing the pinched parts of the nose toward the face.
- Hold this position for five minutes.
- Lean forward to avoid swallowing the blood, and breathe through your mouth. Apply ice — crushed in a plastic bag or washcloth — across the bridge of the nose.

To prevent a nosebleed:
- Be gentle when blowing your nose, and don't try packing your nose with gauze.
- Dry air may make you more susceptible to nosebleeds. Use a humidifier during the winter months.

When to seek medical help for nosebleeds
Call your health care provider if the nosebleed persists, if you have high blood pressure or if it occurs after a head injury.

Numbness in hands
See **Carpal tunnel syndrome**

Overheating
See **Warm, feeling**

Painting
1st, 2nd, 3rd trimesters
Pregnancy is a common time to launch a major redecorating project in

your home. Use caution if you're determined to do painting, stripping, wallpapering or furniture refinishing — or if your job involves painting. Try to avoid exposure, especially during the first trimester, to oil-based paints, lead, mercury (which is present in some latex paints) and other substances that have solvents (chemicals used to dissolve other materials). These substances may increase your risk of miscarriage or cause birth defects.

Most of the studies investigating the risks of these substances to pregnant women involved women who were exposed to paint fumes for long periods because of their occupation. Brief exposure to paints and similar compounds shouldn't pose a significant risk to the fetus. Still, it's best to be cautious. Minimize your exposure to potentially hazardous substances by following these rules:

- Make sure to work in a large, well-ventilated area.
- Wear protective gear, such as gloves and a face mask.
- Don't eat or drink in the work area.
- Consider letting someone else paint that room.
- Use all paints only as directed by the manufacturer. For example, don't use paints labeled for outdoor use indoors.

Pelvic pressure

3rd trimester

In the last weeks of pregnancy, you may feel a sense of pressure, heaviness, soreness or tenderness in your pelvic area. This is caused by the baby pushing into the pelvis and compressing the bladder and rectum. In addition, the baby is likely to compress some veins and cause blood to pool. Finally, the bones of the pelvis are being pushed outward a bit, causing further discomfort.

A feeling of pelvic pressure before the 37th week of pregnancy, however, may be a sign of preterm labor, particularly if the pressure in your pelvis or vagina seems to radiate toward your thighs, or you feel as if the baby is pushing down.

Prevention and self-care for pelvic pressure

If you experience pelvic pressure in the last weeks of pregnancy, you may find some relief by resting with your feet up. Kegel exercises also may help with pelvic soreness: Squeeze the muscles around your vagina tightly, as if you were stopping the flow of urine, for a few seconds, then relax. Repeat 10 times.

When to seek medical help for pelvic pressure

Call your health care provider or go to the hospital if you think you may be experiencing preterm labor. In addition to pelvic pressure, other signs and symptoms of preterm labor include:

- Cramping in the lower abdomen. The cramps may be similar to menstrual cramps and may be continuous or come and go.
- A low, dull backache that radiates to the side or front of your body and isn't relieved by any change in position
- Contractions every 10 minutes or more often
- Clear, pink or brownish fluid leaking from your vagina

You don't have to have all of these symptoms to be in preterm labor. Take action even if you have only one. Your health care provider may ask you to come into the office or go to the hospital, or you may be advised to rest on your left side for an hour. If the symptoms get worse or don't go away after an hour, call your health care provider again or go to the hospital.

Perineal aching
3rd trimester

During the last month of pregnancy, after the baby has dropped into the pelvic cavity, you may feel a sensation of increased pressure or aching in the perineal area — the area between the vulva and the anus. This dropping, referred to as lightening, indicates that the presenting part of the baby, usually the head, is engaged in the upper portion of the pelvis. If this is your first pregnancy, lightening may happen several weeks before labor. If you've had a child before, lightening usually occurs just before labor. (See also **Lightening.**)

In addition to aching or pressure in the perineal area, you may feel sharp twinges when the fetal head presses on the pelvic floor.

Prevention and self-care for perineal aching

Those trusty Kegel exercises can strengthen your perineal muscles and may help with the aching. To do Kegel exercises, squeeze the muscles around your vagina tightly, as if you were stopping the flow of urine, for a few seconds, then relax. Repeat 10 times.

When to seek medical help for perineal aching

Your health care provider may examine you in the last weeks of pregnancy to see if the baby's head is engaged. If perineal aching or pressure grows stronger and is accompanied by a feeling of tightening or contractions, you may be in labor.

Perming your hair
1st, 2nd, 3rd trimesters

Many women wonder if it's safe to perm, dye or use other chemical treatments on their hair when they're expecting. To date, there are no definitive answers. Studies using animals haven't identified any specific risks of birth defects or other problems. But only a few studies in humans have examined the effects of hair care chemicals or treatments on the developing fetus.

Given the lack of human studies, some health care providers advise women to put off having a perm until after the first trimester. The fetus is most vulnerable to adverse effects of exposure to chemicals and other substances during the first trimester. However, one disadvantage of perming your hair in late pregnancy is that often a great deal of hair is lost immediately after delivery, meaning you'll also lose a fairly large portion of the perm.

Perspiration
1st, 2nd, 3rd trimesters
The effects of pregnancy hormones on your sweat glands, along with your need to get rid of all the heat the baby produces, may leave you feeling a little damp. Increased perspiration during pregnancy makes heat rashes more common. Hot summer weather can be quite trying in late pregnancy. If you're pregnant during the summer, you may need to rest, drink cold liquids and take cool showers to avoid overheating. (See also **Warm, feeling.**)

Pica
See **Food cravings**

Pinkeye
1st, 2nd, 3rd trimesters
Pinkeye (conjunctivitis) is an inflammation or infection of the conjunctiva, the moist, delicate membrane that lines the inside of the eyelids and covers the whites of the eyes. Symptoms include redness of the eyes, itchiness or irritation, a gritty feeling in the eyes and watery eyes. In adults, pinkeye is most often a viral or bacterial infection. It can also be caused by allergies, chemical irritants in the eyes or the use of contact lenses, particularly extended-wear lenses. If you get pinkeye while pregnant, it won't affect your fetus.

Newborns can develop conjunctivitis if they're exposed to bacteria during birth. Bacteria from the mother's vagina can pass into the infant's eyes during birth. This condition is most often caused by the sexually transmitted bacteria that cause chlamydia or gonorrhea. Conjunctivitis in infants must be treated immediately to prevent serious eye damage and preserve sight.

To prevent eye infections, newborns are given silver nitrate eyedrops at birth. Irritation from the drops may cause a brief bout of pinkeye. It usually begins six to 12 hours after birth and clears up within two days.

Prevention and self-care for pinkeye

Pregnant women should make sure they have no active sexually transmitted disease that might affect their infant before birth or after delivery.

To help protect yourself from bacterial and viral conjunctivitis, follow these precautions, especially if someone else in your family has pinkeye:
- Keep your hands away from your eyes.
- Wash your hands frequently.
- Don't share washcloths, towels or pillowcases with anyone. Change these items frequently, and wash them in hot water and detergent after use.
- Replace your eye makeup containers and applicators regularly.
- Use and care for your contact lenses properly.

To soothe the discomfort of pinkeye, apply a compress — a clean cloth soaked in warm or cool water — to closed eyes. Warm water works well for bacterial or viral pinkeye, and a cool compress is best for pinkeye caused by allergies. These methods may provide some comfort, but pinkeye needs medical attention to rule out serious causes.

Medical care for pinkeye

Treatment for pinkeye depends on the cause. The bacterial form is treated with antibiotics, usually given as eyedrops or an ointment. Oral antibiotics may be used for certain types of bacteria. Conjunctivitis caused by a virus will disappear on its own after a few days.

Allergic conjunctivitis can sometimes be cured by avoiding the irritant causing the allergy. For example, if you're having an allergic reaction to a substance in a particular brand of contact lens solution, you may be able to solve the problem simply by switching brands.

Flushing out the eyes with water can treat conjunctivitis caused by some types of chemicals. Some cases of chemical conjunctivitis require immediate medical treatment, however. If you've gotten a chemical in your eye, flush the eye gently with cool, running water for at least 15 minutes. After covering the eye with a clean pad, go to a hospital emergency department.

If your infant has pinkeye caused by silver nitrate eyedrops, the signs will typically be very mild and should disappear within a couple of days. Talk to your baby's health care provider if they persist.

Pregnancy test

See **HCG tests**

Ptyalism
■ *1st trimester*
Along with feeling nauseated, you may be experiencing excessive salivation. This is called ptyalism. It's a somewhat unusual side effect of pregnancy, but very real and can be annoying. However, it's not an indication that anything is wrong. It may be that you're not really producing more saliva, but that you're not swallowing as much as usual because of your nausea.

■ *Prevention and self-care for ptyalism*
If you're experiencing ptyalism, it may be helpful to cut back on starchy foods. Otherwise, when your nausea begins to decrease, this problem is likely to ease off as well.

■ *When to seek medical care for ptyalism*
Excessive salivation by itself doesn't require medical care. However, if you have pain with swallowing or difficulty swallowing, tell your health care provider.

Pubic bone pain
■ *3rd trimester*
Some pregnant women are troubled by pain in the pubic bone. The sensation may be mild or sharp and feel like an ache or a bruise. The pain is caused by softening and loosening of your tissues and joints. As the cartilage that connects the two pubic bones in the center of your pelvis softens, your pubic bone may feel very sore when you're moving or walking. Some pregnant women feel this more than others, and some have it only later in their pregnancy. Pubic bone pain should disappear within a few weeks after you give birth.

■ *Prevention and self-care for pubic bone pain*
To ease the discomfort of pubic bone pain, consider wearing a girdle or support pantyhose. It may also help to apply warmth to the area or take a warm bath.

■ *When to seek medical help for pubic bone pain*
Very rarely, pubic bone pain may be caused by an inflammation of the joint that leads to some destruction of the tissues, called osteitis pubis. In this situation, the pain is constant, gets worse and may be accompanied by fever. If these signs and symptoms develop, contact your health care provider.

Puffy face
See **Swelling**

Quickening

■ *2nd trimester*

Quickening is the term for the first movements or kicks you feel from the fetus. In first pregnancies, this exciting development typically occurs by about 20 weeks' gestation, although you might feel the first movements a few weeks earlier or later. The movements might feel like a light tapping or the fluttering of a butterfly. At first you might attribute the sensation to gas or hunger pangs.

It's normal during the second trimester for fetal movements to be somewhat erratic — few and far between at first, or several movements one day and none the next. Later, the kicks and movements usually become stronger and more regular, and you'll be able to feel them by placing a hand on your lower abdomen. Feeling your baby move is a pleasant way to feel connected to your pregnancy. When you and your partner feel movements through your belly, you'll both begin to become more emotionally involved with your baby.

As your pregnancy progresses, you'll probably become aware of your baby's typical movement patterns. Each fetus has its own pattern of activity and development. The most active time is between 27 and 32 weeks. Activity tends to slow down in the last weeks of pregnancy. (See also **Baby movement, decreased.**) If you notice any major changes in your fetus's activity level after 22 weeks — such as an absence or slowdown of movement for more than 24 hours — contact your health care provider.

Rashes

■ *2nd, 3rd trimesters*

Red, itchy skin is probably not the pregnancy glow you had in mind. But some women develop rashes during pregnancy. Heat rashes, sometimes called prickly heat, are most common. They're caused by the increased perspiration and dampness triggered by pregnancy hormones (see also **Perspiration).** Other types of rashes also may appear during pregnancy.

Intertrigo. Increased perspiration can cause a rash called intertrigo, which is particularly common in overweight women. It's typically found in the sweaty skin folds under the breasts or in the groin area — warm, moist areas where fungi can thrive, causing infection with the resulting inflammation. Intertrigo should be treated as early as possible because the longer it goes on, the more difficult it may be to treat.

PUPPP. About one in every 150 pregnant women develop a severe rash with the tongue-twisting name pruritic urticarial papules and plaques of pregnancy (PUPPP). This condition is characterized by itchy, reddish, raised patches on the skin. These itchy bumps are called papules, and the larger raised areas are called plaques. They usually show up first on the abdomen and often spread to the arms, legs and buttocks. In some women, the itching can be extreme. Although PUPPP can be miserable for the mother, it doesn't pose risks to the baby. The signs and symptoms should go away after you deliver.

Although it's not known for certain what causes PUPPP, a genetic factor appears to be involved because the condition tends to run in families. PUPPP is more common in first pregnancies, and it rarely recurs in later ones.

Prevention and self-care for rashes

Most common rashes will improve with gentle skin care. Avoid scrubbing the skin, and use gentle cleansers. Minimize the use of soap. Oatmeal baths or baking soda baths can help relieve itchiness. Heat rash can be soothed by applying cornstarch after bathing, avoiding very hot baths or showers, and keeping the skin cool and dry.

To help prevent intertrigo, wear loosefitting cotton clothing, wash and dry the affected areas frequently — use a gentle cleanser or nonperfumed soap — and apply calamine lotion, baking soda or zinc oxide powder to the affected areas. You can also try blowing a fan or hair dryer on its lowest setting across moist areas.

Medical care for rashes

If self-care measures are ineffective or if your rash persists, worsens or is accompanied by other symptoms, call your health care provider.

If self-care fails to clear up intertrigo, your health care provider may prescribe a steroid, antibiotic or antifungal cream.

Treatment of PUPPP consists of oral medications or anti-itching creams. In particularly severe cases, a steroid cream may be prescribed.

Rectal bleeding

3rd trimester

Rectal bleeding is a very important sign that always requires evaluation. Fortunately, bleeding from your anus rarely indicates a problem with your pregnancy, and because of the age group of pregnant women, it's rarely related to serious colorectal disease either. Most often rectal bleeding is caused by hemorrhoids, which are fairly common during the last trimester and in the weeks following delivery (see also **Hemorrhoids).**

Another possible cause of rectal bleeding is a tiny crack or cracks in the anus (anal fissure). Fissures are usually caused by constipation, another common problem during pregnancy. Anal fissures are usually quite painful.

■ *Prevention and self-care for rectal bleeding*
Hemorrhoids and anal fissures are often caused and irritated by constipation, so your best strategy is to stay regular. For tips on avoiding constipation, see **Constipation.**

■ *When to seek medical help for rectal bleeding*
Always report rectal bleeding to your health care provider. He or she will want to check out the cause of the bleeding and may recommend another treatment for hemorrhoids. Bleeding accompanied by diarrhea with mucus and abdominal pain may indicate the possibility of an inflammatory bowel.

Red palms and soles

■ *1st, 2nd, 3rd trimesters*
Two-thirds of pregnant women find that their palms and the soles of their feet become red. This skin change is more common in white women than in black women. The redness can appear as early as the first trimester and is the result of increased blood flow to the hands and feet. In addition to being red, these areas may itch. Like most skin changes of pregnancy, the redness fades after delivery.

■ *Self-care for red palms and soles*
If your hands and feet itch, moisturizing creams may help.

■ *When to seek medical help for red palms and soles*
If the redness in your palms and soles doesn't fade after delivery, talk to your health care provider. Red palms and soles can also be a sign of cirrhosis of the liver, lupus or an overactive thyroid, although in those cases other signs and symptoms are likely to be present as well.

Rib tenderness

■ *3rd trimester*
In the later months of pregnancy, the fetus runs out of room to stretch and may find it handy to rest his or her feet between your ribs. It's surprising how much those little toes and feet jamming into your rib cage can hurt.

In addition to the pressure the baby is exerting, the shape of your chest is being altered to maintain room for your lungs while the diaphragm is pushed upward by the uterus. This reshaping pushes your ribs outward and can lead to pain between the ribs and the cartilage that attaches them to your breastbone.

If the baby's position is hurting your ribs, try changing your own position. You can do the stretch explained here. Or try this: Take a deep breath while raising one arm over your head, then exhale while you drop your arm. Repeat this movement a few times with each arm. Gently pushing the baby's feet or bottom away from the painful side also is quite safe.

Rib tenderness may disappear after the baby drops into your pelvis, which usually happens two to three weeks before delivery in first pregnancies — but usually not until labor begins in subsequent ones.

Try this stretch: Get down on your hands and knees, with your back relaxed but not sagging. Keeping your head straight and your neck aligned with your spine, round your back upward toward the ceiling. Allow your head to drop all the way down. Gradually release your back and raise your head to the original position. Repeat several times.

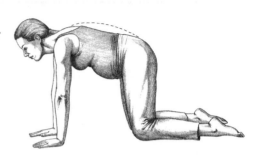

Round ligament pain

2nd, 3rd trimesters

Stretching of the round ligament can cause pain in the abdomen, pelvis or groin during the second and third trimesters. One of several ligaments that hold your uterus in place within your abdomen, the round ligament is a cord-like structure that's less than a quarter of an inch thick before pregnancy. At that time, your uterus is about the size of a pear.

As the uterus grows in size and weight, the ligaments supporting it become longer, thicker and more taut, stretching and tensing like rubber bands. If you move or reach suddenly, the round ligament can stretch, causing a pulling or stabbing pang in your lower pelvic area or groin or a sharp cramp down your side. Round ligament pain can be severe, but the discomfort usually goes away after several minutes. You may wake up at night with this type of pain after rolling over in your sleep. The pain can also be triggered by exercise. Round ligament pain may ease as your pregnancy progresses. It should go away after you have your baby.

Prevention and self-care for round ligament pain

Although round ligament pain is uncomfortable, it's one of the normal changes of pregnancy. The following suggestions may provide relief:

- Change the way you move. Sit down and get up more slowly, and avoid sudden movements.
- Sit or lie down when abdominal pain becomes bothersome.
- Apply heat by soaking in a warm bath or using a heating pad.

■ *When to seek medical help for round ligament pain*
If round ligament pain is severe, call your health care provider. He or she may suggest that you take acetaminophen (Tylenol, others) for pain relief.

Sometimes, abdominal pain is caused by a more serious condition, such as an ectopic pregnancy, ruptured ovarian cyst or appendicitis. Contact your health care provider right away or go to a hospital emergency department if you have any of the following signs and symptoms:
- Fever
- Chills
- Loss of appetite
- Pain when urinating
- Vaginal bleeding

Rupture of membranes
See **Water breaking**

Sciatica
■ *3rd trimester*
Pain, tingling or numbness running down the buttock, back or thigh is called sciatica because it follows the course of the sciatic nerve. It's caused by pressure from the growing uterus, the baby or the relaxed pelvic joints on the sciatic nerve, which is a major nerve that runs from your lower back down the back of your legs to your feet. Lifting, bending and even walking may aggravate sciatica.

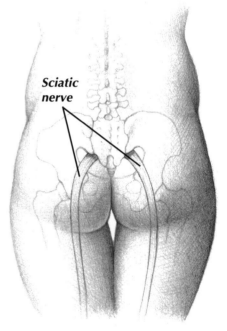

Sciatic nerve

Although sciatica is no fun, it's generally not a cause for concern. When your baby changes position closer to the time of delivery, the pain is likely to ease. Occasionally, the problem is caused by a more serious condition called vertebral disk disease.

■ *Prevention and self-care for sciatica*
Warm baths, a heating pad and switching the side of your body that you sleep on may help with sciatic nerve pain. You may also find relief by changing your position regularly during the day, such as by getting up and moving around once every hour or so.

Swimming is another way to ease the discomfort. Being in the water temporarily takes some of the weight of your uterus off your sciatic nerve.

When to seek medical help for sciatica

Tell your health care provider if you're experiencing sciatica. Seek care if the numbness isn't transient, or if you're tripping when you walk or feel you can't move your foot with equal strength in all directions. He or she will want to rule out other, rarer causes of sciatica that could be more serious. It's fairly common to need physical therapy to help relieve sciatic nerve pain.

Shortness of breath

See **Breath, shortness of**

Skin changes

1st, 2nd, 3rd trimesters

Pregnancy hormones can spur several changes in your skin. For some lucky women, the main change is the famous healthy glow, which happens as a result of increased circulation in the tiny blood vessels just beneath the surface of your skin. But many women notice a variety of other, less desirable skin changes.

Skin darkening. This is one of the most common skin changes, occurring in 90 percent of all pregnant women. The darkening can affect your cheeks, chin, nose, forehead, navel, armpits, inner thighs and the area between your vulva and anus (perineum). In addition, the areas of skin that are already pigmented get even darker, most noticeably on or around your nipples and external labia — the thicker folds of tissue on both sides of your vagina.

When the pale line that runs from your navel to your pubic bone darkens, it's referred to as the linea nigra (see also **Linea nigra).** Skin darkening on the face is referred to as the mask of pregnancy, or melasma (see also **Mask of pregnancy).**

Skin darkening is likely the result of increased melatonin, which has important roles in the developing fetus. It typically fades after you give birth, although some areas of increased pigmentation, such as the nipples and labia, are likely to remain darker than they were before you were pregnant.

Vascular spiders. Vascular spiders (spider nevi) typically appear only during pregnancy. The name comes from the way they look — tiny, reddish spots with raised lines of tiny blood vessels branching out from the center, like spider legs. Caused by increased blood circulation, vascular spiders are most likely to show up on your face, neck, upper chest or arms. They don't cause pain or discomfort, and they usually disappear within a few weeks after you give birth.

Stretch marks. Pink or purplish streaks on the abdomen, breasts, upper arms, buttocks and thighs are common in about half of the pregnant women. (See also **Stretch marks.)**

Acne. You may develop acne when you're pregnant, or your acne may improve. Some topical treatments can be used. (See also **Acne.)**

Moles and freckles. You may get new moles while pregnant, although they're usually not the type that are linked to skin cancer. Existing moles, freckles and skin blemishes may also become darker during pregnancy.

Itchiness. The stretching and tightening of the skin across your abdomen can leave it dry and itchy. Some women also experience itchiness all over their body. Heat rashes and other types of rashes also can cause itchiness. (See also **Itchiness; Rashes.)**

Red palms and soles. Two-thirds of pregnant women find that their palms and the soles of their feet become red. The redness fades after delivery. (See also **Red palms and soles.)**

Perspiration. Pregnant women often perspire more (see also **Perspiration).**

Rashes. Heat rashes are common during pregnancy, due to increased perspiration. Other rashes also may develop (see also **Rashes).**

Skin tags. Small, loose growths of skin may appear under your arms or breasts (see also **Skin growths or tags).**

Soft fingernails. Some women experience problems with their fingernails during pregnancy. This is temporary and not a sign of serious disease.

Self-care for skin changes

If areas of your skin have darkened and it concerns you, avoid getting too much sun. Skin darkening during pregnancy is made worse by exposure to sunlight or other sources of ultraviolet (UV) light. When you're outdoors, wear a sunblock with a sun protection factor (SPF) of at least 15. Remember that the sun's UV rays can still reach your skin even on cloudy or overcast days. You may also want to wear a wide-brimmed hat that shades your face. Makeup can help with areas of skin darkening on your face.

For itchiness, keep your skin lubricated with a good moisturizing cream. Moisturize your nails as well as your hands, and wear rubber gloves when using detergents or cleansers.

When to seek medical help for skin changes

If your skin darkening or itchiness is extreme, talk to your health care provider. A medicated ointment may help the itching. Occasionally, a skin change might be a sign of something more serious. Contact your health care provider if:

- A particular mole changes noticeably in size or appearance. You may want to show any new moles to your health care provider. Even though moles caused by pregnancy are not related to skin cancer, you could develop a melanoma during pregnancy, and it's critical to detect these tumors early.
- Puffy eyelids occur along with a sudden weight increase — 5 pounds or more within a week. Sudden weight gain and puffiness could indicate developing preeclampsia.
- Severe itching develops late in your pregnancy without a rash.

Skin growths or tags

2nd, 3rd trimesters

When you're expecting, you may discover a few new skin growths under your arms, on your neck or shoulders or elsewhere on your body. These tiny, loose protrusions of skin, often called skin tags, are usually painless and harmless. They typically don't grow or change. No one knows what causes them. They often disappear after you give birth. But they're common after midlife.

Generally, skin tags aren't bothersome and don't require treatment. If the growths are irritating or cosmetically displeasing, they can easily be removed. Let your health care provider know if a skin growth changes in appearance.

Sleep, lack of

See **Insomnia**

Smell, sensitive sense of

1st trimester

You normally love the smell of bacon cooking and coffee brewing, but now that you're pregnant these odors make you gag. Your co-worker's perfume makes you feel sick, and you have to fight off nausea when you fill up the gas tank. Research confirms that pregnant women have a sharper sense of smell — they notice odors that they don't normally notice, and previously acceptable smells become repugnant. This heightened sense of smell is also connected to the nausea and vomiting that many pregnant women experience. A variety of odors, such as foods cooking, coffee, perfume, cigarette smoke or particular foods, can trigger nausea.

A sensitive sense of smell may be due in part to the increase in estrogen during pregnancy. Like nausea, this symptom may indicate a rapidly growing placenta and embryo, and that's a good sign. In mice, the fluctuations in smell-controlling brain cells are linked to the hormone prolactin, a hormone which is also found in human pregnancy. Most women find this symptom to tightly parallel nausea in pregnancy, so it usually improves by 13 to 14 weeks.

Self-care for sensitive sense of smell

To keep your overactive olfactory cells from getting the best of you, be aware of the odors that trigger or aggravate your nausea, and avoid them whenever possible. You might have to eat lunch at your desk instead of the cafeteria. Or you may have to ask a co-worker not to wear a particular perfume or cologne until your nausea subsides, usually in the second trimester.

Snoring

1st, 2nd, 3rd trimesters

Up to a quarter of pregnant women snore, compared with about 4 percent of women the same age who aren't pregnant. Because of increased swelling in the nasal passages and nasal congestion during pregnancy, your upper airway is narrower. Narrowing of the upper airway can lead to snoring.

Although snoring is often the subject of jokes, it can have some serious consequences. Snoring can be related to high blood pressure (hypertension), and women who snore during pregnancy are at higher risk of pregnancy-induced high blood pressure (preeclampsia) and of having an infant who is considered small for gestational age. In one study, pregnant women who habitually snored had double the risk for high blood pressure and nearly 3.5 times the risk of slowed fetal growth, compared with nonsnorers.

Snoring may also be a sign of sleep apnea, a sleep disorder in which you stop breathing for short periods during sleep. The lack of oxygen disrupts the mother's sleep and may stress the fetus.

Overweight women may be at particularly high risk of snoring-related problems. In one study involving 502 women who had just given birth, women who reported regular snoring during pregnancy were heavier before becoming pregnant and gained more weight during pregnancy.

▦ *Prevention and self-care for snoring*

To minimize your chance of snoring, follow these tips:

- Sleep on your side rather than your back. Sleeping on your back can cause your tongue and soft palate to rest against the back of your throat and block your airway.
- Nasal strips may help increase the area of your nasal passages and airway.
- Keep your weight gain in check. Avoid gaining more than recommended based on your pre-pregnancy weight.

▦ **When to seek medical help for snoring**

Contact your health care provider if you experience loud snoring, if your partner reports that it's very loud, if your snoring frequently wakes you up or if your partner thinks your snoring is interrupted by periods of stopped breathing. Most people with this problem are excessively sleepy during the day. These signs may indicate obstructive sleep apnea.

If you're diagnosed with sleep apnea, your health care provider may recommend treatment with continuous positive airway pressure (CPAP). This involves wearing a mask that's connected to a machine that gently blows air into your mouth and nose to keep your airway passages open. CPAP can improve sleep, prevent snoring and apnea, and may even improve your blood pressure.

Spotting

See **Vaginal bleeding**

Stretch marks

▦ *2nd, 3rd trimesters*

Get a group of new or expecting moms together, and you're likely to hear something about stretch marks. Stretch marks are pink or purplish streaks that typically appear on the abdomen, breasts, upper arms, buttocks and thighs. About half of the pregnant women get them, especially during the last half of pregnancy.

Stretch marks aren't a sign of excessive weight gain. They're caused by a stretching of the skin along with a normal increase in cortisone, a hormone produced by the adrenal glands. The increase may weaken elastic fibers of the skin. Heredity is thought to play the biggest role in their development. Some women get severe stretch marks even though they've gained little weight during pregnancy.

Stretch marks usually don't disappear altogether, but after delivery they often fade gradually to light pink or white.

■ *Prevention for stretch marks*

Contrary to popular belief, no creams or ointments can prevent stretch marks or make them vanish. Because stretch marks develop from deep within the connective tissue underneath the skin, they can't be prevented by anything applied externally.

Stuffy nose

■ *1st, 2nd, 3rd trimesters*

Nasal stuffiness is a common problem in pregnancy, even if you don't have a cold or allergies. Nasal congestion and nosebleeds are more frequent because of the increased blood flow to the mucous membranes in your body. As the lining of your nose and airway swells, your airway shrinks. Your nasal tissue also becomes softer and more prone to bleeding. This nasal stuffiness is common in pregnancy and isn't inflammation of the mucous membranes of the nose (rhinitis). It can be annoying, however.

Rhinitis — in other words, a runny or stuffy nose caused by inflammation — is the body's strategy for getting rid of foreign invaders. Allergic rhinitis is caused by seasonal or perennial allergies. Nonallergic rhinitis is triggered by factors such as air pollution, smoke and infections.

When blood vessel changes are the cause of nasal congestion or stuffiness along with a very runny nose, the condition is called vasomotor rhinitis. It's often associated with overuse of nasal spray decongestants.

■ *Prevention and self-care for a stuffy nose*

Most pregnant women can tolerate a stuffy nose and other nasal symptoms without taking medications. If there's no accompanying problem such as a cold or allergies, no treatment is generally required. These tips may help keep your stuffy nose clearer:
- Use a humidifier in your home to loosen nasal secretions.
- Place a towel over your head and breathe the steam from a pan of water.
- Sleep propped up with your head elevated.

■ *Medical care for a stuffy nose*

Avoid over-the-counter remedies for your stuffed-up nose. Prolonged use of these medications can cause problems, and your nasal stuffiness may last for nine months. Try to deal with it using conservative means.

For other tips on dealing with nasal congestion related to inflammation, see **Allergies; Colds.**

Swelling

■ *3rd trimester*

At times, you may feel swollen while you're pregnant. Swelling (edema) is common during pregnancy when your body tissues accumulate more fluid due to dilated blood vessels and increased blood volume. Warm weather can aggravate the condition.

During the last three months of pregnancy, about half of the pregnant women notice their eyelids and face becoming puffy, mostly in the morning. This is due to fluid retention and dilated blood vessels, which are expected in pregnancy. In the last few weeks of pregnancy, almost all women have some swelling in their ankles, legs, fingers or face. By itself, swelling is annoying but not a serious complication.

Prevention and self-care for swelling

If you have problems with swelling:

- Use cold-water compresses on swollen areas.
- Don't cut back dramatically on salt, although easing off on pretzels with rock salt might be a good idea. Although you may be advised to limit sodium to help with fluid retention, cutting back drastically on salt will cause your body to conserve sodium and water, which can make swelling worse.
- To relieve swelling in your legs and feet, lie down and elevate your legs for an hour in the middle of the afternoon. Using a footrest also may help.
- Swimming or even standing in a pool may provide some relief. Water pressure will compress your ankles, and your uterus will float just a bit, easing the pressure on your veins.

When to seek medical help for swelling

If you experience a sudden swelling of your face and hands — especially if you find you aren't urinating as often as usual — contact your health care provider immediately. Swelling in the face, especially around the eyes, may occasionally be a sign of preeclampsia.

Tanning

1st, 2nd, 3rd trimesters

If you're a sun worshiper, you may wonder if it's OK to keep tanning while you're pregnant. Tanning can't be endorsed at any time.

Many dermatologists and public health officials caution that there's no such thing as a safe or healthy tan. Ultraviolet (UV) radiation from the sun, tanning beds or sunlamps may cause skin cancer. It can also have a damaging effect on the connective tissues and can lead to premature aging of the skin, giving it a wrinkled, leathery appearance. Most skin cancers are clearly related to UV exposure, including some that cause premature death for thousands every year.

The mask of pregnancy — skin darkening on the face — is made worse by exposure to sunlight and tanning beds (see also **Mask of pregnancy).**

No controlled studies have examined the direct effects of tanning, tanning beds or self-tanning lotions on pregnant women. Although you won't get overheated on a tanning bed, you still have the other risks associated with UV radiation. As for self-tanning creams and lotions, the chemical that produces the tan, dihydroxyacetone (DHA), hasn't been studied in pregnant women. No evidence indicates that self-tanners are harmful, but there's no proof that they're safe, either.

Exposure to sunlight does provide some important benefits, such as increased vitamin D production and a sense of well-being. Sunlight can also affect mental health. There is good evidence that sunshine improves the mood of many healthy people and those suffering with disease. Remember, however, only a small amount of sunlight is needed for the body to manufacture vitamin D — much less sun exposure than it takes to get a suntan.

Tips for avoiding sun damage
- When you're outdoors, always wear a sunscreen with a sun protection factor (SPF) of 15 or greater, and reapply it often when you're outside for longer periods or when you're swimming. Remember that some of the sun's UV rays also reach your skin on cloudy or overcast days.
- Plan your outdoor activities to avoid the sun's strongest rays in the middle of the day. As a general rule, be particularly cautious between 10 a.m. and 4 p.m.
- Reduce your sun exposure by wearing a wide-brimmed hat that shades your face and long-sleeved shirts and pants.
- Wear sunglasses that provide 100 percent UV protection.
- Seek shade, such as at outdoor cafes with umbrellas or under covered porches.
- Drink enough water, and make sure you don't get overheated.
- If you're determined to use a self-tanning lotion, check with your health care provider first. And remember that self-tanners don't provide protection from UV rays.

Thirst

1st, 2nd, 3rd trimesters
You may notice that you're thirstier than normal while you're pregnant. That's perfectly healthy — increased thirst is your body's way of getting you to drink more water and other fluids. Your body needs extra fluids to replenish the amniotic fluid and maintain your increased blood volume.

Drinking more fluids also helps prevent constipation and dry skin and helps your kidneys dispose of the waste products being produced by the fetus.

Prevention and self-care for thirst
Drink at least eight glasses a day of water or other beverages. Caffeinated beverages stimulate urine production and so aren't the best choices. In addition to plain or sparkling water, good choices include a fruit juice fizz made with half juice and half sparkling water, vegetable juice, soup and a fruit shake made with skim milk. You have many fine choices for fluid replenishment in pregnancy. If you have been vomiting or you've had trouble with feeling faint, sports drinks such as Gatorade and Powerade may have some advantage.

When to seek medical help for thirst
Although increased thirst is normal when you're expecting, it can also be a symptom of diabetes. Gestational diabetes generally has no symptoms, but it's possible to develop full-blown diabetes during pregnancy. It can be hard to distinguish the subtle signs and symptoms of diabetes, such as fatigue, excessive thirst or excessive urination, from the typical changes of pregnancy.

Tooth, abscessed
1st, 2nd, 3rd trimesters
An abscessed tooth isn't good news for anyone, and being pregnant provides for no exception.

An abscess starts when a cracked tooth or deep cavity allows bacteria to enter the tooth's soft core (dental pulp), causing an infection. Pus builds up at the root tip of the tooth, located in the jawbone, and forms a pocket of pus — the abscess. An abscess can damage the bone around the tooth as well as lead to a general infection.

Prevention and self-care for an abscessed tooth
An abscessed tooth always requires skilled dental care. The only self-care is prevention by routine dental hygiene and preventive dental care. Preventive dental care is especially important during pregnancy, as oral changes seem to speed up the progress of dental disease. For tips on good dental hygiene, see also **Gum disease.**

Medical care for an abscessed tooth
If you have pain in your tooth or jaw or signs of an infection, such as a fever, call your dentist. A root canal will probably be needed to treat an abscessed tooth, and you may be given an antibiotic. If you need to have

major dental work done during pregnancy, talk to both your dentist and your health care provider about any special precautions that should be taken. Never delay your care because of the pregnancy.

Toxic substances, exposure to

1st, 2nd, 3rd trimesters

It's rare to be exposed to substances that are harmful to a developing fetus. But it can happen. Agents that are known to harm a fetus if a woman is exposed to them during pregnancy are called teratogens. They can cause a miscarriage or birth defects. Some substances may harm an infant through breast-feeding.

Substances known to be harmful include:

- Pesticides
- Heavy metals, such as lead and mercury
- Drugs used to treat cancer, such as methotrexate and aminopterin
- Ionizing radiation (X-rays)
- Some viruses, bacteria and protozoa

Organic solvents such as benzene are suspected to be harmful, although results of studies are inconclusive. Women who work in health care, farming, manufacturing, dry cleaning, printing, crafts businesses such as painting or pottery glazing, or electronics should be aware of the substances they're exposed to at work.

Industries in the United States are required to provide information to employees about hazardous substances in a workplace. As long as you and the company you work for follow Occupational Safety & Health Administration (OSHA) practices, it's unlikely that your fetus will be harmed. Proper clothing and safety measures can reduce or prevent exposure.

Fortunately, few birth defects are caused by environmental agents. Yet, it's best to avoid exposure to known or suspected harmful substances.

Talk to your health care provider about any exposure you have to chemicals, drugs, metals or radiation. You'll also want to tell the health care provider about any equipment in the workplace designed to minimize exposure, such as gowns, gloves, masks and ventilation systems. The health care provider can help determine if a risk exists and, if so, what can be done to eliminate it or reduce it. Although your health care provider will try to be helpful, he or she may not know of the specific use of an agent in a given industry.

It's a good idea to discuss any concerns you may have about being exposed to toxic substances with your employer or union representative. Several federal laws are designed to protect the health, safety and employment rights of pregnant working women. To find out about laws on workplace safety, contact your state or county health department.

Urinary incontinence
2nd, 3rd trimesters

Sometimes, pregnant women and new mothers may pass urine involuntarily, especially when coughing, straining or laughing. During pregnancy, the baby is often resting directly on your bladder, and no one can stay dry with a baby bouncing on her bladder. Sometimes, damage at birth to the pelvic floor muscles and nerves to the bladder will cause urine leakage for a few weeks after birth. Fortunately, this problem usually improves within three months of giving birth. Unfortunately, the problem tends to recur later in life.

Prevention and self-care for urinary incontinence

Research shows that doing Kegel exercises may help prevent urinary incontinence during pregnancy and after childbirth. These strengthening exercises help form a stronger, thicker support for your bladder, urethra and other pelvic organs. To do Kegel exercises, squeeze the muscles around your vagina tightly, as if you were stopping the flow of urine, for a few seconds, then relax. Repeat 10 times.

If you do experience incontinence, wear protective undergarments or sanitary napkins.

Urinary tract infections
1st, 2nd, 3rd trimesters

Many of the normal changes of pregnancy can increase your risk of urinary tract infections (UTIs) — infections of the bladder, kidney or urethra. It's very important to recognize and treat UTIs during pregnancy. These infections are a common cause of preterm labor. What's more, UTIs during pregnancy are more likely to be severe. For example, if you have a bladder infection that goes untreated, it may result in a kidney infection.

You're also more susceptible to UTIs after giving birth. For a time after delivery, you may be unable to empty your bladder completely. The urine that's left provides a breeding ground for bacteria.

Fortunately, bladder infections — even those that cause no signs and symptoms — can usually be found and treated before the kidneys become infected. Several screening methods are used to detect early evidence of infection. When treated early and properly, a UTI won't hurt your baby.

If you have a UTI, you may feel pain or burning when you urinate. You might feel a frequent, almost panicky urge to go, or you might feel like you need to go again right after you've urinated. Other signs and symptoms include blood in the urine, strong-smelling urine, mild fever and tenderness over the area of the bladder. Abdominal pain and backache also may signal an infection.

Prevention and self-care for urinary tract infections
You can help prevent and clear up UTIs in several ways:
- Drink plenty of liquids, especially water.
- Urinate often — don't hold it or wait for long periods of time before you go. Holding in your urine can result in incomplete emptying of the bladder, which can lead to a UTI. Frequent urination is also helpful in clearing up a UTI.
- Lean forward while you urinate to help empty your bladder more fully.
- Always urinate after sexual intercourse.
- After you urinate, wipe from front to back.

Medical care for urinary tract infections
A urinary tract infection is diagnosed by testing a urine sample for bacteria. Treatment includes antibiotics to clear up the infection and acetaminophen to reduce fever. These medications are safe to take during pregnancy, though your health care provider needs to know of your pregnancy to choose the safest antibiotic. If you have a kidney infection, you may be admitted to the hospital for intravenous antibiotics. After your UTI is resolved, your health care provider might recommend that you continue taking antibiotic medication to lessen the chance of recurrence.

Urination, frequent
1st, 3rd trimesters
During the first trimester of pregnancy, your growing uterus pushes on your bladder. As a result, you may find yourself running to the bathroom more often than usual. You may also leak a small amount of urine when you cough, sneeze or laugh. By the fourth month, the uterus expands up out of the pelvic cavity, easing pressure on the bladder. Then, in the last few weeks of pregnancy, you may need to urinate more frequently again, when the baby's head drops into the pelvis, placing renewed pressure on the bladder. Frequent urination almost always goes away after you give birth.

Prevention and self-care for frequent urination
The following suggestions may help:
- Urinate as often as you need to. Holding in your urine can result in incomplete emptying of the bladder, which can lead to a urinary tract infection.
- Lean forward when you urinate to help empty your bladder more fully.
- Avoid drinking anything for a few hours before bedtime so that you have to get up less often during the night. Make sure you're still getting plenty of fluids during the rest of the day, however.

- Try Kegel exercises, which may enhance continence if done several times a day. Squeeze the muscles around your vagina tightly, as if you were stopping the flow of urine, for a few seconds, then relax. Repeat 10 times.
- If you leak urine during the day, wear unscented panty liners.

When to seek medical help for frequent urination
If you are urinating frequently and are also experiencing burning, pain, fever or a change in the odor or color of your urine, you may have an infection (see also **Urinary tract infections**). Contact your health care provider.

Urination with pain and burning
1st, 2nd, 3rd trimesters
Painful urination or a burning sensation when you urinate is often one of the first symptoms of a urinary tract infection (see also **Urinary tract infections**). Contact your health care provider promptly if you experience painful urination.

Vaginal bleeding
1st, 2nd, 3rd trimesters
As many as half of all pregnant women may experience spotting or vaginal bleeding at some point during their pregnancy, especially in the first trimester. Vaginal bleeding in pregnancy has many causes — some are serious and some aren't. The significance and possible causes of bleeding are different in each trimester.

First trimester. Many women have spotting or bleeding in the first 12 weeks of pregnancy. Depending on whether it's heavy or light, how long it lasts and if it's continuous or sporadic, bleeding can indicate many things. It may be a warning sign, but it may also be due to the normal events of pregnancy.

You may notice a small amount of spotting or bleeding very early in pregnancy, about a week to 14 days after fertilization. Known as implantation bleeding, it happens when the fertilized egg first attaches to the lining of the uterus. This type of light bleeding usually doesn't last long.

Bleeding in the first trimester can also be a sign of a miscarriage. Most miscarriages take place during the first trimester, although they can occur any time during the first half of a pregnancy. But bleeding doesn't necessarily mean you're having a miscarriage — at least half the women who bleed in the first trimester don't have miscarriages.

Another problem that can cause bleeding and pain in early pregnancy is ectopic pregnancy, in which the embryo implants outside the uterus, usually in a fallopian tube. An uncommon cause of bleeding in the first trimester is molar pregnancy, a rare condition in which an abnormal mass — instead of a baby — forms inside the uterus after fertilization.

Second trimester. Although miscarriage is less common in the second trimester than in the first, a risk still exists. Vaginal bleeding is the primary sign of miscarriage.

Moderate to heavy bleeding in the second trimester may also indicate a problem with the placenta — placenta previa, in which the placenta lies too low in the uterus and partly or completely covers the uterus, or placental abruption, in which the placenta begins to separate from the inner wall of the uterus before birth. Both of these conditions are more frequent in the third trimester.

If bleeding occurs between 20 and 37 weeks, it may be a sign of preterm labor.

A cervical infection, inflamed cervix or growths on the cervix also can cause vaginal bleeding. Cervical bleeding is usually not a risk to the baby, but if it's caused by cervical cancer, it's very important that the diagnosis be made promptly. Occasionally, light bleeding from the cervix may be a sign of cervical incompetence, a condition where the cervix opens spontaneously, leading to preterm delivery.

Third trimester. Vaginal bleeding in the third trimester may be a sign of a problem with the placenta. In placental abruption, the placenta begins to detach from the inner wall of the uterus. The bleeding from this condition may be scant, heavy or somewhere in between.

In placenta previa, the cervix is partly or completely blocked by the placenta, which is normally located near the top of the uterus. The main sign of placenta previa is painless vaginal bleeding, typically near the end of the second trimester or the beginning of the third. The blood from placenta previa is usually bright red and may be scant but is usually fairly heavy. The bleeding may stop on its own at some point, but it nearly always comes back days or weeks later.

Light bleeding from weeks 20 to 37 may indicate preterm labor. Bleeding in the last weeks of pregnancy may be a sign of impending labor. The mucous plug that seals the opening of the uterus during pregnancy is passed out a few weeks before or at the start of labor. The discharge may have a small amount of blood in it (see **Bloody show).**

When to seek medical help for vaginal bleeding
Sometimes, bleeding in pregnancy is caused by a minor condition or normal process that requires no treatment. Other times, bleeding is a sign of a

serious problem. Be sure to have any bleeding during pregnancy evaluated by your health care provider. That's especially true after the first trimester.

Call your health care provider if you have slight spotting or bleeding, even if it goes away within a day. Contact him or her immediately or go to a hospital emergency room if you have:

- Any bleeding in the second or third trimester
- Moderate to heavy bleeding
- Any amount of bleeding accompanied by pain, cramping, fever, chills or contractions

You may need to be admitted to the hospital to find the cause of the bleeding. Treatment will depend on the cause.

Vaginal discharge

1st, 2nd, 3rd trimesters

Many women have increased vaginal discharge throughout pregnancy. This discharge, called leukorrhea, is thin, white and mild smelling or odorless. It's caused by the effects of hormones on the vaginal lining, which must grow dramatically during the pregnancy. It may increase throughout the pregnancy, becoming quite heavy. The high acidity of the discharge is thought to play a role in suppressing growth of harmful bacteria.

In the last few weeks of pregnancy, you may have a discharge that's blood tinged or a thick or stringy mass. This is probably the mucous plug that protects the cervix during pregnancy (see also **Bloody show).**

You'll also have a temporary vaginal discharge after giving birth. This discharge, called lochia, is caused by hormone shifts and will occur whether you had a vaginal or Caesarean birth. The discharge varies in amount, appearance and duration. Initially it's bloody, then it becomes paler or brownish after about four days and white or yellowish after about 10 days. You may occasionally pass a blood clot. This postpregnancy discharge can last from two to eight weeks. The amount should gradually diminish.

A discharge may also be a sign of a vaginal infection, which can be triggered by pregnancy hormones or medications such as antibiotics. If your vaginal discharge is greenish, yellowish, thick and cheesy, strong smelling or accompanied by redness, itching or irritation of the vulva, you may have a vaginal infection. Bacterial vaginosis is one common type of vaginal infection. It causes a foul-smelling gray to greenish discharge, and it's associated with preterm labor. It's treated orally or vaginally with metronidazole (Flagyl, MetroGel). Two other common types of vaginal infection during pregnancy are candidiasis (see also **Yeast infections)** and trichomoniasis. Neither presents a direct hazard to your baby, and both can be treated during pregnancy.

A steady or heavy watery discharge may be a sign that your membranes have ruptured (your water has broken). A vaginal discharge that's bloody or thick and mucus-like may indicate a problem with the cervix.

Prevention and self-care for vaginal discharge

To deal with the normal increased discharge of pregnancy, you might want to wear panty liners or a light sanitary pad. To reduce your risk of getting an infection:

- Do not douche. Douching can upset the normal balance of microorganisms in the vagina and can lead to a vaginal infection called bacterial vaginosis.
- Wear cotton underwear.
- Wear comfortable, loosefitting clothing. Avoid fabrics that don't breathe, tight slacks, exercise pants and leotards.
- There's some evidence that you can reduce your risk of yeast vaginal infection by eating 1 cup a day of yogurt containing live *Lactobacillus acidophilus* cultures.

When to seek medical help for vaginal discharge

Contact your health care provider if:

- You have abdominal pain or fever with a discharge.
- The discharge becomes greenish, yellowish or foul smelling.
- The discharge is thick and cheesy or curd-like.
- The discharge is accompanied by soreness, redness, burning or itching of the vulva.
- You have a steady or heavy discharge of watery fluid.
- The discharge is bloody or unusually thick.
- You've just had amniocentesis, and you have an increased vaginal discharge. This could indicate an amniotic fluid leak.

If you've already given birth, call your health care provider in the following situations:

- You're soaking a sanitary napkin every hour for four hours — don't wait the four hours if you become dizzy or notice increasing blood loss; call right away or go to the emergency room.
- The discharge has a foul, fishy odor.
- Your abdomen feels tender or your bleeding increases, and you're passing numerous clots.

Varicose veins

2nd, 3rd trimesters

The circulatory changes that support the growing fetus during pregnancy can also produce the unfortunate side effect of varicose veins. About 20 percent of pregnant women develop them. To accommodate the increased blood flow during pregnancy, blood vessels often become larger. At the same time, blood flow from your legs to your pelvis may be decreased. This can cause the valves in the veins in your legs to fail, leading to dilated, bulging veins. Vein problems may also show up as fine bluish, reddish or purplish lines under the skin, most often on the legs and ankles. Varicose veins tend to run in families. An inherited weakness in the valves of veins can make you more susceptible.

Varicose veins may cause no symptoms, or they may be painful or uncomfortable, causing sore, aching legs. The size of the veins usually decreases somewhat after birth.

Prevention and self-care for varicose veins

These measures can help prevent varicose veins, keep them from getting worse or ease the discomfort from them:
- Avoid standing for long periods.
- Don't sit with your legs crossed. This position can aggravate circulatory problems.
- Elevate your legs as often as you can. When sitting, rest your legs on another chair or a stool. When lying down, raise your legs and feet on a pillow.
- Exercise regularly to improve your overall circulation.
- Wear support stockings from the time you wake up until you go to bed. These stockings help improve the circulation in your legs. Ask your health care provider to recommend a good brand.
- Wear loose clothing around your thighs and waist. Socks and tight clothing on the lower legs are fine, but don't wear clothes that constrict the upper legs, such as underwear with tight leg holes. This can impede the return of blood from your legs and worsen varicose veins.

Medical care for varicose veins

Varicose veins generally don't require treatment. In severe cases, they can be removed surgically, but the procedure isn't normally done while you're pregnant.

Vomiting

1st trimester

Nausea and vomiting are common during early pregnancy and can occur at any time of day (see also **Morning sickness; Nausea throughout the day**). But sometimes vomiting is so severe that a pregnant woman can't eat or drink enough to maintain proper nutrition and stay hydrated. This condition is called hyperemesis gravidarum, the medical term for excessive vomiting in pregnancy.

Hyperemesis gravidarum affects about one in every 300 pregnant women. It's characterized by vomiting that's frequent, persistent and severe. You may also feel faint, dizzy or lightheaded. If not treated, hyperemesis can keep you from getting the nutrition and fluids you need. You may become dehydrated, which is the most serious complication of this condition. Rarely, the loss of fluids and salts from vomiting can be severe enough to threaten the fetus.

The exact causes of hyperemesis aren't known, but it seems to occur more frequently when the pregnancy hormone human chorionic gonadotropin (HCG) is very high, as in multiple pregnancy and molar pregnancy (a rare condition in which an abnormal mass — instead of a baby — forms inside the uterus after fertilization). It's more common in first pregnancies, young women and women carrying multiple fetuses.

Prevention and self-care for vomiting
If you're vomiting only occasionally or about once a day, follow the self-care measures listed under **Morning sickness.**

When to seek medical help for vomiting
Contact your health care provider if:
- You have nausea and vomiting so severe that you can't keep any food down
- You're vomiting more than two or three times a day
- Vomiting persists well into the second trimester
- You have some of the signs and symptoms of early or mild dehydration, which include:
  - Flushed face
  - Extreme thirst
  - Small amounts of dark yellow urine
  - Dizziness that's worse when you stand
  - Cramps in your arms or legs
  - Headache
  - Dry mouth with thick saliva

Before treating you for hyperemesis, your health care provider will rule out other possible causes of vomiting, such as molar pregnancy, gastrointestinal disorders and thyroid problems.

Warm, feeling

2nd, 3rd trimesters
Overheated? It's not just because you're getting bigger or because the

weather is warm. During pregnancy, your metabolism — the rate at which your body expends energy at rest — speeds up. And you're probably perspiring more as a result of needing to lose all the heat your baby is making. This can leave you feeling too warm, even in winter.

Prevention and self-care for feeling warm
It's important to avoid getting overheated while you're pregnant. Follow these tips to keep cool:
- Drink plenty of water and other fluids. Carry a water bottle with you.
- Dress lightly in breathable fabrics such as cotton.
- Avoid exercising outside in the warmest part of the day. Take a walk before breakfast or after dinner, or go to a fitness center.
- Stay out of the sun as much as possible.
- Go for a swim, or take a tepid or cool shower or bath.
- When the temperature is over 90 F, stay in air-conditioned environments as much as possible.

Water breaking (rupture of membranes)
3rd trimester
When the amniotic sac leaks or breaks before labor begins, the fluid that has been cushioning the baby comes out in a trickle or gush. This dramatic event is known as the water breaking, or the rupture of membranes. Only about 10 percent of women experience this, however, and it usually occurs at home, often in bed. Your membranes are more likely to rupture sometime during labor, often during the second stage. When it happens, labor usually starts or becomes more intense.

Contact your health care provider if your water breaks. Most health care providers want to evaluate you as soon as it happens because there's a risk of infection after the membranes rupture. There are no deadlines, but generally, unless the baby is very immature, it's best that the baby is born within about 24 hours. Let your health care provider know if the fluid is anything other than clear and odorless. A greenish or foul-smelling fluid could be a sign of uterine infection.

If you're uncertain whether the leaking fluid is amniotic fluid or urine, have it checked by your health care provider. Many pregnant women leak urine during the later stages of pregnancy. In the meantime, don't do anything that could introduce bacteria into your vagina, such as having sex or using tampons.

Weepiness
See **Mood swings**

Yeast infections

1st, 2nd, 3rd trimesters

Yeast infections (candidiasis) are caused by the organism *Candida albicans,* which is found in small amounts in the vagina in about 25 percent of women. Normally, various organisms in the vagina tend to keep one another in check. But increased estrogen levels during pregnancy cause changes in the vaginal environment, which may throw off the natural balance and allow some organisms to grow faster than others.

Candida may be present without causing signs and symptoms, or it may cause an infection. Signs and symptoms of infection include a vaginal discharge that is thick, white and curd-like, itching, burning and redness around the vagina and vulva, and painful urination.

Although a yeast infection is unpleasant for you, it won't hurt your baby, and it can safely be treated during pregnancy.

Prevention and self-care for yeast infections

To help prevent yeast infections:

- Eat yogurt that contains live *Lactobacillus acidophilus* cultures — most yogurt does. It may help keep the right mix of bacteria flourishing in your body.
- Wear underwear or pantyhose with cotton crotches, as well as loose-fitting pants.
- Avoid wearing wet bathing suits or exercise clothes for long periods of time, and wash them after each use.

Medical care for yeast infections

Candidiasis is treated during pregnancy with a vaginal cream or a suppository containing an antifungal cream. These medications are available without a prescription, but don't use one without consulting your health care provider first. Your health care provider needs to confirm the diagnosis before you start treatment. Although oral preparations are available for treating yeast infections, most health care providers recommend topical treatment during pregnancy.

Once you've had a yeast infection while pregnant, it can be a recurring problem until after delivery, when it usually subsides. It may be necessary to treat yeast infections repeatedly throughout your pregnancy.

PART 4

complications of pregnancy and childbirth

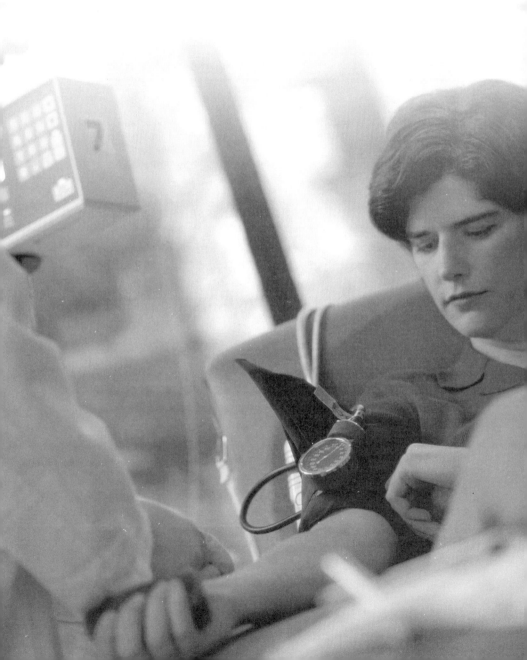

Every woman wants a problem-free pregnancy. But at times, problems develop. If you have or develop a medical condition, it can change how your pregnancy proceeds. "Complications of Pregnancy and Childbirth" explains some of the problems that can develop, how they might affect your pregnancy, and how you and your health care provider can manage the situation.

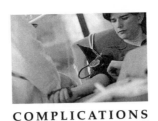

maternal health problems and pregnancy

When you have an existing health condition and become pregnant, it can change the way your pregnancy proceeds. The good news is, with the help of your health care provider, most problems can be managed in a way that's safe for both you and your baby. This section explains how pregnancy might interact with some health conditions.

Asthma

Asthma occurs when the main air passages of the lungs (bronchial tubes) become inflamed and constricted. When the muscles of the bronchial walls tighten, extra mucus is produced, further causing the airways to narrow. This can lead to everything from minor wheezing to severe difficulty breathing.

Asthma can develop at any age. Your chances of developing it increase if one or both of your parents had it and if you're sensitive to allergens or irritants in the environment. Obesity, gastroesophageal reflux disease (GERD) and exposure to secondhand smoke also may increase the risk. Although asthma attacks can be life-threatening, asthma is a highly treatable condition. With the right self-care and medication, problems can be prevented during pregnancy.

Managing asthma during pregnancy

If your asthma is well managed during pregnancy, there's little chance you and your baby will have an increased risk of health complications. Talk with your health care provider about what steps to take. If medications are needed, they aren't likely to affect your fetus — and remember, if you can't breathe well, that can hurt your unborn child.

If you don't use a peak flow meter, you may want to ask your health care provider about using one during pregnancy. A peak flow meter allows you to measure day-to-day variations in your breathing. It can help you identify asthma triggers and determine whether further care is needed.

Left uncontrolled, asthma can cause problems for both you and your baby. If it causes low oxygen levels in you, it will also decrease oxygen available to the fetus. This could result in a slowdown in fetal growth and even fetal brain damage. If you have severe episodes of asthma during pregnancy, you're likely to be treated with oxygen. During an attack, you may have pulmonary function tests or arterial blood gas studies performed. Your health care provider may also look more closely for anemia, which would pose an added stress for women with asthma.

If you have asthma, it's especially important that you have a flu (influenza) vaccination, at least after your first trimester of pregnancy. Illnesses such as the flu can make breathing more difficult. Your health care provider may also want to review any prescription and nonprescription medications you're taking. To control your signs and symptoms, it's important to continue taking medications as directed. Don't stop any medication for asthma unless directed to do so by your health care provider.

It's hard to predict how pregnancy might affect your asthma. It can stay the same, worsen or improve. For some pregnant women, asthma worsens in the second and third trimesters. In rare cases, it can worsen during labor. Medications for asthma are safe in pregnancy, so it's very likely your asthma can be controlled even if it does worsen a bit during pregnancy.

Cancer

One in 1,000 pregnancies is complicated by cancer. No evidence indicates that a woman's risk of cancer increases during pregnancy. However, a number of cancers can occur in women of childbearing age. These include breast cancer, cervical cancer, ovarian cancer and a form of skin cancer called melanoma.

Cancer is the name of a wide variety of diseases whose common characteristic is the overgrowth of one kind of cell in the body. Under normal circumstances, cells grow and divide to produce more cells needed by the body. Sometimes, cells keep dividing and form extra cells that become a mass of tissue. These masses are called growths (tumors).

Benign tumors are not cancerous. They rarely pose a threat to life. In fact, they often can be removed and cause no future problems. Malignant (cancerous) tumors contain cells that divide uncontrollably. They can spread to other parts of the body (metastasize), causing tissue and organ damage that can become life-threatening.

If you are being treated for cancer or have a history of it, you may be advised to delay becoming pregnant. Women diagnosed with breast cancer, for example, usually are encouraged to use birth control until after treatment. Those who have had breast cancer in the past also may be advised to wait and see if there's a recurrence before trying to conceive. The greatest risk of recurrence is during the first two or three years following treatment.

In some cases, previous treatment of cancer may impair fertility. With ovarian cancer, one or both ovaries, which provide a woman's eggs, may be removed surgically. If the cancer has advanced, the fallopian tubes, uterus and cervix also may need to be removed. In these cases, it isn't possible for a woman to conceive.

Managing cancer during pregnancy

If you receive a diagnosis of cancer after you become pregnant, treatment will be based on several factors. These include the type of cancer you have, how far it has advanced, what the best treatment would be and how far along you are in pregnancy. Various treatments may be considered.

Chemotherapy, a common cancer treatment, is most dangerous during the first trimester of pregnancy. During that time, it has a risk of causing birth defects. During the second and third trimesters, chemotherapy may lower your baby's birth weight. The degree of risk for other problems varies according to the medications used.

Radiation might or might not affect your baby. It depends on the strength of exposure, the location of the radiation site and the gestational age of the fetus. Radiation applied to your chest or abdominal area is almost certain to affect the fetus. Large doses of radiation exposure can cause problems with organ abnormalities, mental retardation or fetal growth restriction, depending on when the baby is exposed. The most vulnerable period for a fetus is between eight and 15 weeks of gestation.

Surgery is usually possible while you're pregnant. If surgery is needed for cancer and it doesn't involve the uterus, it's probably best to do the surgery during the pregnancy rather than waiting. However, if surgery causes inflammation or infection in the abdomen, it increases the risk of preterm labor.

If certain treatments are performed during pregnancy, they can lead to complications. For example, if it's necessary to remove cancerous tissue from the cervix while a woman is still pregnant, the risk of bleeding, preterm birth or miscarriage may increase.

In addition, cancer that spreads to other parts of the body can put the fetus in danger. In rare cases, malignant melanoma can metastasize to the placenta or the fetus. Advanced cases of cancer also may threaten the life of the mother if treatment is suspended or delayed in order to continue a pregnancy.

It's not clear whether pregnancy directly affects the progression of cancer. However, in many cases it can complicate treatment or reduce certain treatment options, which may affect final outcomes. This is particularly true in cases of advanced breast cancer, cervical cancer and lymphoma.

If you receive a diagnosis of breast cancer while you're pregnant, the prognosis generally is the same as that of women with a similar cancer who aren't pregnant. It's important that treatment begins, however, and delays in diagnosis and treatment during pregnancy are common. Women diagnosed with advanced disease in pregnancy may not have the same treatment options as other women if they choose to continue their pregnancies. Radiation, for example, isn't generally used because it might affect the baby when directed near the uterus. Depending on the extent of the disease, surgery and chemotherapy may be recommended.

Even though treatments could put a fetus at risk, advanced breast cancer typically must be treated promptly to improve the mother's outcome. Delaying or modifying treatment could reduce survival rates. The same is true of advanced or invasive cervical cancer.

Ovarian cancer seldom causes signs and symptoms in the early stages of the disease. As a result, it's commonly diagnosed at an advanced stage, leading to a poorer prognosis. The incidence during pregnancy is low because ovarian cancer is more common among older women.

When an ovarian tumor is discovered during pregnancy, it may be in an earlier stage and is accidentally discovered during a routine ultrasound. In addition, surgery can be performed to remove a diseased ovary during pregnancy. In some cases, the procedure might be delayed until a baby can be born, but in most cases delay isn't necessary or advisable. Benign tumors of the ovary are much more common in pregnancy than is ovarian cancer.

Malignant melanoma is an aggressive cancer that begins in the cells of a skin mole (nevus). Survival in malignant melanoma depends on the location and size of the cancerous lesion. Pregnancy appears to have no influence on how the disease progresses, but it may delay diagnosis. Surgery is the primary treatment of malignant melanoma, and skin surgery presents very little risk to the developing baby. Suspicious skin lesions should be removed when discovered, even if you're pregnant.

Before, during and after pregnancy, be sure to have regular medical exams that screen for cancers. It's especially important if you have a family history of these illnesses or other risk factors for a particular disease. For instance, during pregnancy, most women are advised to continue doing breast self-exams as well as check for irregular moles that could be a sign of malignant melanoma.

Cancer in pregnancy is rare, but cancers that aren't detected until they reach a late stage are more difficult to treat. It's important that you and your doctor don't delay any appropriate diagnostic tests and treatments during pregnancy.

High blood pressure

Blood pressure is the force with which blood pushes against the walls of the arteries. This pressure adjusts to meet the requirements of the body as it changes with position or activity. When the pressure becomes too high, the condition is called high blood pressure (hypertension).

Chronic hypertension, which can occur before pregnancy, can develop for various reasons. Heredity, diet and lifestyle are thought to play a role in the condition, but other chronic conditions can account for its development. These conditions may include kidney disease, thyroid dysfunction, Cushing's syndrome and sleep apnea. The primary underlying reason for high blood pressure can have a great impact on the way the condition is managed. No matter the cause, high blood pressure can lead to heart attack, stroke, kidney failure and premature death. It's important that high blood pressure is treated.

Managing high blood pressure during pregnancy

Most women with high blood pressure can have healthy pregnancies. However, the condition does require close observation and careful management throughout the pregnancy. Chronic hypertension can worsen significantly, leading to problems for both the mother and baby. This is particularly true when the unique hypertensive disease of pregnancy — preeclampsia — is added to chronic high blood pressure. Possible complications for the mother can include congestive heart failure, seizures, impairments of kidney or liver function, vision changes and stroke. Severe hypertension in pregnancy can become life-threatening. Many women with hypertension also develop problems during subsequent pregnancies.

Possible fetal problems related to high blood pressure include growth impairment (intrauterine growth restriction), greater risk of breathing problems before or during labor, greater risk of the placenta separating from the uterus before labor (placental abruption) and possible effects from medications used to treat the mother's hypertension.

If you have chronic hypertension, it's best to see your doctor before trying to become pregnant so that he or she can see if your condition is under control and review your medications. Some medications used to lower blood pressure are safe to take during pregnancy, but others, such as angiotensin-converting enzyme (ACE) inhibitors, can harm your baby. For that reason, your doctor may want to change the type or dosage of medications you take during pregnancy.

Blood pressure usually changes as part of the adaptation of the body to pregnancy. High blood pressure that existed before pregnancy can worsen during pregnancy, especially in the last trimester. The long-term course of high blood pressure is unaffected by pregnancy, but potentially serious complications can arise during pregnancy and childbirth. In some cases, pregnancy can reveal previously unrecognized hypertension.

Treatment is important for the mother during pregnancy. It appears that the developing baby also must be monitored closely, no matter how well controlled the mother's blood pressure is. To monitor the baby's health and development, frequent visits and repeated ultrasounds will usually be done to assess fetal growth and the distribution of blood flow within the baby. In the last trimester, testing can be done to keep a close eye on the baby's well-being. In most cases, women with high blood pressure will need to deliver a few weeks before their due dates to avoid complications.

Depression

Depression is a serious mental health condition. It can interfere with the ability to eat, sleep, work, interact with others and enjoy life. It may be a one-time problem, triggered by a stressful event such as the death of a loved one, or it may be a chronic condition. The illness often runs in families, which indicates that genetics play a part. Experts think this genetic vulnerability, along with environmental factors such as stress, may trigger an imbalance in brain chemicals and result in depression.

Depression is much more than a case of the blues. Left untreated, depression can lead to disability, dependency and suicide. Counseling, medications and other therapies are used to treat depression.

Managing depression during pregnancy

Depression can strike anyone. But women of childbearing age have a high risk of depression. The good news is, with proper medical care, most women with depression have normal pregnancies.

Pregnancy can, however, affect depression. During pregnancy, women go through many changes. For a woman with depression, pregnancy can trigger a wide range of emotions that can make coping more difficult. Physical changes during pregnancy and labor can also lessen or change the effectiveness of antidepressant medications. In addition, women with histories of major depression can have repeated episodes of it during and after pregnancy. This is especially true if they decide to stop using their antidepressant medications during pregnancy.

If you have depression and are trying to conceive or are pregnant, discuss your situation with your health care provider. If you're using medications, you may review the type and dosage used to treat depression with your health care provider. If you have mild depression, you may be able to stop using your antidepressant. If you have major depression or a recent history of depression, you'll probably be encouraged to continue your treatment.

Research has been done on the safety of antidepressants during pregnancy. Studies of fluoxetine (Prozac, Sarafem, others), sertraline (Zoloft) and paroxetine (Paxil) didn't show evidence of increased risk of birth defects. In addition, the medication bupropion (Wellbutrin) hasn't been shown to cause birth defects. However, the effects these medications may have on an unborn child's future behavior is unknown.

The use during pregnancy of an older class of drugs known as tricyclic antidepressants does cause concern. Because other, more effective medications are now available, there's rarely a need to consider using these drugs during pregnancy.

It's important to take proper care of depression during pregnancy. If you don't, you may put your health at risk, which can harm both you and your baby. Depression may result in your not eating well or not gaining enough weight. It can also lead to the abuse of alcohol or drugs or other risky behaviors. Severe depression can result in your trying to injure yourself or take your own life.

In addition, untreated depression during pregnancy may affect your baby's well-being. Some studies have associated signs and symptoms of maternal depression to preterm birth, lower birth weight and a lower score on the Apgar test, which is done to assess a baby's well-being right after birth.

If you are being treated for depression or have a history of it, follow your health care provider's advice on how to best manage it during pregnancy. Check with your health care provider before starting, stopping or changing the dosage of any medication. In addition, alert your health care provider if a previous case of depression appears to be returning.

Diabetes

Diabetes is a disease that affects the regulation of blood sugar (glucose), the body's main source of energy. Foods you eat are broken down to glucose and absorbed into the bloodstream minutes to hours later. Insulin, a hormone secreted by the pancreas, then helps glucose enter your cells for energy use or storage.

In people with diabetes, this system goes awry. Instead of the glucose being transported into the cells, it accumulates in the bloodstream and is eventually excreted in the urine. Over time, exposure to high levels of glucose in the blood can damage the nerves, kidneys, eyes, heart, blood vessels and immune system.

The two main varieties of diabetes, type 1 and type 2, differ significantly:

Type 1 diabetes (formerly called juvenile or insulin-dependent diabetes) arises when your pancreas makes little if any insulin or your muscles and tissue cells become resistant to insulin. Insulin must be given by injection daily.

Type 2 diabetes (formerly called adult-onset or noninsulin-dependent diabetes) arises when your pancreas doesn't make enough insulin or develops a resistance to it. When your cells develop a resistance to insulin, they refuse to accept insulin as the key that unlocks the door for sugar. As a result, sugar stays in your bloodstream and accumulates.

Diabetes affects 16 million adults and children in the United States. During pregnancy, some women develop a temporary condition known as gestational diabetes. It resembles type 2 diabetes, but goes away after the pregnancy ends.

The risk of developing type 2 diabetes increases as you get older and is associated with a family history of the disease. It's also more common in blacks, Hispanics and American Indians. For type 2 diabetes, certain behavioral factors can increase your risk, including excess weight and an inactive lifestyle. Currently, there is no cure for diabetes. But blood sugar can be controlled with proper medication and lifestyle management, which includes eating right, maintaining a healthy weight and getting plenty of exercise.

Managing diabetes during pregnancy

If you have diabetes and your blood sugar levels are kept under control before conception and during pregnancy, you're likely to have a healthy pregnancy and give birth to a healthy baby. When your diabetes isn't under control, you're at higher risk of having a baby with a birth defect of the brain or spinal cord, heart or kidneys. The risk of miscarriage and stillbirth also increases significantly.

Poor control of your diabetes also puts you at increased risk of having a baby that weighs 10 pounds or more. That's because when blood sugar becomes too high, the baby receives a higher-than-normal glucose load and produces extra insulin to break down the sugar and store the fat. The fat tends to accumulate and produce an infant that's larger than normal — a medical condition known as macrosomia. Monitoring your baby's growth during pregnancy can give advanced warning of its being adversely affected by the diabetes. Because of the risk of stillbirth in women whose diabetes is poorly controlled, often labor is induced before their pregnancies are full-term.

Still, an early birth poses a risk because babies of women with diabetes are particularly susceptible to respiratory distress syndrome and jaundice. The babies of mothers with uncontrolled diabetes, especially those who are very large, also may be born with low blood sugar levels and require intravenous (IV) glucose or tube feedings shortly after birth.

Insulin requirements tend to increase for pregnant women with diabetes because hormones from the placenta impair the normal response to insulin. In fact, some women may need two to three times their usual dose of insulin to control their blood sugar. Most women taking insulin before pregnancy will require multiple daily doses of insulin or an insulin pump. Frequent adjustments of insulin dosage will likely be needed.

If you're not taking insulin for your diabetes, your doctor will likely want to review the type of medication you're taking to control blood glucose. If you take oral medications, you may be advised to switch to insulin before conception and during pregnancy because some oral medications may pose a risk of birth defects.

During pregnancy, maintaining a proper diet to control blood sugar can pose a challenge, especially when nausea complicates early pregnancy. Eating properly throughout pregnancy is an important part of diabetes care.

Many complications of diabetes must be guarded against during pregnancy. Ketoacidosis occurs when there isn't enough insulin, and cells become so starved for energy that your body begins to break down fat, producing toxic acids called ketones. Complications such as eye abnormalities due to diabetes (retinopathy) also can worsen during pregnancy, requiring intensive treatment and repeated examinations. However, this worsening seems to be related to control of diabetes and blood pressure rather than to pregnancy itself.

If you're pregnant and have kidney problems related to diabetes (diabetic nephropathy), you'll need careful monitoring because you can develop high blood pressure and deterioration in kidney function. In addition to endangering your health, these complications can put the fetus at greater risk of birth defects and poor fetal growth (intrauterine growth restriction). You may also need to have the baby early if the baby's risks in pregnancy outweigh the risks of preterm birth.

Even if you're experienced with and educated about diabetes, pregnancy can create new medical challenges. It's important to work closely with your doctor to protect your own health and the health of your baby. It's extremely important to plan your pregnancy if you have diabetes. If you are in good control when you conceive and take supplemental folic acid, the chances that your baby and your pregnancy will be normal are very good.

Epilepsy

Epilepsy is a seizure disorder that results from abnormal electrical activity in the brain. These abnormal signals may cause temporary changes in sensation, behavior, movement or consciousness. In some cases, seizures may have a known cause, such as a disease or an accident that affects the brain. In others, they may occur for no apparent reason.

Anti-epileptic drugs can eliminate or reduce the amount and intensity of seizures in the majority of people with epilepsy. In cases where seizures can't be controlled with medication, surgery may be an option.

Managing epilepsy during pregnancy

The majority — more than 90 percent — of women with epilepsy who become pregnant will have successful pregnancies. Still, epilepsy does appear to increase the risk of vaginal bleeding and placental abruption, in which the placenta separates from the uterus. Women with a seizure disorder may also have a higher risk of premature rupture of the membranes and pregnancy-induced high blood pressure (pregnancy-induced hypertension), and a slightly higher risk of having a baby with a birth defect. The risk of birth defects seems to be related to the medications used to control seizures, but for many patients those medications are absolutely necessary.

Even though some medications taken during pregnancy can affect the fetus, it's important to continue treatment to control seizures. Seizures can injure the baby. In rare cases, they may also cause a miscarriage. Before you conceive, talk with your doctor about your treatment. Some newer anti-seizure medications appear to be less risky for babies. Although many of these drugs are promising, they haven't been on the market long enough for doctors to be completely confident in their safety for pregnant women.

To protect you and your baby, don't stop taking medications or change the dosages without the advice and supervision of your doctor. Most women should continue taking the same medications they used before becoming pregnant because changing medications increases the risk of new seizures. It's best to work with your doctor to select the optimal treatment before you conceive.

Some anti-epileptic drugs affect the way the body uses folic acid, an important source of protection against birth defects. Therefore, your doctor may ask you to take a high-dose folic acid supplement with your other medications.

Because your blood volume increases during pregnancy and your kidneys can remove medications faster, you may need to increase your medication dosage. Be sure to follow doctor's orders.

It's difficult to predict how pregnancy will affect seizures. About half the time, seizure frequency is unaffected. About one-fourth of pregnant women with epilepsy have a decrease in seizures, and about one-fourth have an increase in seizures. The increase is mostly during the first trimester and is thought to be due to changes in body chemistry. In addition, severe nausea and vomiting during early pregnancy may interfere with the ability of some women to take anticonvulsant medication, increasing the risk of seizures.

During pregnancy, the blood levels of many medications used to treat epilepsy tend to decrease. As a result, your medications may need more frequent adjustments, and you may need more blood tests to check your medication levels.

Gallstones

The gallbladder is a small, pear-shaped sac. It lies under your liver and on the right side of your upper abdomen. Its job is to store bile, a fluid produced in your liver, until it's needed to help digest fats in your small intestine. If this bile contains too much cholesterol or other substances that don't easily dissolve, hard, solid deposits form in your gallbladder or nearby bile ducts. These deposits, called gallstones, can be as small as a grain of sand or as large as a golf ball.

Although 10 percent of people have gallstones, many don't even know it until these deposits are discovered during medical tests. Sometimes, however, gallstones may block the flow of bile from the liver to the intestine. This can cause symptoms such as indigestion or pain in your upper abdomen. Intense and constant abdominal pain that begins suddenly and lasts several hours can signal a gallbladder attack. Nausea and vomiting also may occur. If gallbladder attacks are severe or recurrent, your gallbladder may need to be surgically removed.

Managing gallstones during pregnancy

Women are more than twice as likely to have gallstones as men are. Much of that increased risk is related to pregnancy, because the gallbladder empties more slowly and less completely in response to pregnancy hormones. The resulting pooling of bile promotes the formation of stones. Pregnancy can further increase the risk because some women gain too much weight during pregnancy, which in turn increases the cholesterol content in the bile. Although you can't entirely prevent gallstones from forming, you can lower your risk by maintaining a healthy weight during pregnancy, exercising regularly and eating a low-fat, high-fiber diet that emphasizes fresh fruits, vegetables and whole grains.

Most pregnancies won't be affected by gallbladder attacks, even if a woman received a diagnosis of gallstones before she became pregnant. If an attack does occur, management of it is the same whether a woman is pregnant or not. Ultrasound examinations are preferred for the evaluation of gallstones in pregnant women, however, so X-ray procedures typically used to evaluate gallstones often are put off until after pregnancy.

An operation to remove the gallbladder is needed in about one in 1,000 pregnancies. If it's necessary, it can be done safely for both the mother and fetus, especially during the second trimester. If you experience signs and symptoms of a gallbladder attack, contact your doctor.

Heart disease

Heart disease can include a range of different conditions, including everything from coronary artery disease to congenital heart problems and valve disease. Although some conditions are more serious than others, all can affect how the heart and circulation function.

Until recently, many women with a history of heart problems were advised not to become pregnant. Now, it's thought that many women with cardiovascular problems can be monitored closely during pregnancy to minimize the risks to them and their babies. However, some heart problems — such as cyanotic congenital heart disease, pulmonary hypertension and severe aortic stenosis — may need to be corrected first to reduce the health risks they can pose to both mother and child during pregnancy. It's always best to consult your doctor about the specifics of your condition before becoming pregnant and to work with the proper specialist during pregnancy to manage your condition.

Managing heart disease during pregnancy

Pregnancy can put additional stress on the heart and circulatory system. In fact, the workload on your heart increases even in the first trimester of pregnancy. During labor, and particularly during pushing, abrupt changes occur in the dynamics of blood flow and pressure. Then, immediately after birth, the decrease in blood flow through the uterus puts an increased load on the heart.

Women with congenital heart disease have a greater risk of giving birth to babies with heart defects. If you're taking medications for heart disease, such as anticoagulants, talk with your doctor before you become pregnant so that he or she can consider whether to adjust the dosage or make a substitution before or during your pregnancy, to minimize risks to the fetus or newborn. He or she may also make drug adjustments to allow for changes in circulation due to pregnancy.

During your pregnancy, you may need fetal ultrasound tests so that your doctor can look for heart abnormalities in the fetus.

You'll be closely monitored during pregnancy for possible worsening of your underlying condition. This may mean more frequent tests and exams. In addition, some of the normal changes accompanying pregnancy may be of special concern for you. Anemia, for example, poses greater risks for people with some types of heart conditions. Fluid retention also may be more difficult to manage or might indicate a worsening of the underlying heart problem.

When in labor, you may require very close monitoring or specialized technology, such as pulmonary or arterial pressure catheters and echocardiography. During labor, pain relief medications are used, in part, to decrease stress on the mother's circulation. Epidural or spinal anesthesia is commonly used. In addition, forceps are more likely to be used during a vaginal birth to minimize prolonged pushing, which also puts stress on circulation.

Labor might even be avoided by planning a Caesarean birth, but most often vaginal delivery is preferable. During the first few weeks after delivery, you may continue to be closely monitored because major changes in circulation occur after birth.

Pregnancy can also pose a risk of endocarditis, a potentially life-threatening bacterial infection of the membrane that lines the interior of the heart's four chambers and valves. If you have a malformed heart or heart valves or if your valves are scarred, the inner surface of your heart is roughened. This provides infecting organisms with an area where they can congregate, multiply and potentially spread to other parts of the body. Because bacteria can easily enter your bloodstream during childbirth, women at risk of endocarditis are usually treated with antibiotics just before and after the birth to minimize the risk of infection.

Minor abnormalities in heart rhythm, such as occasional extra atrial or ventricular beats, are common during pregnancy and are usually not a cause for concern. Other pregnancy-related complications may increase a woman's risk of cardiovascular illness and death in the future. Recent studies have shown that mothers who experience preeclampsia (pregnancy-induced high blood pressure) or multiple miscarriages should pay close attention to their heart health over the course of their lives.

Hepatitis B

Hepatitis B is a serious liver infection caused by the hepatitis B virus (HBV). It's transmitted in the blood and body fluids of someone who is infected — the same way the human immunodeficiency virus (HIV), the virus that causes AIDS, spreads. HBV is much more infectious than HIV. More than 1 billion adults and children worldwide are infected with HBV.

Women with HBV can pass the infection to their babies during childbirth. Newborn babies can also become infected with the virus from contact with an HBV-positive mother.

In some people, HBV can cause liver failure. It also increases the risk of liver cancer. Most people infected with HBV as adults recover fully. Infants and children are much more likely to develop a chronic infection. Early signs and symptoms of HBV infection can range from mild to severe. They can be mistaken for the flu.

Many adults and children infected with HBV never develop signs and symptoms, or develop them weeks after infection. As a result, many people may carry the virus and not know it. In the United States, pregnant women who receive prenatal care are screened for HBV.

Managing hepatitis B during pregnancy

Pregnant women with hepatitis B infection have an increased risk of giving birth prematurely. But the greatest risk is that of infecting the baby with HBV. If you have evidence of HBV, your newborn can be given an injection of antibodies against the virus after birth.

Vaccination against HBV is a common, and in some states a mandatory, part of the series of immunizations given to children during infancy. The hepatitis B vaccination may be given to newborns as well as to premature infants.

Herpes

Herpes is a contagious disease caused by the herpes simplex virus. The virus comes in two forms: herpes simplex virus type 1 (HSV-1) and herpes simplex virus type 2 (HSV-2). Type 1 causes cold sores around the mouth or nose, but it may also involve the genital area. Type 2 causes painful genital blisters that rupture and become sores. Both types are passed on through direct contact with an infected person.

The initial (primary) infection may be obvious with signs and symptoms lasting a week or more. In other cases, the primary infection may not even be recognized. After the initial outbreak, the virus remains dormant in infected areas, periodically reactivating. These episodes last about 10 days. They may start with tingling, itching or pain before sores become visible. Herpes is contagious whenever sores are present.

Managing herpes during pregnancy

Antiviral drugs can help reduce the number of reactivations or shorten their length. Sometimes, they're used to help avoid recurrences in late pregnancy.

If you have genital herpes, your baby potentially can become infected with the virus on the way through the birth canal. The most serious risk for a newborn exists when the mother has her first (primary) herpes infection just before labor. A recurring episode of herpes at childbirth poses much less risk to the baby.

Preventing newborn herpes infection can be difficult. In the majority of newborn infections, the mother has no signs or symptoms suggesting herpes during labor or birth. Still, prevention is important because herpes infection can be life-threatening for a newborn. In addition, newborns who contract herpes can develop serious infections that damage the eyes, internal organs or brain, despite treatment with antiviral drugs.

If you have had genital herpes, your baby is unlikely to have a serious infection acquired at birth. Women who have had the disease develop antibodies that they pass to their babies and provide some temporary protection. Nevertheless, the risk isn't quite absent. If sores are present, Caesarean birth might lessen this very small risk of newborn infection and is the current standard of care in the United States. If the mother is having a new primary infection, the Caesarean birth may be lifesaving for the baby.

After birth, a baby can be infected with herpes by direct contact with someone with a cold sore. Anyone with a cold sore should avoid kissing a baby. Hand washing before handling a baby also is important. If you have a cold sore when you give birth, keep your baby away from your face and wash your hands often.

HIV/AIDS

Acquired immunodeficiency syndrome (AIDS) is a chronic, life-threatening condition. It's caused by the human immunodeficiency virus (HIV). When HIV infects a person, the virus can lie dormant for years. During that time, the person shows few or no signs and symptoms of the disease. It's not until the virus becomes active and weakens the body's immune system that the condition becomes known as AIDS.

HIV is most commonly spread by sexual contact with an infected partner. It can also spread through infected blood and shared needles or syringes contaminated with the virus. Untreated women with HIV can pass the infection to their babies during pregnancy and delivery or through their breast milk.

Managing HIV/AIDS during pregnancy

Before or during pregnancy, consider having your HIV status tested. Many women go undiagnosed because they don't fit the category of individuals at high risk of the disease. Although a positive diagnosis can be devastating, treatments now are available that can greatly reduce a mother's risk of passing

HIV to her baby. Drug treatments begun before or during pregnancy can also improve the health and prolong the life of most women.

HIV infection or AIDS doesn't directly influence pregnancy. However, poor health or infection in advanced AIDS would pose added risks for a mother in later pregnancy, during labor and at birth. In addition, certain antibiotics used to treat infections in people with AIDS may pose risks to the fetus.

For pregnant women with HIV or AIDS, the biggest risk is that of passing the infection to their babies. About 15 percent of HIV-infected babies develop serious signs and symptoms of the disease or die in the first year of life. Close to half don't live past age 10.

If you have HIV or AIDS, inform your doctor. A doctor who knows about your condition can help monitor you and help you to avoid procedures that could increase your baby's exposure to your blood. Your medical treatment can greatly influence the risk of transmission to your baby. Your doctor can also make sure your baby is promptly tested for infection after birth. Early testing can make it possible for infants diagnosed with HIV to be treated with HIV-fighting drugs, which have been shown to slow the progression of the disease and improve survival rates.

Hyperthyroidism

The thyroid is a butterfly-shaped gland located at the base of your neck, just below your Adam's apple. The hormones it produces regulate your metabolism, which is related to everything from your heart rate to how quickly you burn calories. Using radioactive iodine can be of great benefit in the diagnosis and management of thyroid disease, but these agents can't be used in pregnancy. Fortunately, there are other options.

When your thyroid gland produces too much of the hormone thyroxine, it can cause hyperthyroidism (overactive thyroid disease). This can prompt your body's metabolism to speed up. This may lead to sudden weight loss, a rapid or irregular heartbeat, and nervousness or irritability.

Women are more likely to have hyperthyroidism than men are. Although this disease can lead to serious complications if it isn't treated, effective medications and other treatments can reduce or eliminate your signs and symptoms.

Managing hyperthyroidism during pregnancy

Most pregnancies proceed normally in women with hyperthyroidism. But if the disease is difficult to control, there's a higher risk of preterm birth, slowed growth for the baby and high blood pressure for the mother. In addition, some medications commonly used to treat hyperthyroidism may need to be avoided or readjusted during pregnancy or while breast-feeding. For example, radioactive iodine medications can't be used during pregnancy.

If you have hyperthyroidism or a history of the condition, review your medication with your doctor. He or she can monitor it throughout your pregnancy. Overuse of medication can cause hypothyroidism (underactive thyroid disease) in the baby, with serious side effects. Therefore, careful management of your condition is important for the health of both you and your baby. You can help by following instructions carefully and reporting signs and symptoms that return or worsen.

During pregnancy, hyperthyroidism sometimes worsens during the first trimester. It can improve during the second half of pregnancy. In some women, hyperthyroidism develops after birth (postpartum thyroiditis). It can cause excessive fatigue, nervousness and increased sensitivity to heat. Sometimes, it's mistaken for other problems, such as postpartum depression. Report such symptoms to your health care provider, even if you've already completed your postpartum examination.

Hypothyroidism

The thyroid is a butterfly-shaped gland located at the base of your neck, just below your Adam's apple. The hormones it produces regulate your metabolism, which is related to everything from your heart rate to how quickly you burn calories.

Hypothyroidism occurs when the thyroid doesn't produce enough hormones. When the thyroid is underactive, you may feel tired and sluggish. If it's left untreated, signs and symptoms can include increased sensitivity to cold, constipation, pale and dry skin, a puffy face, weight gain, a hoarse voice, elevated blood cholesterol levels and depression.

Managing hypothyroidism during pregnancy

The signs and symptoms of hypothyroidism can be masked by the fatigue of early pregnancy. The diagnosis may be missed if your provider isn't alerted to your signs and symptoms. Yet once this condition is identified, it can — and should — be treated with medication.

Women with hypothyroidism may have difficulty becoming pregnant. If they do become pregnant and their hypothyroidism is left untreated, they'll have an increased risk of miscarriage, preeclampsia (pregnancy-induced high blood pressure), problems with the placenta and slowed growth for their babies. Babies born to women with thyroid disease may have a higher risk of birth defects than do babies born to healthy mothers. Proper thyroid hormone replacement is required for the normal development of a baby's brain.

Checking thyroid function is part of preventive care. If your provider has any suspicions about your having this condition, he or she will probably test for hypothyroidism in early pregnancy. Hormones of early pregnancy influence thyroid tests, so results must be interpreted with care. If you have hypothyroidism, your dosage of replacement hormone will likely change over the course of the pregnancy. Most likely the dose will need to be increased. Your care provider can check your thyroid levels throughout pregnancy, perhaps each trimester or monthly. It never hurts to help your provider remember that you need these tests done.

Immune thrombocytopenic purpura

Immune thrombocytopenic purpura (ITP) is a disease that results in an abnormally low number of platelets in the blood. Platelets are a type of blood cell essential to clotting, which stops bleeding from cuts or bruises. If the level of platelets becomes too low, bleeding can occur even after minor injury or even through normal wear and tear.

Common other causes of low platelet counts include viral and severe bacterial infections, certain medications, and the diseases lupus and rheumatoid arthritis. In addition, platelet count may decrease somewhat during pregnancy.

ITP is a special form of low-platelet-count disease is immune thrombocytopenic purpura. This is a disease in which the body destroys platelets due to a malfunction of the immune system. The result is very low counts and a resulting skin condition called purpura.

Treatment of low platelets depends on the underlying cause of the problem, but medications are available to treat the condition. Intravenous immunoglobulin (IVIG) and corticosteroids may be used. In some cases, the spleen may be surgically removed to increase the number of platelets. This condition is more common in women than in men and occurs at young ages.

Managing ITP during pregnancy

Pregnancy itself doesn't affect the course or severity of ITP. But the antibodies that can destroy platelets occasionally cross the placenta and can decrease the platelet count in your baby. Unfortunately, the baby's platelet count can't be predicted by your platelet count or even by the length of time you've had a low platelet level. The baby's platelet count may be low even if yours is fine. For that reason, doctors have been interested in tests to determine the baby's platelet count near the time of birth or during labor. However, testing the baby's count can be risky because invasive methods are used. The possibility that a Caesarean birth would protect the baby from harm has long been considered. Neither the testing nor the Caesarean births have been very successful.

Because the risk of bleeding in the baby is actually very low, Caesarean birth isn't routine for this condition. Efforts should be made to provide the baby with appropriate treatment at delivery with a team approach including an obstetrician and a pediatrician.

If your platelet count is very low, it's less likely that spinal or epidural anesthesia would be offered during labor and birth. If Caesarean birth is necessary, you may be given platelet transfusions.

Other causes of low platelet counts in pregnancy may complicate delivery. Pregnancy-induced high blood pressure (preeclampsia), the placenta separating from the uterus (placental abruption), uterine infections and a severe form of preeclampsia can result in lowered platelet counts. These conditions may cause problems for the mother but won't lower the baby's platelet count.

Inflammatory bowel disease

Inflammatory bowel disease (IBD) causes chronic inflammation of the digestive tract. Ulcerative colitis and Crohn's disease are the two most common forms of IBD. Both can cause repeated episodes of fever, diarrhea, rectal bleeding and abdominal pain. No one knows exactly what causes IBD. Heredity, environment and the immune system may play a role.

Crohn's disease can occur anywhere in the digestive tract. It can spread into layers of the affected tissue, which can cause ulcers, intestinal obstructions and difficulty with eating and absorbing nutrients. Ulcerative colitis usually affects only the innermost lining of the large intestine (colon) and rectum.

Although there is no cure for ulcerative colitis or Crohn's disease, medications and other treatments are available. IBD conditions can begin during pregnancy. But the diagnosis is more likely to be made before pregnancy.

Women whose IBD has affected their weight or nutritional condition may have difficulty getting pregnant. Women with active Crohn's disease may also have gynecologic problems that affect their ability to conceive. They may be at increased risk of giving birth prematurely. Still, if women have IBD conditions under control before and during their pregnancies, they're likely to have healthy pregnancies and full-term deliveries.

Managing IBD during pregnancy

In general, if you have IBD, you can work with your doctor to manage any problems it may cause with your pregnancy. Pregnancy won't significantly affect your treatment. Most of the medications commonly used to treat IBD don't harm the fetus. Improving your condition is likely to benefit both mother and baby, outweighing potential concern for a drug's effect on the fetus.

However, some immunosuppressive medications used to treat certain cases of IBD might cause harm to the fetus. If you use one of these medications, discuss it with your doctor. Also discuss the use of anti-diarrheal medications, especially their use during the first trimester of pregnancy.

If you have Crohn's disease and it was inactive before pregnancy, it's likely to stay inactive while you're pregnant. When it's active, it's likely to remain active or even worsen during pregnancy. With ulcerative colitis, about one-third of the women who become pregnant while the disease is in remission will experience a flare-up. If the colitis is active when you become pregnant, it's likely to remain active or possibly worsen. A flare-up of ulcerative colitis is most likely to occur during the first three months of pregnancy.

If an operation becomes necessary to deal with IBD during pregnancy, it most likely can be done safely. Extra precautions may be necessary to minimize risk to the fetus. Diagnostic tests such as sigmoidoscopy, rectal biopsy or colonoscopy can be safely performed during pregnancy. Diagnostic X-rays usually are postponed until after birth, but in case of serious illness, their benefit may far outweigh the risk.

Lupus erythematosus

Lupus erythematosus is a condition that can result in chronic inflammation of many organ systems. It can affect skin, joints, kidneys, blood cells, heart and lungs. The disease, which affects about 14 million Americans, commonly results in a rash and arthritis of varying severity. Other, more serious problems can arise, including kidney failure or seizures.

Several types of lupus exist. The most common type is systemic lupus erythematosus (SLE), which can cause the most difficulties. The cause of lupus is unknown, but women are much more likely to develop the disease than men are. A family history of the condition also increases the risk. Currently, no cure exists for lupus, but treatments can ease the signs and symptoms and reduce the complications.

Lupus sometimes shows up for the first time during pregnancy or shortly after giving birth. Women who already have lupus often have worse signs and symptoms during pregnancy — even if the condition hasn't been active. If lupus is active at the start of pregnancy, there is a much higher risk of it worsening during pregnancy. Fortunately, the problems experienced during pregnancy improve after birth in the majority of affected women.

Managing lupus during pregnancy

If you have active lupus during your pregnancy, you're at risk of several problems. You have a higher risk of miscarriage, stillbirth or pregnancy complications. In addition, you're at higher risk of high blood pressure or preeclampsia developing, especially if your lupus has affected your kidneys. At times, it can be difficult for medical professionals to determine whether problems such as high blood pressure and protein in the urine are caused by preeclampsia or by lupus. You'll likely want to work with a specialist to sort out any problems that develop.

Your baby may have poor fetal growth (intrauterine growth restriction) or develop an unusually low heart rate, a condition called fetal heart block. Both of these conditions can be identified through monitoring during pregnancy.

A small percentage of babies born to women with lupus have neonatal lupus. It's characterized by a rash and abnormal blood counts. Typically, this condition disappears within six months. Yet, about half the babies with neonatal lupus will be born with a permanent heart condition that will need treatment.

Although you may have active signs and symptoms of lupus during pregnancy, you may need to adjust the use of certain medications that can cause harm to your baby. Work closely with your doctor before and during pregnancy to take proper care of your health and to protect that of your baby.

Phenylketonuria

Phenylketonuria (PKU) is an inherited disease. It affects how the body processes protein. More specifically, it affects how the body processes phenylalanine, one of the amino acids that are building blocks of proteins. Phenylalanine is found in milk, cheeses, eggs, meat, fish and other high-protein foods. If the level of phenylalanine in the bloodstream becomes too high, it can cause brain injury. A special diet low in phenylalanine can prevent or minimize brain damage in those with PKU.

Healthy women with PKU have been successfully treated as children. They may no longer be following a diet that regulates their blood phenylalanine levels. In the United States, an estimated 3,000 women of childbearing age have the disease.

Managing PKU during pregnancy

If you have PKU and it's been kept under control both before and during pregnancy, you can have a healthy baby. If your blood levels of phenylalanine are not well regulated, you're likely to give birth to an infant with mild to severe mental retardation. Affected infants may also be born with an abnormally small head and congenital heart disease.

If you have a family history of the disease or were treated for PKU as a child, tell your doctor. Ideally, you'll have your blood levels of phenylalanine measured before trying to conceive. If necessary, you can begin a special diet to keep levels low and prevent birth defects.

During pregnancy, the dietary restrictions needed to keep down the levels of phenylalanine can be hard to manage. If you have PKU, you'll need regular blood tests. Your diet may be reviewed and adjusted if phenylalanine levels are too high. You may be referred to a doctor who specializes in managing PKU. Most of the experts in this disease are pediatricians.

Rheumatoid arthritis

Rheumatoid arthritis is a disease that causes chronic inflammation of the joints. Commonly affected joints include the wrists, hands, feet and ankles. The disease can also involve the elbows, shoulders, hips, knees, neck and jaw. Problems can vary from occasional flares of pain to serious joint damage.

The condition, which affects more than 2 million Americans, can strike at any age. It's most common in women between the ages of 20 and 50. Currently, there is no cure. The condition can be managed with proper medical treatment and self-care.

Managing rheumatoid arthritis during pregnancy

If you have rheumatoid arthritis, it's unlikely to affect your pregnancy. But the medications you may use to treat the condition may need to be adjusted. Aspirin is one drug that can help relieve both the pain and inflammation of rheumatoid arthritis. However, it can cause bleeding or other problems for your baby. Your doctor may recommend that you use other anti-inflammatory medications during your pregnancy instead.

While you're pregnant, you may experience some improvement with your rheumatoid arthritis. This may result from a change in your immune system while you're carrying a child. Still, signs and symptoms of almost all women who have improvement will return after pregnancy.

Sexually transmitted diseases

If sexually transmitted diseases (STDs) aren't diagnosed and treated, they can affect the health of a pregnant woman and her unborn baby. Unfortunately, many STDs have mild signs and symptoms that may go unnoticed. Many women may be unaware they have been infected until problems arise.

Chlamydia is the most common bacterial STD in the United States. About 75 percent of women and 50 percent of men who contract it have no signs or symptoms. The infection occurs most frequently in people under 25. If left untreated in women, it can result in pelvic inflammatory disease (PID). PID is an infection of the uterus and fallopian tubes that can cause infertility and chronic pelvic pain. Chlamydia may also result in eye infections and blindness if infectious secretions are transferred to the eye. This kind of infection can be transferred to a baby at birth.

Like chlamydia, gonorrhea is a common and highly contagious STD. It, too, often has no clearly recognizable signs and symptoms. Often, the only clue that a person may have gonorrhea is that a past or current sexual partner develops signs and symptoms of the disease. Sometimes, there's a slight increase in vaginal discharge. In females, gonorrhea occurs most frequently between the ages of 15 and 19. If not detected, it can result in PID and infertility in adult women.

Syphilis was once a prominent STD. The number of new cases is rising again, but it remains much less common than other STDs. Syphilis is a serious bacterial infection that, if left untreated, can result in anything from serious neurologic or cardiovascular problems to death in adults. Syphilis can easily be passed from a woman to her unborn baby during pregnancy. Signs and symptoms of syphilis occur in stages, which may make early detection possible. The most common sign is painless sores on the genitals that may occur 10 days to six weeks after exposure.

There are many kinds of genital warts, some invisible and some hard to miss. Genital warts can appear one month to several years after sexual contact with an infected person. They appear in the moist areas of the genitals and may look like small, flesh-colored bumps. Several warts close together can take on a cauliflower shape. Genital warts may cause itching or burning in the genital area. In some cases, warts can develop in the mouth or throat after oral sexual contact with an infected person. Although genital warts can be treated, they're a serious health concern. The virus that causes them — called the human papillomavirus (HPV) — has been strongly associated with cervical cancer. It has also been linked with other types of genital cancers.

Managing STDs during pregnancy

STDs in pregnancy can cause premature births and complications during and after delivery. When a mother passes on an infection to her fetus or newborn infant, the infection can result in serious and sometimes fatal problems for the baby.

If you have untreated chlamydia, you may face an increased risk of miscarriage and premature breaking of the water (rupturing of the membranes) surrounding your baby in the uterus. It's also possible for you to spread chlamydia from your vaginal canal to your child during delivery. This can cause pneumonia or an eye infection in the child, which may lead to blindness.

Gonorrhea, like chlamydia, can increase your risk of miscarriage and premature rupture of the membranes if the disease is left untreated. In addition, you can infect your infant during vaginal delivery. A baby who becomes infected can develop a severe eye infection. Because gonorrhea can go undetected in mothers and poses a serious risk to a newborn's eyes, all newborns are given medication at birth to prevent development of this eye infection.

If you have syphilis, it can easily pass from you to your infant, causing a serious and often fatal infection. Prematurity and stillbirth are more common in babies born to mothers with syphilis. In syphilis-infected infants, problems can develop in the eyes, ears, liver, bone marrow, bones, skin and heart — if the baby doesn't receive prompt treatment with antibiotics. Even if you were treated for syphilis during your pregnancy, your newborn child may need antibiotic treatment.

If you have genital warts, they can enlarge during pregnancy, which may make it more difficult to urinate. In addition, a large amount of genital warts can bleed profusely or even obstruct the birth canal. Your doctor may remove these warts using one of several procedures, including surgery. Often, though, the warts go away after delivery and it's not necessary to have them removed unless the outbreak is extensive. In extremely rare cases, an infant born to an infected mother may develop warts in the throat and voice box, which may require surgery to prevent obstruction of the airway.

Many STDs can be successfully treated if caught at an early enough stage. To protect you and your baby, get screened for STDs, even if you've been screened for them in the past. Screening is a routine part of prenatal testing for some infections, but your doctor may not test for all the most common STDs unless you ask him or her to do so. You might want to have your partner screened, too.

If you aren't in a monogamous relationship during your pregnancy, use a latex or polyurethane condom during intercourse. It can help protect you from contracting STDs and passing them on to your baby.

Sickle cell disease

Sickle cell disease is an inherited blood disease. It can cause anemia, pain, frequent infections and damage to vital organs. It's caused by a defective form of hemoglobin, a substance that enables red blood cells to carry oxygen from the lungs to all parts of the body. In people with the disease, red blood cells sickle, changing from healthy, round cells to crescent-shape cells. These unusual cells can block blood flow through blood vessels.

Sickle cell disease typically is diagnosed in infancy with a screening test. Anyone can inherit the disease, which affects millions. In the United States, it most commonly affects blacks, Hispanics and American Indians. Although there's no cure for sickle cell disease, treatments are available to reduce pain and prevent problems.

Women with sickle cell disease can pass on the disease or the trait for the disease to their unborn children. To have the condition, children must receive a sickle cell gene from both their mother and father. If they receive only one gene, they become carriers. That means they may pass the gene on to their own children.

Managing sickle cell disease during pregnancy

Women with sickle cell disease have a greater risk of developing serious pregnancy-related complications, such as pregnancy-induced high blood pressure. In addition, they have an increased risk of preterm labor and of delivering a low-birth-weight baby. During pregnancy, infections can occur more frequently and lead to painful sickle cell crises. These infections may include urinary tract infection, pneumonia and uterine infection.

Women with sickle cell disease may need to have a team of medical specialists involved in their prenatal care. This team may include an obstetrician, a perinatologist experienced in the care of women with sickle cell disease, a hematologist and a neonatologist. Pregnant women with sickle cell disease may also need to be monitored for complications of the disease, such as seizures, congestive heart failure and severe anemia. Anemia is likely to be most severe during the final two months of pregnancy. It may require blood transfusions.

If the mother has a sickle cell crisis or another complication, the baby's health can be monitored closely. If Caesarean birth is needed, it's likely to be done with the use of an epidural rather than general anesthesia for the mother.

Uterine fibroids

Uterine fibroids are noncancerous tumors of the uterus that are common in women in their childbearing years. In fact, these fibroids are found in one out of every four or five women over the age of 35.

Uterine fibroids can appear on the inside or outside lining of the uterus, or within its muscular wall. It's not clear why they occur. They usually develop from a single smooth muscle cell that continues to grow. Some can be as small as a pea. Others can grow as large as a grapefruit. Most cause no symptoms and are discovered only during a routine pelvic exam or during prenatal care.

When symptoms do occur, they may include abnormally heavy or prolonged menstrual bleeding, abdominal or lower back pain, pain during sexual intercourse, difficult or more frequent urination, and pelvic pressure. Drug therapy or surgery may be recommended to shrink or remove fibroids that cause discomfort or could result in complications such as heavy blood loss or infertility.

Managing uterine fibroids during pregnancy

Fibroids can sometimes increase the risk of miscarriage during the first and second trimesters or increase the likelihood of preterm labor. In some cases, they can also obstruct the birth canal, complicating labor and delivery. Rarely, uterine fibroids can interfere with the ability of a fertilized egg to implant on the uterine lining, making it hard to become pregnant.

Fibroids tend to enlarge during pregnancy, possibly because of the increased levels of estrogen in the body. Occasionally, larger fibroids bleed or lose their blood supply, resulting in pelvic pain. If you experience pelvic pain or abnormal bleeding, contact your doctor immediately. If the fibroids are painful, they can be treated with medications.

If fibroids lead to preterm labor, the treatment is usually bed rest. If fibroids result in bleeding, treatment may include hospitalization, monitoring of the baby's condition and, if needed, a blood transfusion. During pregnancy, surgery for fibroids is generally avoided because it can lead to preterm delivery and extensive blood loss.

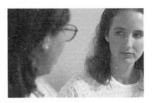

problems during pregnancy

If you face a problem during your pregnancy, you may be concerned, confused and frightened. This section describes some of the problems pregnant women may face and explains how health care providers might manage those conditions.

Preterm labor

A full-term pregnancy is defined as one in which birth occurs between weeks 37 and 42 of pregnancy. Preterm labor refers to contractions that begin opening the cervix before the end of the 37th week.

About 11 percent of births in the United States are preterm. Babies who are born this early often have low birth weight, defined as less than 5 1/2 pounds. Their low weight, along with various other problems associated with preterm birth, puts them at risk of several health problems.

Preterm labor sometimes occurs between weeks 20 and 28. It more often occurs between weeks 29 and 37. No one knows exactly what causes preterm labor. In many cases, it occurs among women who have no known risk factors.

Health care providers and scientists have identified factors that seem to increase your risk. These include:
- A previous preterm labor or birth
- A pregnancy with twins, triplets or other multiples
- Previous miscarriages or abortions
- An infection of the amniotic fluid or fetal membranes
- Excess amniotic fluid (hydramnios)
- Abnormalities in your uterus
- Problems with your placenta
- Pre-existing medical conditions, especially serious illness or disease
- Bleeding during your current pregnancy
- A dilated cervix

- Other infections, including urinary tract infections
- Preeclampsia, a condition characterized by high blood pressure after your 20th week of pregnancy

Signs and symptoms

For some women, the clues that labor is starting are unmistakable. For others, they're more subtle. You may have contractions that feel like a tightening in your abdomen. If the contractions aren't painful, you may be able to tell you're having them only by feeling your abdomen with your hand. Some women go into preterm labor without feeling any sensation of uterine contractions.

Women sometimes attribute contractions to gas pain, constipation or movement of the fetus. In many cases, the contractions aren't painful. Other signs of preterm labor may include the following:

- You have pain in the abdomen, pelvis or back.
- It feels as if your baby is pressing down, creating pelvic pressure.
- You're urinating more frequently.
- You have diarrhea.
- You're having menstrual-type cramps or abdominal cramps.
- You have light vaginal spotting or bleeding.
- There's a watery discharge from your vagina.

If you have a watery discharge, it may be amniotic fluid, a sign that the membranes surrounding the fetus have ruptured (your water has broken). If you pass the mucous plug — the mucus that builds in the cervix during pregnancy — you may notice this as a thick discharge tinged with blood.

If you have any concerns about what you're feeling — especially if you have vaginal bleeding along with abdominal cramps or pain — call your health care provider or your hospital. Don't be embarrassed about the possibility of mistaking false labor for the real thing.

Treatment

If your health care provider suspects that you may be having early labor, you'll need to be examined. Your health care provider may look to see whether your cervix has begun to dilate and whether your water has broken. A cervical exam may be needed to make these determinations.

In some cases, a uterine monitor may be used to measure the duration and spacing of your contractions. Or ultrasound imaging may be used to monitor your cervix. In addition, a sampling of the cervical canal for the presence of a glue-like tissue lost with labor (fetal fibronectin) may help guide your treatment. A salivary estrogen test may be used to detect preterm labor, although this test is being used less often than previously.

Unless birth seems imminent, your health care provider will probably make every attempt to help you continue your pregnancy, giving your baby an opportunity to mature fully. Factors that might have brought on early labor can be carefully considered, as can your general physical condition.

Your health care provider might begin by reviewing your medical history and doing a physical exam. During your pelvic exam, your health care provider can take a look at your cervix, checking to see if it's opening (dilating) or thinning (effacing).

Tests may be done to evaluate the health of your baby. You may have an ultrasound exam. A prenatal test called amniocentesis may be done to obtain a sample of amniotic fluid. This test can be useful in several ways. One of the biggest problems facing premature infants is underdeveloped lungs. By analyzing a sample of amniotic fluid, experts can predict the maturity of a baby's lungs. Testing can also indicate whether the amniotic fluid is infected, which would indicate the baby might be better served by delivery.

Most women in preterm labor receive fluids through an intravenous (IV) tube and are asked to rest in bed. Sometimes, these measures alone will stop preterm labor. In fact, if contractions decrease and your cervix isn't dilating, you may simply be sent home and may be advised to remain on bed rest to reduce the chances of another episode of preterm labor.

If contractions continue and your cervix dilates, your health care provider will probably recommend a medication called a tocolytic to help stop your preterm labor and an injection with potent steroid medications. This is especially true if you and your baby seem to be healthy and if you're less than 34 weeks along in your pregnancy. Tocolytic medications have been shown to be effective at stopping labor only for a short time. Most commonly, they're used to allow time for the baby to gain the benefits of the steroid injection, which can help a baby's lungs move toward maturity in as little as 48 hours.

In some cases, your health care provider may recommend that your baby be delivered early. This may happen if contractions can't be stopped, your baby's health is threatened before your pregnancy runs its normal course, or you develop a health problem, such as severe high blood pressure (hypertension). Sometimes, the baby is delivered by Caesarean birth, but most often labor is started (induced).

To induce labor, your health care provider will probably give you a medication called oxytocin. With oxytocin you may begin to have contractions within half an hour, but most likely it will take longer. Sometimes a medication is given to soften (ripen) the cervix. This, too, helps imitate the natural onset of labor.

Most premature births follow a course similar to that of a normal birth. It's very beneficial for your preterm baby when a team of pediatric experts is immediately available at the time of birth. These health care providers can assess your baby's condition at birth and give help as needed.

If you've had one premature birth, you have a 25 percent to 50 percent chance of going into premature labor again. Research continues on methods

MAKING THE BEST OF BED REST

Your health care provider has prescribed bed rest due to complications of your pregnancy. For the first few hours, it seems wonderful. You have permission to rest, and your family is waiting on you hand and foot.

Then reality sets in. You can't go to work, weed your garden or play tag with your children. You can't shop for groceries, take a walk around the block or meet your friends at the movies. How can you make the best of the situation? Start by focusing on the fact that you're doing what's best for you and your baby. Your health care provider wouldn't suggest bed rest otherwise. Total bed rest can:

- Decrease the pressure of the baby on the cervix and reduce cervical stretching, which may cause premature contractions and miscarriage.
- Increase blood flow to the placenta, helping your baby receive maximal nutrition and oxygen. This is particularly important if the baby isn't growing as rapidly as he or she should.
- Help your organs, especially your heart and kidneys, to function more efficiently, improving problems with high blood pressure.

Work closely with your health care provider to understand exactly what your restrictions are. Ask questions, such as:

- What position should I use while lying down?
- Can I sit up at times? If so, for how long at any one time?
- Can I get up to use the bathroom? Is any other type of physical activity allowed?
- Can I take a bath or shower?
- Is sexual activity off-limits?
- Are there any exercises I should do while in bed?

Tips for bed rest

To make bed rest tolerable, try these tips:

- Set up your bedroom so that everything you need is within reach from the bed.
- Organize your day. Schedule specific times to phone the office, connect with your spouse, watch television, read, and so on.
- Take up a new hobby, such as making a scrapbook, painting or knitting.
- Learn relaxation and visualization techniques. They'll help not only during bed rest but also during labor and delivery.
- Work on crossword puzzles.
- Write e-mails or letters to friends or call them on the phone.
- Help your family stay organized. Record schedules on a calendar, make weekly menus, or pay bills and balance the checkbook.
- Read. Try books, magazines or newspapers you don't usually buy.
- Plan for your baby's arrival by buying any necessities, either online or from catalogs.
- Learn about newborn care — how to bathe, dress, breast-feed, handle and soothe your baby.
- Prepare a list of tasks so that when friends and family call to offer help, you can offer them something specific to do for you or your family.

for preventing preterm labor. Recent studies using weekly injections of the hormone progesterone for the prevention of preterm labor have shown promise. However, much is yet to be learned on using this approach.

Pregnancy loss

Your pregnancy has ended without the dreamed-of outcome. You have no new baby to hold in your arms.

If this is your situation, it's likely a time of grief, confusion and fear. While understanding why a pregnancy loss occurs won't stop the emotional pain, it may help you understand why your health care provider recommends certain types of care and provide a tiny step toward healing.

Pregnancy loss can take many forms, including miscarriage, ectopic pregnancy, molar pregnancy, cervical incompetence and stillbirth. Each has different causes and treatments.

Miscarriage

When a woman has a pregnancy loss before 20 weeks of gestation, this is known as a miscarriage. In medical terms, a pregnancy that's lost due to natural causes is called a spontaneous abortion.

It's estimated that 15 percent to 20 percent of known pregnancies end in miscarriage. The actual number of miscarriages, however, is probably higher. Many miscarriages occur very early in pregnancy, before a woman even knows she's pregnant.

Among known pregnancies, miscarriages typically occur between the seventh and 12th weeks. By the 12th week of pregnancy, more than 80 percent of miscarriages have occurred. Miscarriage early in pregnancy can occur as many as several weeks after the embryo or fetus has died.

If you've had a miscarriage or are worried about having one, it's important to know what *doesn't* cause it. Except for the use of some illicit drugs, your actions can't cause a miscarriage. Miscarriage isn't caused by exercising, having sex, working or lifting heavy objects. Nausea and vomiting in early pregnancy, even if it's severe, won't cause a miscarriage. Finally, there's no evidence that a fall, a blow or a sudden fright can cause miscarriage. The fetus is unlikely to be harmed by an injury unless the injury is serious enough to threaten your own life.

At least half of early pregnancy losses are thought to be caused by chromosome abnormalities in the fetus. Typically, these chromosome problems aren't inherited from the baby's parents. Rather, they're the result of errors that occur by chance as the embryo divides and grows. A miscarriage caused by a chromosome defect is a situation in which there was never a chance that the fetus would survive.

Other causes of miscarriage may be factors related to the mother's health or physical condition. Miscarriage from these causes usually occurs later in pregnancy. These causes are also associated with stillbirth, when a baby dies late in pregnancy. They include:

- Severe high blood pressure
- Uncontrolled diabetes
- Problems with the immune system (autoimmune diseases)
- Tendency toward blood clots (thrombophilia)
- Problems with the uterus or cervix (cervical incompetence)

The risk of miscarriage is higher in women over age 35 and in women with a history of three or more previous miscarriages. Lifestyle factors such as smoking, heavy drinking and illicit drug use also increase the risk. In addition, a recent study suggests that pregnant women with low blood levels of the vitamin folate are more likely to have early miscarriages than are pregnant women with enough folate.

Signs and symptoms

Vaginal bleeding is the warning sign that precedes nearly all pregnancy losses. However, vaginal bleeding doesn't always signal a miscarriage. As many as 40 percent of all pregnant women have bleeding at some point during pregnancy. Of these women, about half will have a miscarriage.

Bleeding that precedes a miscarriage may be light or heavy. It may be constant, or it may come and go. Bleeding may be followed by cramping, abdominal pain or lower backache. If you have heavy bleeding or pain in pregnancy, contact your health care provider promptly.

If you go to your health care provider's office with bleeding, he or she will likely perform a pelvic exam to check whether your cervix has begun to dilate. Today, an ultrasound also is commonly performed to assess the status of the pregnancy. Bleeding without dilation of the cervix is called a *threatened abortion*. Frequently, these pregnancies proceed without any further problems until the baby is born.

If your cervix is dilated and tissue is coming out of your vagina, then a miscarriage can't be stopped. This is referred to as *inevitable abortion*. If you have passed tissue, your health care provider may suspect that a miscarriage already has occurred. If the tissue is available, your health care provider may examine it to see whether it contains any fetal tissue or is a clot or a piece of placenta.

An ultrasound exam often is used to try to determine whether a live fetus is inside the uterus. With this test, your health care provider can examine you for the presence of an embryo that is alive, growing according to schedule and the appropriate size in relation to its yolk sac and amniotic sac. If the fetus isn't alive but hasn't been passed out of your body, this is called a *missed abortion*. Because of the use of ultrasound in bleeding complications of early pregnancy, this diagnosis is being made much more frequently.

Treatment

In cases of threatened abortion, rest may be prescribed until the bleeding or pain has passed. In rare cases, when bleeding or pain is severe, hospitalization is recommended. Some health care providers may also recommend avoiding exercise and abstaining from intercourse. However, studies have shown that bed rest or the avoidance of usual or vigorous activities doesn't improve a woman's chances of keeping the pregnancy. Staying close to good health care resources until the bleeding has disappeared is wise, though.

RECURRENT PREGNANCY LOSS

Recurrent pregnancy loss is the consecutive loss of three or more pregnancies in the first trimester or very early in the second trimester. As many as one couple in 20 experiences two pregnancy losses in a row. Up to one in 100 has three or more consecutive losses. Losses after the first weeks of the second trimester are much less common.

In the rare circumstance where more than two miscarriages have occurred, a specific cause can sometimes be identified and treated. Possible causes include:

- **Chromosomal alterations.** One of the parents may have a chromosomal makeup that's altered, resulting in changes in the fetus that lead to miscarriage. This problem could be addressed with donor sperm or donor egg procedures.
- **Problems with the uterus or cervix.** If the woman has an unusually shaped uterus or weakened cervix, it may lead to miscarriage. Surgery may be able to correct some problems with the uterus and cervix.
- **Blood-clotting problems.** Some women are more likely to form blood clots, which can result in poor placental function and miscarriage. Testing can determine whether a woman carries anticardiolipin antibodies or antiphospholipid antibodies or factor V Leiden, all of which may cause miscarriage through increased blood clotting. A variety of approaches to anticoagulation have been used in these cases to reduce the risk of miscarriage.

A wide range of other factors have been suggested as causes of recurrent miscarriages. Possible causes include progesterone deficiency in early pregnancy, problems with implantation of the placenta and even a variety of infections. However, there's no firm evidence that treating these problems affects the outcome of subsequent pregnancies.

At least half of the time, no cause for the pregnancy losses can be found. But even in those cases, there is hope. According to the American College of Obstetricians and Gynecologists, about 60 percent of couples who have unexplained recurrent pregnancy losses and who don't receive medical treatment go on to have a successful pregnancy.

When the cervix is dilated or some tissue has passed, a miscarriage will occur soon afterward. Rarely, bleeding is so heavy or the pain so intense that this process needs to be completed quickly. In this case, placental tissue must be removed from the uterus. In these circumstances, a minor operation called dilation and curettage (D and C) is performed.

In a D and C, the cervix is gradually dilated, if necessary, and the tissue is gently suctioned (aspirated) out of the uterus. D and C is also typically required after a missed or incomplete spontaneous abortion to make sure no fetal tissue remains in the uterus. After a miscarriage, medications can be used to stop bleeding promptly.

After a pregnancy loss or a procedure to remove fetal tissue, continue to monitor any vaginal bleeding. Call your health care provider right away if you have heavy bleeding, fever, chills or severe pain. These could signal an infection.

In a missed abortion, where it has been determined that a fetus has died or was never even formed within the uterus, you're faced with several possible courses of action. In time, nature will cause a spontaneous miscarriage, though it's impossible to know how long that will take. Waiting for this to happen is safe, but psychologically it can be very hard for a woman. D and C can be done at any time, but it has a few small risks associated with it. Some anesthesia is required, and there's always some risk of an adverse reaction to medications. Also, stretching the cervix is part of the D and C, and poses a small risk of weakening the cervix, which could predispose a woman to future miscarriages. Rarely, an instrument can pierce the wall of the uterus, leading to bleeding. Another option is to use medications to provoke a miscarriage, but this approach isn't always effective with the first dose, and a D and C may be necessary to complete the procedure anyway. Each woman sees the options differently, and there's no consensus regarding which approach is best.

Future pregnancies

Most women who have had a miscarriage go on to have successful pregnancies later. Health care providers usually advise women to wait awhile before becoming pregnant again so that they can heal physically and emotionally. Talk with your health care provider about when the best time would be for you to attempt pregnancy after a miscarriage. Your health care provider may be able to help you find the emotional support you need to help cope with your loss.

Ectopic pregnancy

An ectopic, or tubal, pregnancy is one in which the fertilized egg attaches itself in a place other than inside the uterus. More than 95 percent of ectopic pregnancies occur in a fallopian tube. They can also occur in the abdomen, ovary or cervix.

Because the fallopian tube is too narrow to hold a growing baby, ectopic pregnancies can't proceed normally. Eventually, the walls of the fallopian tube stretch and burst, putting the woman in danger of life-threatening blood loss.

Ectopic pregnancies occur in about one in every 60 pregnancies. There are strong associations between fallopian tube abnormalities and ectopic pregnancy. Factors known to increase the risk of tubal pregnancy include:

- An infection or inflammation of the tube that has caused it to become partly or entirely blocked
- Previous surgery in the pelvic area or on the fallopian tubes
- A condition called endometriosis, in which the tissue that normally lines the uterus is found outside the uterus, causing blockage of a fallopian tube
- An abnormality in the shape of a fallopian tube

The major risk factor for ectopic pregnancy is pelvic inflammatory disease (PID), an infection of the uterus, fallopian tubes or ovaries. The risk of ectopic pregnancy is also higher in women who have had any of the following:

- A previous ectopic pregnancy
- Surgery on a fallopian tube
- Infertility problems
- A medication to stimulate ovulation

Signs and symptoms

At first, an ectopic pregnancy may seem like a normal pregnancy. Early signs and symptoms are the same as those of any pregnancy — a missed period, breast tenderness, fatigue and nausea.

Pain is generally the first sign of an ectopic pregnancy, but abnormal bleeding is also usually present. You may feel sharp, stabbing pain in your pelvis, abdomen or even your shoulder and neck. It may come and go, or get better and worse. Other warning signs of ectopic pregnancy include gastrointestinal symptoms, dizziness and lightheadedness. If you experience any of these symptoms, contact your health care provider right away. Although there may be other reasons for them, your health care provider is likely to want to rule out ectopic pregnancy as a cause.

Treatment

If your health care provider suspects an ectopic pregnancy, he or she will probably first perform a pelvic exam to locate pain, tenderness or a mass in the region of the tube and ovary next to your uterus. Unless your condition is obvious or you're clearly in an emergency situation, lab tests and ultrasound are almost always used to confirm the diagnosis.

The narrow fallopian tubes aren't designed to hold a growing embryo. As a result, the fertilized egg can't develop normally. It usually must be removed to prevent the rupture of the tube and other complications. If you receive a diagnosis of an ectopic pregnancy, you need to have care from a doctor.

Surgery is the most common treatment method. It's often possible to remove an ectopic pregnancy using a surgical technique called laparoscopy. In this procedure, a small incision is made in the lower abdomen, near or in the navel. The surgeon then inserts into the pelvic area a long, thin instrument called a laparoscope. It allows him or her to see the ectopic pregnancy and repair or remove the affected fallopian tube.

In certain circumstances, an oral medication called methotrexate can be used to treat an early ectopic pregnancy. Strict guidelines must be followed when treating tubal pregnancy with methotrexate. For example, the doctor must consider pregnancy hormone levels and the size of the ectopic gestation as revealed by ultrasound.

After treatment, your doctor will likely want to recheck your level of a pregnancy hormone called human chorionic gonadotropin (HCG) until it reaches zero. If the level remains high, it could indicate that the ectopic tissue wasn't entirely removed. In that case, you may need additional surgery or medical management with methotrexate.

COPING WITH THE LOSS OF A BABY

In rare situations, a baby dies during the course of late pregnancy. This is called an intrauterine fetal death, and the result is stillbirth.

When a baby dies, the loss is immense and the grief is hard to overcome. The baby that you've carried for many months, dreamed about and planned for is suddenly gone. There's possibly no greater pain than that inflicted by such a loss.

You may feel as if your world has come crashing down. Maybe you can't even think of life continuing as normal. Yet you can do some things to make the future more bearable and to ease your pain. It may help you to:

Say goodbye to the baby

Grieving is a vital step in accepting and recovering from your loss. But you may not be able to grieve for a baby you've never seen, held or named. It may be easier for you to deal with the death if it's more real to you. You may feel better if you arrange a funeral or burial for the child.

Save a memento of the baby

Experts say it helps to have a photo or memento from someone who has died so that you have a tangible reminder of him or her to cherish now and in the future. Ask well-intended family and friends not to clear out the baby's nursery, if you want and need more time to process the loss.

On rare occasions, a health care provider may recommend no treatment except observation to see if an ectopic pregnancy will end on its own, through spontaneous abortion, before any damage is done to the fallopian tube.

Future pregnancies

After you've had one ectopic pregnancy, you're more likely to have another. In women who've had one ectopic pregnancy, about 10 percent of subsequent pregnancies will be ectopic. If you've had two ectopic pregnancies, your chance of having a normal pregnancy is less than 50 percent.

Although the chances of having a successful pregnancy are lower if you've had an ectopic pregnancy, they're still good if one of the fallopian tubes has been spared. Even if one tube has been removed, an egg can be fertilized in the other one. If one or more ectopic pregnancies have significantly injured both fallopian tubes, *in vitro fertilization* may be an option.

In vitro fertilization is a commonly used form of assisted reproductive technology. It involves retrieving mature eggs from a woman, fertilizing them with sperm in a petri dish in a laboratory and implanting the fertilized eggs in her uterus two days later.

If you've had an ectopic pregnancy, talk to your health care provider before becoming pregnant again so that together you can plan your care.

Grieve

Cry as often and for as long as you need to. Talk about your feelings and allow yourself to experience them fully. It's best not to avoid the mourning process.

Seek support

Lean on your spouse, family and friends for support. Although nothing can banish the hurt you're feeling, you may gain strength from others who love you and support you. You likely could benefit from professional counseling after the loss of a child or from joining a support group of parents who have experienced a loss.

You and your husband or partner will likely wonder why you had to experience loss. You will never have a satisfactory answer to that philosophical question. But it may help you to learn about the physical causes of the death of the fetus or newborn so that you have some understanding of what happened. You may want to discuss the findings from the autopsy with your health care provider, after the initial shock has passed. Knowing a cause of death or details of what transpired may help you better accept the loss.

For more help on dealing with the loss of a baby, visit the Web site for March of Dimes at *www.marchofdimes.com* and go to the pregnancy and newborn loss section of the pregnancy and newborn center.

Molar pregnancy

Molar pregnancy occurs when the tiny, finger-like projections that attach the placenta to the uterine lining (chorionic villi) don't develop properly. The result is an abnormal mass — instead of a baby — forming inside the uterus after fertilization. This mass is a tumor of placental tissue and arises from abnormal chromosomes in the fertilized ovum.

Relatively rare, molar pregnancy occurs in only one of every 1,000 to 1,200 reported pregnancies in the United States.

Signs and symptoms

The main sign of molar pregnancy is bleeding by the 12th week of pregnancy. Often, the uterus is much larger than expected, given the length of the pregnancy. Severe nausea and other problems of pregnancy are common. If you think you have the signs and symptoms of a molar pregnancy, contact your health care provider right away. Molar pregnancies are diagnosed with ultrasound, which have a high level of reliability.

Treatment

A molar pregnancy is removed from the uterus using suction curettage. In this procedure, an anesthetic is given, then the cervix is dilated and the contents of the uterus gently removed by suction.

Once tissue from a molar pregnancy is removed, your health care provider will likely want to monitor your levels of the pregnancy hormone HCG for an extended time. Occasionally, this tumor will take on a malignant character. Invasive disease usually is marked by an HCG hormone level that remains high or increases after the tumor has been removed. For this reason, your health care provider will probably want to test your HCG level on a regular basis. If abnormal cells become malignant following a molar pregnancy, they'll need to be treated with chemotherapy. This is one of the greatest success stories in cancer medicine — with appropriate chemotherapy, these malignancies are usually cured.

Future pregnancies

Women who have had a molar pregnancy are advised not to become pregnant again for at least a year. Once you've had a molar pregnancy, you're at greater risk of a second, but the likelihood is that future pregnancies will be normal.

Cervical incompetence

Cervical incompetence is the medical name for a cervix that begins to thin and open before a pregnancy has reached full term. Instead of happening in response to uterine contractions, as in a normal pregnancy, these events occur because the connective tissue of the cervix can't withstand the pressure of the growing uterus.

Cervical incompetence is relatively rare. It occurs in only 1 percent to 2 percent of all pregnancies. However, it's thought to cause as many as one in four pregnancy losses in the second trimester. You're more likely to develop cervical incompetence if you've had a previous operation on your cervix or you have a damaged cervix due to a previous difficult delivery or a malformed cervix due to a birth defect. You're also at increased risk if you're carrying more than one baby or have excessive amniotic fluid in your current pregnancy.

Signs and symptoms

Cervical incompetence occurs without pain, but it causes many of the other signs and symptoms of miscarriage and preterm labor. These include spotting or bleeding, vaginal discharge that's bloody, thick or mucus-like, and a feeling of pressure or heaviness in your lower abdomen.

Treatment

If you have any of the signs and symptoms noted above in the second trimester, call your health care provider immediately. If you develop cervical incompetence and it's caught early, your health care provider may be able to stitch your cervix shut, which may save your pregnancy. This procedure, called cerclage, is most successful if it's performed before the 20th week of pregnancy.

Future pregnancies

If you've had a previous pregnancy loss due to cervical incompetence, you'll probably have the cerclage procedure done early in subsequent pregnancies — at about 12 to 14 weeks, which is after the pregnancy is well-established but before its weight is taxing the cervix.

You may also be interested in reading "Decision Guide: Trying again after a pregnancy loss," page 315.

Depression

Most everyone experiences a depressive episode once in a while. But long-term, inappropriate depression is a mental disorder. It can interfere with your ability to eat, sleep, work, interact with others and enjoy life.

Depression has no single cause. The illness often runs in families. Experts think that this genetic vulnerability combined with factors such as stress or illness may trigger an imbalance in brain chemicals that results in depression.

Depression is a common problem for women during pregnancy, and it can occur after pregnancy (postpartum) as well. One study revealed that almost 25 percent of cases of postpartum depression start during pregnancy.

During pregnancy, many factors can contribute to depression, including:
- Bodily changes you're experiencing
- Health difficulties during pregnancy
- An unexpected pregnancy
- A previous pregnancy loss
- Pressure on family finances
- Unrealistic expectations of childbirth and parenting
- Insufficient social or emotional support
- Unresolved issues from your own childhood

Depression can affect pregnant women of all ages, races and socioeconomic levels. Certain personality traits and lifestyle choices can make you more vulnerable. For instance, having low self-esteem and being overly self-critical, pessimistic and easily overwhelmed by stress can put you at increased risk of depression. Alcohol and drug abuse as well as nicotine use also may contribute to depression. Finally, a diet that is deficient in folate and vitamin B-12 may cause symptoms of depression.

Signs and symptoms

Two symptoms are key to establishing a diagnosis of depression. They are:
- **Loss of interest in normal daily activities.** You lose interest in or pleasure from activities you once enjoyed.
- **Depressed mood.** You feel sad, helpless and hopeless and may have crying spells.

Other common signs and symptoms of depression often can be mistaken for common problems of pregnancy. That can make depression during pregnancy easy to overlook. For a health care provider to diagnose depression, most of the following must be present most of the day, nearly every day for at least two weeks:
- Sleep disturbances
- Impaired thinking or concentration
- Significant and unexplained weight gain or loss due to increased or decreased appetite
- Agitation or slowing of body movements
- Fatigue
- Low self-esteem
- Loss of interest in sex
- Thoughts of death

Depression can cause a wide variety of physical complaints as well. These can include itching, blurred vision, excessive sweating, dry mouth, headache, backache and gastrointestinal problems. Many people with depression also have symptoms of anxiety, such as persistent worry.

If you think you may be depressed, it's important to talk with your health care provider about it. Your health care provider may take a detailed history of your signs and symptoms. Tests may be done to rule out other conditions that can cause depression-like symptoms.

Treatment

If you're diagnosed with depression, follow your health care provider's advice. Depression is a serious disease that requires treatment. Ignoring this diagnosis can put you and your baby at risk.

During pregnancy, depression most often is treated with counseling and psychotherapy. Antidepressant medications may be used as well. Many of these medications appear to pose little risk to developing babies, and it's best to use medication if your depression is severe.

Consult with your health care provider to discuss your treatment options and how you can best manage your depression during pregnancy. He or she can help you find support and develop an individualized treatment plan. If medication is recommended, your health care provider can determine which one is the safest for you to take during pregnancy.

Realize that having depression during pregnancy can increase your risk of postpartum depression. Untreated depression can become a chronic condition that can return before or during subsequent pregnancies. As with any other illness, depression needs to be treated, whether it occurs before, during or after pregnancy.

Gestational diabetes

Diabetes is a condition in which the levels of blood sugar (glucose) aren't properly regulated. The condition is related to a hormone called insulin, which controls glucose levels. When diabetes develops in a woman who didn't have the condition before pregnancy, it's called gestational diabetes. This condition is thought to result from metabolic changes brought about by the effects of hormones in pregnancy. About 3 percent to 5 percent of pregnant women in the United States develop this form of diabetes.

The risk of developing gestational diabetes is higher in some women, particularly those who:

- Are older than 30 years
- Have a family history of diabetes
- Are obese
- Had a previous complicated pregnancy

If you have had a stillbirth, a large baby or gestational diabetes in a previous pregnancy, you're at higher risk of developing the condition. For reasons that aren't clear, black, Hispanic and American Indian women are at increased risk of developing gestational diabetes.

Although gestational diabetes isn't usually a threat to the mother's health, health care providers test for it because it poses some risks for the baby. The major risk for babies of women with gestational diabetes is excessive weight at birth (macrosomia). Most health care providers define macrosomia as a birth weight of 9 pounds, 14 ounces or more.

These large babies are at greater risk of birth injury than are others. This is largely due to shoulder dystocia, which occurs when the head is delivered through the birth canal, but the shoulders are too big to come through, preventing the baby from being born. Other problems that may develop as a result of gestational diabetes include low blood sugar (hypoglycemia) in the baby shortly after birth, jaundice and respiratory distress syndrome, which is a condition that makes breathing difficult.

If gestational diabetes goes undetected, the baby has an increased risk of stillbirth or death as a newborn. But when the problem is properly diagnosed and managed, your baby is at no greater risk than is a baby whose mother doesn't have gestational diabetes.

Signs and symptoms

Generally, gestational diabetes doesn't cause any symptoms. Because the condition can't be diagnosed on the basis of the mother's signs and symptoms, glucose testing must be done to detect it.

A glucose tolerance test generally is performed at 26 weeks to 28 weeks of pregnancy. It may be performed earlier if your health care provider thinks that you're at high risk of developing gestational diabetes. About half the women who develop diabetes during pregnancy have no risk factors for the condition. For that reason, many health care providers choose to check all women for gestational diabetes, regardless of their age or risk factors.

For the glucose tolerance test, you'll be asked to drink a glucose solution. After an hour, a sample of your blood is drawn and the glucose level is checked. About 15 percent of pregnant women who are given this test will have abnormal levels of blood glucose. If this is the case, a second test, called an oral glucose tolerance test, is done.

For the follow-up test, you fast overnight and then are given another glucose solution to drink. Blood tests are taken again during a three-hour period and your blood glucose is measured several times. Of the women whose first test result was abnormal, gestational diabetes will be diagnosed in roughly 15 percent of those who take this follow-up test.

Treatment

Controlling your blood sugar level is the key to managing gestational diabetes. In most cases, this can be done through a carefully planned diet, plenty of exercise and regular testing of the blood glucose level.

Today, most health care providers will ask you to monitor your glucose at home on a regular basis to assure adequate control of glucose levels. This is usually done first thing in the morning before you've eaten and again after meals to see how high glucose levels climb after eating.

If, despite diet and exercise, your blood glucose level remains too high, further treatment is required. Treatment in this situation usually includes insulin injections. Insulin doesn't cross the placenta to reach the baby, but it does effectively control the mother's blood sugar levels.

An oral medication called glyburide may be used before adding insulin to try and control blood sugars. There has been less experience with this approach, but it appears to be safe for the baby and effective for many women.

In addition to helping you maintain a normal blood glucose level, your health care provider may advise regular monitoring of the baby during the last weeks of pregnancy. Ultrasound can be used to evaluate the growth of the fetus. It's good to remember that ultrasound has a significant error rate in estimating fetal weight. It's a useful tool for assessing trends of growth, but less so in pegging the baby's exact birth weight.

There's little risk to the baby before term, but most health care providers try to deliver the baby by the due date. With the risk of a large baby, some options to aid vaginal delivery aren't used in women with gestational diabetes because of the risk of shoulder dystocia. A Caesarean birth is a common outcome.

If labor hasn't begun on its own by 40 weeks, it may be started (induced). If delivery is planned before 39 weeks, amniocentesis is usually performed beforehand to determine whether the baby's lungs are mature enough for delivery.

Shortly after delivery, gestational diabetes almost always disappears. To make sure that your glucose level has returned to normal, your health care provider may check it once or twice on the day after delivery. The glucose test may be repeated six weeks after delivery.

If you have had gestational diabetes in one pregnancy, your risk of developing it in another pregnancy is increased. You're also more likely to develop type 2 diabetes (formerly called adult-onset or noninsulin-dependent diabetes) in the future. About half the women with gestational diabetes eventually develop a nongestational form of diabetes. For this reason, it's important to follow your health care provider's advice concerning diet and exercise after delivery and to have your glucose level checked at least yearly.

Hyperemesis gravidarum

Nausea and vomiting in early pregnancy are common. But at times, vomiting in pregnancy becomes excessive. This is known as hyperemesis gravidarum, defined as vomiting that's frequent, persistent and severe.

Hyperemesis gravidarum affects about one in every 300 women. The cause of this condition isn't known for certain, but it appears to be linked to higher-than-usual levels of the pregnancy hormones human chorionic gonadotropin (HCG) and estrogen. It's more common in first pregnancies, young women and women carrying more than one baby.

Signs and symptoms

Persistent excessive vomiting is the main sign of hyperemesis gravidarum. In some cases, it can be so severe that a pregnant woman may experience weight loss, become lightheaded or faint, and show signs of dehydration.

If you have nausea and vomiting so severe that you can't keep any food or liquids down, or if it persists past the 20th week of your pregnancy, contact your health care provider. Do so right away if vomiting is accompanied by fever or you have persistent pain after you vomit.

If it's not treated, hyperemesis gravidarum can keep you from getting the nutrition and fluids you need. If it lasts long enough, it can threaten your baby.

Before treating you for the condition, your health care provider may want to rule out other possible causes of the vomiting. He or she may check to see if you're carrying more than one baby. Other possibilities include gastrointestinal disorders, diabetes or a rare condition in which an abnormal mass, instead of a normal embryo, forms inside the uterus (molar pregnancy). Evaluations may include blood, urine and ultrasound studies.

Treatment

Mild cases of hyperemesis gravidarum are treated with reassurance, avoidance of foods that trigger problems, over-the-counter medications, and small, frequent feedings. Severe cases often require intravenous (IV) fluids and prescription medications. Very severe cases may require a hospital stay and IV feeding.

Women with hyperemesis gravidarum who work with their health care providers to make sure they're getting adequate nutrition and fluids shouldn't experience any serious complications for themselves or their babies.

Intrauterine growth restriction

Intrauterine growth restriction (IUGR) is a term used to describe a condition in which babies don't grow as fast as they should inside the uterus. These babies are smaller than normal during pregnancy. At birth, they weigh less than the 10th percentile for their gestational age.

Each year in the United States, as many as 40,000 babies are born at term with a birth weight of less than 5½ pounds. IUGR may be caused by problems with the placenta that prevent it from delivering enough oxygen and nutrients to the fetus. This situation can be caused by:

- High blood pressure (hypertension) in the mother
- Cigarette smoking
- Severe malnutrition or poor weight gain in the mother
- Drug or alcohol abuse
- Chronic disease in the mother, such as complicated type 1 diabetes (formerly called juvenile or insulin-dependent diabetes); heart, liver or kidney disease; rheumatologic diseases such as lupus; or antibody disorders such as red blood cell antibodies
- Preeclampsia or eclampsia
- Placental and cord abnormalities
- Multiple fetuses
- Antiphospholipid antibody syndrome, a rare immune system disorder

IUGR may also occur because of a problem with the fetus in which the nutrition sent by the placenta may be adequate but the fetus is restricted in growth by disease. Examples include:

- Infections such as rubella, cytomegalovirus and toxoplasmosis
- Birth defects or chromosome abnormalities

IUGR can also occur without a known cause.

Medical advances have greatly reduced the risks for growth-restricted infants. However, these babies are still at risk of problems. These smaller infants have low stores of body fat and glycogen, a type of carbohydrate that's readily turned into glucose, an energy source. As a result, they're unable to conserve heat. They may develop a below-normal body temperature (hypothermia). Stillbirth and fetal distress also are more common in growth-restricted fetuses. Because of their low energy stores, they may have low blood sugar (hypoglycemia) after birth. Finally, when the placenta is unable to deliver adequate oxygen and energy sources, these fetuses are less able to tolerate the stress of labor than are infants of normal size.

Signs and symptoms

If you're carrying a growth-restricted baby, you may have few, if any, signs and symptoms. But during your pregnancy, your health care provider can check regularly to see if your baby is growing normally.

Your health care provider may measure your uterus at each of your prenatal visits, in part to detect IUGR at an early stage. By looking at how this measurement increases over time, the health care provider may be alerted to IUGR.

If IUGR is suspected, an ultrasound exam likely will be done to measure the baby's size. The width and circumference of the baby's head, the length of the thigh bone, the size of the abdomen and the amount of amniotic fluid may be measured.

If you're pregnant with twins, IUGR can affect both babies to the same degree. Or it may affect one twin more than the other. Your health care provider may determine the difference in the growth rate is significant if it's more than 15 percent.

Treatment

To treat growth restriction, the first step is to identify and reverse any contributing factors, such as smoking, drug use or poor nutrition. Sometimes, hospital admission or bed rest is recommended.

You and your health care provider can continue to watch the baby's condition. You may be asked to keep a daily record of the baby's movements. Ultrasound exams generally are done every three to four weeks to track the baby's growth and the volume of amniotic fluid. Your health care provider may do tests t6 assess the baby's health.

Amniocentesis might be performed to check for chromosome abnormalities or infection. In this situation, the chromosomes are often assessed by fluorescence in situ hybridization (FISH) as well as full testing to get a rapid analysis. Rarely, fetal blood analysis is needed. If it is, a blood sample is obtained from the umbilical cord. This procedure is known as percutaneous umbilical blood sampling (PUBS).

Your health care provider may discuss the pros and cons of these techniques with you if these tests are being considered. If tests and ultrasounds show that the baby is growing and isn't in danger, the pregnancy may be continued until labor begins on its own. But if test results indicate that the fetus may be in danger or isn't growing properly, your health care provider may recommend an early delivery.

Depending on circumstances, labor may be induced for a vaginal birth or the baby may be born by Caesarean birth. If labor is induced, the baby can be monitored closely. If the fetal heart rate pattern or other tests indicate the baby isn't tolerating labor, a Caesarean birth may still be necessary.

No matter how a growth-restricted baby is born, there are still risks posed to the infant's health. A growth-restricted baby may need to be given fluid with sugar (glucose) soon after birth. The baby's temperature can be monitored to make sure he or she remains warm enough.

If you've had one growth-restricted baby, you're at increased risk of having another undersized infant. Fortunately, careful monitoring and early intervention often can lessen some of the dangers faced by growth-restricted babies. In some cases, growth restriction can even be reversed. In addition, a focus on good prenatal care, including getting excellent nutrition and eliminating smoking and alcohol use, will increase your chances of having a healthy baby.

Even if you do have a growth-restricted baby, size at birth may not be an indication of how well he or she will grow and develop. Many growth-restricted babies tend to catch up to their normal counterparts by 18 to 24 months. Unless these babies have serious birth defects, the chances are good for most of them to have normal intellectual and physical development in the long term.

Iron deficiency anemia

Iron deficiency anemia is a condition marked by a decline in the number of red blood cells in your body. It results when your body isn't getting the iron it needs to fuel red blood cell production. Iron deficiency anemia develops most often in the second half of pregnancy, after the 20th week. That's because for the first 20 weeks of pregnancy, as your body makes more and more blood, you make the fluid portion of blood (plasma) more quickly than you make red blood cells. This results in lower red blood cell concentrations overall.

Statistics indicate that up to 20 percent of all pregnant women are iron deficient. That means they don't get the recommended 30 milligrams of iron each day — a risk factor for developing iron deficiency anemia. When you're pregnant, it's a challenge to keep your iron stores at an adequate level through diet alone. That's why many health care providers prescribe iron supplements during the second half of pregnancy. If you're getting regular prenatal care and taking a daily prenatal vitamin, you'll generally be able to steer clear of iron deficiency anemia.

Signs and symptoms

If you have a mild case of iron deficiency anemia, you may not even notice any problems. If, however, you have a moderate or severe case, you may be pale, excessively tired and weak, short of breath, and dizzy or lightheaded. Heart palpitations and fainting spells also are signs and symptoms of iron deficiency anemia.

An unusual but frequent symptom of iron deficiency anemia is the desire to consume unusual things. Common targets of this craving include ice chips, cornstarch and even clay. If you have any of these signs and symptoms, contact your health care provider.

If you're diagnosed with iron deficiency anemia, don't be alarmed. Although iron deficiency anemia can make you tired and more susceptible to illness, it's unlikely to hurt your baby unless it's severe. It's also readily treatable.

Treatment

Treatment consists of taking in enough iron, which is prescribed in capsule or tablet form. Very rarely, blood transfusions may be required. But this is used only if a pregnant woman is severely anemic and has an ongoing source of blood loss.

Placental abruption

Placental abruption occurs when your placenta separates from the inner wall of the uterus before delivery. It can cause life-threatening problems for you and your baby. You can go into shock from blood loss. Your baby can be deprived of oxygen-rich blood he or she needs to survive. Placental abruption occurs in about one of every 150 births. Its cause is unknown.

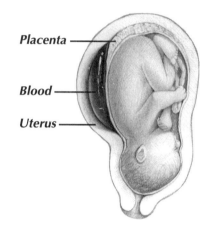

The most common condition associated with placental abruption is high blood pressure (hypertension) in pregnancy. That's true whether the high blood pressure first developed during pregnancy or was present before conception.

Placental abruption also appears to be more common in black women, women who are older — especially those older than 40 — women who have had many children, women who smoke, and women who abuse alcohol or drugs such as cocaine during pregnancy.

Placental abruption has also been associated with the presence of abnormalities in the mother's blood-clotting system. Very rarely, trauma or injury to the mother may cause placental abruption.

Signs and symptoms

In the early stages of placental abruption, you may not have signs and symptoms. When they do occur, the most common one is bleeding from the vagina. The bleeding may be light, heavy or somewhere in between. The amount of blood doesn't necessarily correspond to how much of the placenta has separated from the inside of the uterus. Other signs and symptoms that may be caused by placental abruption include:
- Back or abdominal pain
- Uterine tenderness
- Rapid contractions
- A hard and rigid feel to the uterus

To diagnose placental abruption, your health care provider will likely try to exclude other possible causes of vaginal bleeding. An ultrasound will probably be done to assure the bleeding isn't from placenta previa. Placental abruptions only rarely are seen on ultrasound.

Treatment

If placental abruption is suspected, treatment depends largely on the condition of the mother and baby and the stage of the pregnancy. Electronic monitoring is usually used to look at patterns of the baby's heart rate. If the monitoring shows no signs that the baby is in immediate trouble and the pregnancy hasn't reached a safe time for the baby to be born, the mother may be hospitalized so that her condition can be monitored closely for several days.

If the baby has reached maturity and placental abruption is minimal, a vaginal delivery is possible. If an abruption progresses and signs indicate that the mother or baby is in jeopardy, an immediate delivery, usually by Caesarean, will most likely be necessary. In addition, a mother who experiences severe bleeding may need blood transfusions.

There is a one in 10 chance that placental abruption will recur in a subsequent pregnancy. Some of the possible causes — such as high blood pressure, maternal-clotting disorders or substance abuse — may be treated before the next pregnancy.

Abruption is a serious complication. Prompt and expert care is required to avoid serious complications for mother and baby. In rare cases, an abruption can occur so rapidly and extensively that a baby can't be saved from injury.

Placenta previa

In some pregnancies, the placenta is located low in the uterus. It may partly or completely cover the opening of the cervix. This condition is known as placenta previa. It poses a potential danger to the mother and baby because of the risk of excessive bleeding before or during delivery.

Placenta previa occurs in about one in 200 pregnancies and may take one of several forms, including:

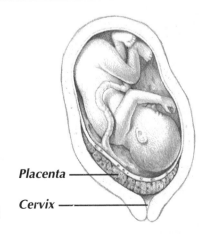

Placenta ——
Cervix ——

- **Marginal.** With this, the edge of the placenta is at the margin of the cervical opening. As the cervix dilates during labor, the edge of the placenta may be disrupted but allow the baby to enter the pelvis. Vaginal delivery may be possible under certain conditions.

- **Partial.** In partial placenta previa, the placenta partly covers the cervical opening. To avoid significant bleeding, a Caesarean birth is done.
- **Total.** Here, the placenta completely covers the cervical opening, making vaginal delivery impossible because of the risk of massive bleeding.

The cause of placenta previa isn't known. But like placental abruption, it's more common in women who have had children before, older women and women who smoke. Previous uterine surgery, such as a dilation and curettage (D and C), in which the lining of the uterus is scraped for medical reasons, seems to increase the risk. Caesarean birth scars also seem to significantly increase the risk.

Signs and symptoms

Painless vaginal bleeding is the main sign of placenta previa. This bleeding most often occurs near the end of the second trimester or the beginning of the third. The blood is usually bright red, and the amount may range from light to heavy. The bleeding may stop, but it nearly always recurs days or weeks later. Any bleeding in the third trimester should be reported to your health care provider immediately.

Almost all cases of placenta previa may be detected by an ultrasound exam before any bleeding has occurred. Because even the gentlest cervical exam can cause hemorrhage, this type of exam is done only when delivery is planned and only when an immediate Caesarean birth can be performed. Hemorrhaging as a result of placenta previa is quite uncommon, as either ultrasound or magnetic resonance imaging (MRI) can define the location of the placenta. If you know from a prior ultrasound you may have this condition, tell any health care provider you see during your pregnancy before he or she considers a vaginal exam. In addition, don't have intercourse until your health care provider has told you any question of placenta previa has been resolved.

Treatment

The treatment for placenta previa depends on several factors, including whether the fetus is mature enough to be born and whether you are experiencing vaginal bleeding.

If the placenta is close to but not covering the cervix and there's no bleeding, you may be allowed to rest at home — with instructions to call your health care provider or hospital immediately if bleeding starts. Early in the pregnancy, medications may be given to stop premature labor.

Usually after an initial bleeding episode, women with placenta previa are kept in the hospital and a Caesarean birth is planned for as soon as the baby can safely be delivered.

If bleeding starts and can't be controlled, an immediate Caesarean birth probably is necessary for the sake of the baby, even if the birth is premature.

Women who have had placenta previa in a previous pregnancy have a 4 percent to 8 percent chance of experiencing it in a future pregnancy. In most cases, however, placenta previa can be detected accurately before a fetus is in significant danger. However, if the placenta lies over the area in the uterus of a prior Caesarean birth scar, the next Caesarean may be much more complicated.

Preeclampsia

Preeclampsia is a disease that produces an increase in blood pressure in pregnant women. It's characterized by:

- High blood pressure
- Swelling of the face and hands
- Protein in the urine after the 20th week of pregnancy

The condition used to be called toxemia because it was once thought to be caused by a toxin in a pregnant woman's bloodstream. It's now known that preeclampsia isn't caused by a toxin. But its true cause isn't known.

Preeclampsia is a relatively common disorder. It affects 6 percent to 8 percent of all pregnancies. Eighty-five percent of all cases occur in the first pregnancy.

Other risk factors include carrying two or more fetuses (multiple pregnancy), diabetes, chronic high blood pressure (hypertension), kidney disease, rheumatologic disease such as lupus, and family history. Preeclampsia is more common in teenagers and in women older than 35.

Signs and symptoms

Women with preeclampsia have had the disease since very early in the pregnancy, but it doesn't become obvious until much later in pregnancy. By the time obvious signs and symptoms — high blood pressure, a swollen face and hands, and protein in the urine — do appear, preeclampsia is in an advanced state.

In some women, the first sign of preeclampsia may be a sudden weight gain. Typically, that means more than 2 pounds in a week or 6 pounds in a month. This weight gain is due to the retaining of fluids rather than the buildup of fat. Headaches, vision problems and pain in the upper abdomen may occur.

Health care providers monitor a woman's blood pressure throughout her pregnancy. The diagnosis of preeclampsia typically begins when blood pressure is consistently elevated over a period of time. A single high blood pressure reading doesn't mean you have preeclampsia. Normal blood pressure readings for pregnant women are less than 130/85 millimeters of mercury (mm Hg). In pregnant women, a blood pressure reading of 140/90 mm Hg or more is considered above the normal range.

Preeclampsia has various degrees of severity. If the only sign you have is elevated blood pressure, your health care provider may call your condition gestational hypertension.

Preeclampsia is also diagnosed by testing urine samples for protein. Your health care provider may also want to do some blood tests to see how well your liver and kidneys are functioning. Blood tests can confirm if the number of platelets in your blood is normal. Platelets are necessary for blood to clot.

There's also a severe form of preeclampsia known as HELLP syndrome. It's distinguished from other milder forms of the condition by elevated liver enzyme values and a low blood platelet level.

Treatment

The only cure for preeclampsia is delivery. Medications to treat high blood pressure in pregnancy are sometimes used, but other measures are usually preferred.

A mild case of preeclampsia may be managed at home with bed rest and regular monitoring of your blood pressure. Your health care provider may want to see you a few times a week to check your blood pressure, urine protein levels and the status of your baby.

A more severe case of preeclampsia often requires a stay in a hospital. Testing of the baby's well-being with nonstress tests or biophysical profiles can be done regularly. In addition, an ultrasound exam is often used to measure the volume of amniotic fluid. If the amount is too low, it's a sign that the blood supply to the baby has been inadequate and delivery may be necessary.

Left untreated, preeclampsia can result in eclampsia. With eclampsia, seizures can occur, and this severe complication has significant risks for both mother and baby. Your health care provider will likely treat preeclampsia vigorously to avoid those complications.

Many cases of preeclampsia become apparent close enough to the mother's due date that they can be managed by inducing labor when recognized. In more severe cases, though, it may not be possible to consider the baby's gestational age. In those cases, labor may need to be induced or a Caesarean birth performed to protect the life of the mother and the baby. Magnesium sulfate is a drug that may be given intravenously to the mother with preeclampsia to increase uterine blood flow and to prevent seizures.

A pregnancy complicated by known preeclampsia usually isn't allowed to go beyond 40 weeks because of the increased risk to the fetus. The readiness of the cervix — whether it's beginning to open (dilate), thin (efface) and soften (ripen) — also may be a factor in determining whether or when labor will be induced.

After delivery, blood pressure usually returns to normal within several days or weeks. Blood pressure medication may be prescribed when you're dismissed from the hospital. If blood pressure medicine is necessary, its use usually can be gradually stopped a month or two after delivery. Your health care provider may want to see you frequently after you go home from the hospital in order to monitor your blood pressure.

The risk that preeclampsia will happen in a subsequent pregnancy depends on how severe it was during the first pregnancy. With mild preeclampsia, the risk of recurrence is low. But if preeclampsia was severe in a first pregnancy, the risk in future pregnancies may be as high as 25 percent to 45 percent.

Rhesus factor incompatibility

Rhesus (Rh) factor incompatibility occurs when a pregnant mother and her fetus have a different Rh blood type. Rh factor is a type of protein sometimes found on the surface of red blood cells. Those with Rh factor are called Rh positive. Those without it are called Rh negative.

Eighty-five percent of whites are Rh positive. Among blacks, the percentage is slightly higher, and virtually all American Indians and Asians are Rh positive. About 15 percent of whites and 7 percent of blacks are Rh negative, which means their blood cells lack the Rh antigen.

When you're not pregnant, your Rh status has no effect on your health. If you're Rh positive, you have no cause for concern during pregnancy either. But if you're Rh negative and your baby is Rh positive — which can happen if your partner is Rh positive — a problem called Rh factor incompatibility results. Your body sees the Rh-positive factor in your baby's blood as a foreign substance to be destroyed and starts making antibodies to combat it. The result can be a destruction of red blood cells in your baby (fetal anemia). If left untreated, this can cause mild or severe damage to your baby. In very rare cases, it can cause death.

On the bright side, if you're Rh negative, your partner is Rh positive and this is your first pregnancy, Rh incompatibility isn't likely to be a problem for you. That's true even if your baby turns out to be Rh positive. It usually takes one Rh-incompatible pregnancy for your body to build up enough antibodies to the point they could harm your baby. Your risk, if untreated, will be higher during any future pregnancies.

Signs and symptoms
If you tested Rh-negative early in your pregnancy, you'll probably have a blood test for Rh antibodies at about 28 or 29 weeks into your pregnancy. If results show that you're not yet producing any Rh antibodies, your health

care provider can give you an injection of Rh immunoglobulin (RhIg) into a muscle. The RhIg injection will destroy any Rh-positive cells that may be floating around in your bloodstream. With no Rh factor to fight, antibodies will not form. Think of it as a pre-emptive strike against the formation of Rh antibodies. Because of the development of RhIg, fetal Rh disease is now rare.

If you're one of the few women who do have Rh antibodies, you can be tested on a regular basis throughout the second trimester to determine the level of antibodies in your blood. Further testing may be recommended to monitor the health of the fetus. These tests may include ultrasound measurements of blood flow, which is related to fetal anemia, or the use of amniocentesis to measure the amount of fetal blood destruction.

If the level of antibodies becomes too high, measures can be taken to prevent harm to the baby. These measures may include blood transfusions to the fetus while still in the uterus or, in some cases, early delivery. After birth, the baby may have anemia and may develop jaundice that requires treatment.

One other important note: If you're Rh negative and your fetus is Rh positive, it's not necessary to carry a pregnancy to term to develop Rh antibodies. Antibodies can form even during an Rh-incompatible pregnancy that ended in miscarriage or abortion. They can also form during an ectopic or molar pregnancy. If you become pregnant again and haven't been treated to prevent the development of Rh antibodies, an Rh-positive fetus is at risk.

While Rh antibodies are the most common type, many other rare types of red blood cell antibodies can need similar detection. Unfortunately, for these irregular antibodies, no preventive treatments are available. For this reason, blood type and antibody screening tests are done for each pregnancy.

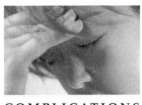

Infections during pregnancy

Pregnancy doesn't make you immune from everyday infections and illnesses. It may, however, change the way an infection is managed by your health care provider. This section explores how pregnancy might be affected by various infections.

Chickenpox

Chickenpox (varicella) is caused by the varicella-zoster virus. It's a common and highly contagious childhood illness characterized by red, itchy spots on the skin. About 4 million Americans, mostly children, contract the illness each year. Adults also can have chickenpox.

A vaccine to prevent chickenpox became available in 1995. Now, children are routinely vaccinated against the illness, and the number of current and future cases is expected to decline. Those who had chickenpox or were vaccinated against it are typically immune to the virus. If you're not sure whether you're immune, your health care provider can perform a blood test to find out.

The vaccine isn't approved for women who are pregnant. But if you're susceptible to the illness and still haven't conceived, your health care provider may recommend getting vaccinated and putting off pregnancy for a month or more. In childhood, chickenpox is generally a mild disease. However, in adults — and especially in pregnant women — it can be serious. If not treated, it can lead to complications such as pneumonia.

Managing chickenpox during pregnancy

Chickenpox early in pregnancy very rarely results in birth defects. The greatest threat to the baby is when a mother develops chickenpox the week before birth. It can cause a serious, life-threatening infection in a newborn. Usually, an injection of a drug called varicella-zoster immune globulin (VZIG) can lessen the severity of the infection if a baby is treated quickly after birth.

Pregnant women exposed to chickenpox also need protection with this drug to diminish the severity of the disease. Treating an expectant mother with VZIG within 72 hours of exposure appears to reduce the risk of pneumonia and other serious complications.

Cytomegalovirus

Cytomegalovirus (CMV) is a common viral infection. In healthy adults, almost all CMV infections go unrecognized. However, infected adults sometimes experience signs and symptoms such as a fever, a sore throat, aching muscles and fatigue.

Up to 85 percent of all adults in the United States are infected with CMV by age 40. An infection can recur, but recurrences are likely to go unnoticed. After you've been infected by CMV, you can shed the virus for years in saliva, urine or breast milk.

Managing cytomegalovirus during pregnancy

CMV can be passed from one person to another through infected body fluids. A pregnant woman with CMV can infect her baby with the virus before birth, during delivery or while breast-feeding. In the United States, CMV is the viral infection most frequently passed from mother to child before birth.

When a woman has a recurrent infection of CMV during pregnancy, less than 1 percent of fetuses are infected. Those who do contract CMV rarely develop any serious problems related to the infection.

Women who contract CMV for the first time during pregnancy have a greater risk of passing a severe congenital infection on to their babies. Often, CMV infections go unnoticed in infants because they have no signs of it at birth. However, CMV may have serious effects on these children. A small number may have neurologic problems such as learning disabilities. Up to 10 percent will have some degree of hearing loss.

About 1 percent of infants show signs and symptoms of CMV at birth. These include severe liver problems, seizures, blindness, deafness and pneumonia. Up to 20 percent of these babies die. The majority of those who live have serious neurologic defects.

An amniocentesis can test for infection in the fetus if CMV is diagnosed in a pregnant woman. Your health care provider may recommend a series of ultrasounds to see if the fetus develops structural problems related to the infection. No treatment currently exists for congenital CMV, but new vaccines are being studied.

Fifth disease

Fifth disease (erythema infectiosum) is a contagious infection common among school-age children. This condition is caused by the human parvovirus B19. Sometimes, it's also called slapped-cheek disease because the most noticeable part of the infection in children is the bright red rash on the cheeks. A lacy red rash may also be seen on the legs, trunk and neck. Many children with fifth disease feel well. Other children may have a mild fever, upset stomach and other flu-like symptoms.

In adults, the most noticeable symptom is joint soreness, which may last from days to weeks. Adults are much less likely to develop the telltale rash than are children. Infection can also occur without signs or symptoms in either children or adults. For this reason, many adults may not know if they had the infection in childhood. Once you've had the infection, you're generally immune from getting it again.

Fifth disease is contagious for up to a week before the onset of the facial rash, so it's difficult to stop its spread. The time between exposure and development of the disease ranges from four to 14 days. Currently, no vaccine exists to prevent fifth disease. Antiviral therapy hasn't yet been shown to benefit women with the infection.

Managing fifth disease during pregnancy

Between one-fourth and one-half of pregnant women remain susceptible to the B19 virus during pregnancy, so it's not uncommon for expectant women to contract the disease. The great majority of these women will have healthy babies.

In rare cases, however, fifth disease in the mother can cause severe, even fatal, anemia in the fetus. The anemia can cause congestive heart failure in the fetus, manifested by a severe form of swelling (edema) called fetal hydrops. If a fetus develops this complication, it may be possible to give the fetus a blood transfusion through the umbilical cord.

If a pregnant woman has been exposed to fifth disease or is suspected of having it, blood tests can help determine immunity or confirm infection. If the blood tests show immunity, there's no cause for concern. If the tests show evidence of fifth disease, additional ultrasounds might be done for up to 12 weeks to watch for possible signs of anemia and congestive heart failure in the fetus.

Group B streptococcus

Up to 35 percent of adults in the United States carry a bacterium known as Group B streptococcus (GBS). For women with GBS, it's normal for the organism to reside in their colons and rectums. Typically, GBS lives harmlessly in the body. However, pregnant women who harbor GBS may pass it to their babies during labor and delivery. Babies who acquire this infection may become seriously ill.

Managing group B streptococcus during pregnancy

Only a small number of babies born to women carrying group B strep become ill. However, it's now clear that using antibiotics during labor to treat women who carry the bacterium will prevent most of these infections. Women who carry GBS don't show symptoms, so all women should be screened for it.

If GBS infects a newborn, the resulting illness can take one of two forms: early-onset infection or late-onset infection. In early-onset infection, a baby typically becomes sick within hours after birth. Problems can include infection of the fluid in and around the brain (meningitis), inflammation and infection of the lungs (pneumonia) and a life-threatening condition called sepsis, which can cause fever, difficulty breathing and shock. Up to 20 percent of babies with early-onset GBS infection have long-term problems or die, even with immediate treatment. Using antiobiotics during labor to treat pregnant women who carry GBS can prevent the majority of these infections.

Late-onset infection occurs within a week to a few months after birth. It usually results in meningitis. Although meningitis is serious, the death rate isn't as high as in the early-onset form.

Children who survive either type of infection can have long-term neurologic problems.

Listeriosis

Listeriosis is an illness caused by a type of bacteria called *Listeria monocytogenes*. Most infections result from eating contaminated foods. Commonly involved are processed foods such as deli meats and hot dogs, unpasteurized milk and milk products such as soft cheeses.

Most healthy people exposed to listeria don't become ill. But at times the infection can cause flu-like problems such as fever, fatigue, nausea, vomiting and diarrhea. These problems are somewhat more likely during pregnancy.

Managing listeriosis during pregnancy

If you contract listeriosis during pregnancy, the infection can be passed from you to your fetus through the placenta. It can lead to premature delivery, miscarriage, stillbirth or the death of the baby shortly after birth.

It's important to make every effort to prevent exposure to listeria during pregnancy. Listeria contamination events are usually recognized, and warnings are often reported in the news. If you're pregnant, heed these warnings. In addition, always avoid consuming unpasteurized dairy products.

German measles

German measles (rubella) is a viral infection. It causes fever, swollen lymph nodes, aching joints and a rash. Rubella is sometimes confused with measles (rubeola), but each of these illnesses is caused by a different virus.

Rubella is extremely rare in the United States. Most young children are vaccinated against it with the measles-mumps-rubella (MMR) vaccine. As a result, most women in their childbearing years are immune to rubella. Long-term immunity develops in at least 95 percent of the people who receive the vaccine.

However, small outbreaks of rubella continue to occur in the United States. That means it's possible for you to become infected during pregnancy if you aren't immune.

Managing German measles during pregnancy

German measles is a mild infection. However, if you contract it while you're pregnant, it can be dangerous. The infection can cause miscarriages, stillbirths or birth defects. Birth defects may include growth retardation, mental retardation, cataracts or other eye problems, deafness, congenital heart defects and defects in other organs. The highest risk to the fetus is during the first trimester, but exposure to rubella during the second trimester also is dangerous.

Early in pregnancy, women are routinely tested for rubella immunity. If you're pregnant and found not to be immune, avoid contact with anyone who may have been exposed to German measles. The MMR vaccines isn't recommended during pregnancy. However, you can be vaccinated after childbirth so that you will be immune to rubella in future pregnancies. If you're not pregnant and choose to receive the vaccine, you'll be advised to wait at least three months before becoming pregnant.

Toxoplasmosis

Toxoplasmosis is a parasitic infection that's carried by rodent-eating cats. The risk of infection from cleaning an indoor cat's litter box is low. Outside soil or sandboxes may contain the parasite from outdoor cats, especially in warm climates.

The most likely route to acquiring the infection is through contaminated foods. Good food preparation practices are the most effective route to prevent this infection.

In many cases, toxoplasmosis causes no signs and symptoms. It often goes undiagnosed. When signs and symptoms occur, they're often similar to what you would experience with the flu, such as swollen lymph glands, fatigue, muscle aches and fever.

An active infection usually occurs just once. It generally results in immunity to the disease. Pregnant women who have immunity won't pass the infection to their babies. However, women who contract toxoplasmosis for the first time during pregnancy have about a 40 percent chance of infecting their babies.

If you're unsure about whether you're immune, use these tips to help avoid infection:

- Eat only thoroughly cooked meat.
- Wash your hands well after food preparation.
- Wear gloves when gardening or handling soil.
- If you have a cat, have someone else clean its litter box.

Managing toxoplasmosis during pregnancy

Infection with toxoplasmosis during pregnancy can lead to problems. It may result in miscarriage, growth problems for the fetus or preterm (before the 37th week) labor. The majority of fetuses who acquire toxoplasmosis develop normally. However, the disease may cause problems in babies, including blindness or impaired eyesight, an enlarged liver or spleen, jaundice, seizures and mental retardation.

Women aren't routinely screened for toxoplasmosis during pregnancy in most areas. If an infection is suspected, your health care provider can check with a blood test. If the test indicates a current infection, prenatal tests, such as amniocentesis and ultrasound, may help determine if there's a fetal infection. To diagnose toxoplasmosis in a baby after birth, a health care provider may study the placenta, test the spinal fluid and have your baby undergo a computerized tomography (CT) scan of the head.

Treating toxoplasmosis during pregnancy can be difficult. It isn't clear whether the medications used to treat it are effective for the fetus, and the mother rarely requires treatment. Treatment will depend on your circumstances.

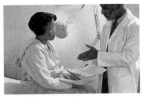

problems of labor and childbirth

Even if you're doing everything right as you go through labor and child-birth, complications can occur. If something does go wrong, trust your health care provider to do the best for both you and your baby. If you aren't comfortable before birth with the care you're receiving, that's the time to make a change. It's important to trust your health care team when problems arise in labor because treatment usually must begin quickly. That's not the time to doubt your provider's skill.

If things start to go wrong, it's easy to feel out of control. Often, it's best to be as flexible as you can. Your health care provider can explain concerns and discuss possible outcomes and new courses of action. Together, you can make a decision about what the next step should be.

Labor that fails to start

Sometimes, labor won't start on its own. If this happens to you, your health care provider may decide to start (induce) your labor by artificial means, through medical intervention.

Signs and symptoms
Your health care provider may induce labor for a variety of reasons. He or she may recommend labor induction if your baby is ready to be born but contractions haven't started yet or if there's concern for the health of you or your baby. Some situations in which you may be induced include:
- Your baby is overdue. You're beyond 42 weeks, or in some cases 41 weeks, pregnant.
- Your water has broken (membranes have ruptured), but your labor hasn't started.
- There's an infection in your uterus.
- Your health care provider is concerned that your baby is no longer thriving because your baby's growth has slowed or stopped, the baby

isn't active enough, there's a decreased amount of amniotic fluid, or your placenta is no longer nourishing the baby.

- You have high blood pressure resulting from your pregnancy (preeclampsia).
- You have diabetes or complications of lung disease, kidney disease or other pre-existing medical conditions that may put you or your baby at risk.
- The placenta has started to separate from the wall of your uterus.
- You have rhesus (Rh) factor complications, which means that your blood and that of your child may not be compatible.

You may be induced for other reasons, such as if you live a long way from the hospital or if you had a rapid delivery the last time you had a child.

If you were planning on a natural delivery but your health care provider wants to induce labor, try to view it as a positive. Making an appointment to have your baby can be much more convenient than waiting for nature to take its course. Induction may allow you to be more prepared, mentally and physically, when you go to the hospital.

Treatment

Your health care provider can induce labor in several ways. But before labor can be induced, your cervix must be softening (ripening) and opening (dilating). If it isn't doing so naturally, your health care provider can give you certain medications — known as cervical-ripening medications — to get things started.

Synthetic forms of prostaglandins, the natural chemicals that trigger contractions in your uterus, can be used to soften and dilate your cervix. Misoprostol (Cytotec) is one such drug. Dinoprostone (Cervidil, Prepidil) is another. These medications often work to begin labor as well, and they may reduce the need for other labor-inducing agents, such as oxytocin. In addition, they tend to decrease the time between induction and delivery.

All medications that induce labor carry one major risk: They might cause exaggerated contractions that may affect your baby's oxygen supply. Because of this risk, your health care provider may monitor your baby's heart rate while any of these agents are being administered. That way the dose can be adjusted in response to any unwanted effects.

In addition to prostaglandin preparations, other means can be used to soften and dilate the cervix. One way is to place into the uterus by way of the cervix a small catheter with a water-filled balloon. The uterus is irritated by the balloon and expels it through the cervix, softening and opening it somewhat. Another technique is to place into the cervix small cylinders of dried leaves of the laminaria plant. The cylinders draw in water and get thicker, thereby slightly dilating the cervix.

If you need to have your cervix ripened, you may go to the hospital the night before your labor is induced to give the medication time to work.

To induce labor, your health care provider may use one or both of these techniques:

Artificial breaking of your water
When your water breaks, the amniotic sac that envelops your baby is ruptured and the fluid begins to flow out. Normally, this signals that the baby isn't too far behind. One of the results of this rupture is an increased production of prostaglandins in your body, leading to increased uterine contractions.

One way of inducing or accelerating labor is to artificially rupture the amniotic sac. To do this, your health care provider inserts a long, thin plastic hook into the cervix and creates a small tear in the membranes. This procedure will feel just like a vaginal exam, and you'll probably sense the warm fluid coming out. It isn't harmful or painful to you or your baby.

Having your health care provider break your water can shorten the duration of your labor. It also gives your health care provider a look at your amniotic fluid, which can be examined for the baby's first bowel movement (meconium). Feces from the baby in the amniotic fluid stains the fluid a greenish-brown and demands that a few precautions be taken. If meconium is found, your labor will likely be monitored a bit more closely.

Administration of oxytocin
Oxytocin is a hormone that your body produces at low levels throughout pregnancy. These levels rise in active labor. Your health care provider may use a synthetic version of oxytocin (Pitocin) to induce labor. Usually, oxytocin is administered after your cervix is dilated somewhat and thinned (effaced).

Oxytocin is administered intravenously. An intravenous (IV) catheter is inserted into a vein in your arm or on the back of your hand. Connected to your IV is a pump that delivers small, regulated doses of oxytocin into your bloodstream. These doses may be adjusted throughout your induction, in case your contractions become too strong or not frequent enough. Contractions usually begin after 30 minutes if you're at or close to full-term, and they are generally more regular and more frequent than are those of a naturally occurring labor.

Oxytocin is one of the most commonly used drugs in the United States. It can initiate labor that may not have started otherwise, and it can also speed things up if contractions stall in the middle of labor and progress isn't being made. Uterine contractions and your baby's heart rate are monitored closely to reduce the risk of complications.

If labor induction is successful, you'll begin to experience signs of active, progressive labor, such as longer-lasting contractions that are stronger and more frequent, dilation of your cervix and rupture of your amniotic sac — if it hasn't broken or been broken already.

Induction of labor should be done only for good reasons. If the health of you or your baby is in question and an induction is unsuccessful, your doctor may decide to take further intervention, such as a Caesarean delivery.

Labor that fails to progress

If your labor isn't progressing, a condition called dystocia, it's usually due to a problem with one or more components of the birth process. Progress in labor is measured by how well your cervix opens (dilates) and the descent of your baby through the pelvis. Good progress is the progressive dilation of your cervix and descent of your baby. This progress requires the following:
- Strong contractions
- A baby that can fit through the mother's pelvis and is in the correct position for descent

ASSISTED BIRTH

If labor is prolonged or complications develop, you may require some assistance (medical intervention). For example, instruments — such as forceps or a vacuum extractor — may be needed to help you deliver if your cervix is fully dilated but your baby fails to make progress down the birth canal. An assisted delivery may also be necessary if your baby's head is facing the wrong direction and is wedged in your pelvis or if your baby is large. If your baby is in distress and must be delivered quickly or you're too exhausted to push any longer, your health care provider may have to intervene medically with a forceps- or vacuum-assisted birth.

Forceps-assisted birth

Forceps are shaped like a pair of spoons that, when hooked together, resemble a pair of salad tongs. The health care provider gently slides one spoon at a time into your vagina and around the side of the baby's head. The two pieces lock together, and the curved tongs cradle the baby's head. While your uterus contracts and you push, the health care provider gently pulls on the forceps to help the baby through the birth canal, which sometimes happens on the very next push.

Forceps may look intimidating, but you may welcome their use if they help you avoid a Caesarean birth. Many health care providers will try the judicious use of forceps when they feel it can be done safely.

Forceps are used today only when the baby's head has descended well into the mother's pelvis or is in the pelvic outlet. If the baby's head isn't well positioned, a Caesarean birth becomes necessary.

Vacuum-assisted birth

An instrument known as a vacuum extractor is sometimes used instead of forceps. The doctor presses a rubber or plastic cup against the baby's head, creates

- A pelvis that's roomy enough to allow for the passage of the baby

If your contractions aren't forceful enough to open the cervix, you may be offered a medication to make your uterus contract. Contractions can sometimes start regularly but then stop halfway through your labor. If this happens and the progress of your labor halts for a few hours, your health care provider may suggest breaking your water — if it hasn't already broken — or artificially stimulating your labor with oxytocin.

Signs and symptoms
Problems that can develop during labor include:

Prolonged early (latent) labor
This occurs when your cervix isn't dilating even to 3 centimeters (cm) — after about 20 hours of labor if you're a first-time mother or after 14 hours if you've delivered before. Sometimes, progress is slow because you're not in true labor.

suction with a pump and gently pulls on the instrument to ease the baby down the birth canal while the mother pushes.

The vacuum extractor cup does not take as much room as forceps delivery and is associated with fewer injuries to the mother. But it's likely that a vacuum-assisted birth is slightly riskier for the baby.

What to expect from an assisted delivery
An assisted delivery doesn't take very long, but it may take 30 to 45 minutes to ready you for the procedure. You may need an epidural or spinal anesthetic. Someone on your health care team may insert a thin, plastic tube (catheter) in your bladder beforehand to empty it of urine. You may be moved to an operating room, if there's a chance that the intervention won't be successful and you'll need a Caesarean birth. Your health care provider may make a cut to enlarge the opening of the vagina (episiotomy) to ease the way of the baby.

Will the use of forceps or a vacuum extractor hurt your baby? Forceps may leave bruises or red marks on the sides of your baby's head. A vacuum extractor may leave a bump on the top of the head. Bruises take about a week to go away. Red marks or a bump disappear within a few days. Serious damage with either technique is rare.

If you have any questions about assisted birth, don't hesitate to ask them. The use of instruments to deliver babies is common practice today and is generally considered safe, although they're associated with increased tearing or extension of the episiotomy. The choice of which approach to use — forceps or a vacuum extractor — is best left to your health care provider. Experience with the instrument is the greatest defense against complications.

The contractions you feel are those of false labor (Braxton-Hicks contractions), and they're not effective at opening your cervix. Certain medications for pain relief given during labor can have the unintended consequence of slowing down labor, especially if they're given too early.

Prolonged active labor

Your labor may go smoothly during the early phase, only to slow down during the second, active phase of labor. That's the case if your cervix doesn't dilate at the rate of 1 cm or greater an hour, after your cervix reaches 3 or 4 cm in diameter. The cause may be dwindling or irregular contractions.

Prolonged pushing

At times, efforts to push the baby through the birth canal aren't effective, which can result in exhaustion on the mother's part.

Treatment

For prolonged early (latent) labor

Whatever the cause of your prolonged early labor, if your cervix is still fairly closed when you arrive at the hospital or birthing center and your contractions aren't very strong, your health care provider may suggest options to accelerate labor. You may be told to walk or to return home and rest. Often, the most effective treatment for a prolonged early phase is rest. A medication may be given to help you rest.

For prolonged active labor

If you're making some progress in active labor, your health care provider may allow your labor to continue naturally. He or she may suggest that you

WILL YOU NEED A BLOOD TRANSFUSION DURING LABOR?

Blood transfusions are required in a very small percentage of births. Women do lose some blood during a routine labor and delivery. But it's not a lot — generally not enough to warrant a blood transfusion.

Women at high risk of needing a blood transfusion are those who have a known blood-clotting disease, have had bleeding problems with past births or have placenta previa. Placenta previa is a condition in which the placenta is near or blocks the opening of the cervix. Sometimes, a blood transfusion is necessary if you have a Caesarean birth. Certainly, the small percentage of women who experience major blood loss (hemorrhage) during or after labor and delivery may need a transfusion.

If you're worried about the possibility of needing blood during delivery, discuss your questions and fears with your health care provider. Be assured, though, that the risk of contracting a disease from a transfusion in the United States today is very low.

walk or change positions to assist in labor. You'll likely be given fluids intravenously, to keep you hydrated, if you're having a long labor.

However, if you've been in active labor and you haven't made any progress for several hours, your health care provider may start oxytocin and rupture your membranes — if your water hasn't broken already — in an attempt to move things along. These steps may be enough to restart labor and allow you to deliver naturally.

Your health care provider may consider the possibility that your baby's head is too large to pass through your pelvis. That may mean that you need a Caesarean birth.

For prolonged pushing
Your health care provider may consider a Caesarean birth if you haven't made good progress after pushing for two to three hours or longer. However, if you're able to continue and the baby isn't showing signs of distress, you may be allowed to push for a longer time. Sometimes, near the end of your labor, the baby's head can be eased out with the gentle use of forceps or a vacuum extractor. You may be asked to try a semisitting, squatting or kneeling position, which can help to push the baby out.

Complications with the baby

Abnormal position of the baby

Your labor and delivery may become complicated if your baby is in an abnormal position within your uterus — making vaginal delivery difficult or, sometimes, impossible.

At around the 32nd to 34th week of pregnancy, most babies settle into a head-down position for descent into the birth canal. As your due date nears, your health care provider may determine the position of your baby simply by feeling your abdomen for external clues as to the baby's placement, by doing a vaginal exam or, sometimes, by using ultrasound. Occasionally, an ultrasound is done while you're in labor to determine the baby's presentation.

If your baby isn't in position for an easy exit through your pelvis during labor, problems can develop. Several positions can cause problems.

Signs and symptoms
Your baby is facing upward
Your pelvis is widest from side to side at the top (inlet). The baby's head is widest front to back. Ideally, the baby's head should turn to one side once engaged at the top of the pelvis. The chin is then forced down to the chest so

that the more narrow back of the head leads the way. After descending to the midpelvis, the baby needs to turn either facedown or faceup to align with the lower pelvis. Most babies turn facedown, but when a baby is facing up, progress in labor can be slowed. Health care providers call this the occiput posterior position. Intense back labor and prolonged labor may accompany this position.

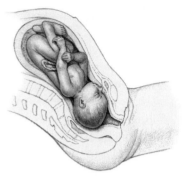

Occiput posterior position

Treatment

Most babies will turn on their own, if there's enough room. Sometimes, changing positions can help rotate the baby. Your health care provider might have you get on your hands and knees with your buttocks in the air. This position can cause your uterus to drop forward and the baby to rotate.

If this doesn't work, your health care provider might try to rotate the baby manually. By reaching through your vagina and using his or her hand as a wedge, he or she can encourage the baby's head to turn facedown. If this technique isn't successful, your health care team can monitor your labor to determine whether your baby is likely to fit through your pelvis faceup or whether a Caesarean birth would be safer. Most babies can be born faceup, but it may take a bit longer.

Signs and symptoms

Your baby's head is at an awkward angle

When a baby's head enters the pelvis, ideally the chin should be pressed down onto the chest. If the chin isn't down, a larger diameter of the head has to fit through the pelvis. However, a baby can enter the birth canal presenting with the top of the head, the forehead or even the face — none of which are preferred positions for descent.

If your baby's head moves through your pelvis at an awkward angle, it can affect the location and intensity of your discomfort and the length of your labor.

Treatment

Your doctor may have to consider a Caesarean birth if your baby isn't making progress down the birth canal or shows signs he or she isn't tolerating labor.

Signs and symptoms

Your baby's head is too big to fit through your pelvis

When a baby's head is too big to fit through the pelvis, the problem is called cephalopelvic disproportion. The problem may be that the baby's head is too big, or the mother's pelvis is too small. Or it may be more that the baby's head isn't properly aligned and the smallest width isn't leading the way. No matter what's causing the problem, labor can't progress beyond a certain point, and the cervix won't continue to dilate. The result is prolonged labor.

Treatment

You may expect your health care provider to have an idea ahead of time whether your baby will fit through your pelvis. With an ultrasound exam, your baby's size can be estimated. But it's nearly impossible to predict the course a labor will take. The forces of labor can temporarily mold a baby's head, even when poorly positioned, to fit through the pelvis, and loosened ligaments allow the bones of the pelvis to move. Because of these variables, the best way for your health care provider to find out whether your baby's head is a match to the roominess of your pelvis is to monitor your labor as it progresses. If necessary, the baby can be delivered by Caesarean birth.

Signs and symptoms

Your baby is breech
A baby is in the breech presentation when the buttocks or one or both feet enter the pelvis first.

Breech presentation poses potential problems for the baby during birth, and those problems can, in turn, create complications for you. A prolapsed umbilical cord is serious and more common in breech births. In addition, it's impossible to be certain whether the baby's head will fit through the pelvis. The head is the largest and least compressible part of the baby to travel through the birth canal, and it may become trapped even though the body was born easily.

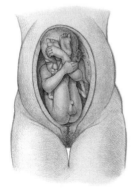 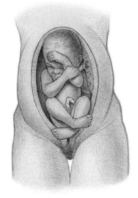 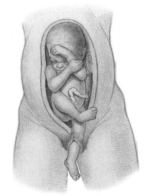

Three examples of breech presentation

Treatment

Your health care provider may try to turn the baby into the proper position, usually a few weeks before your due date. This technique is called an external version. If the baby isn't too far down in the pelvis, your health care provider might be able to move the baby into a head-down position simply by pushing on the baby through your abdomen.

If the external version doesn't work, your health care provider will likely discuss with you the option of a Caesarean birth. Although most babies born breech are fine, current evidence indicates that a Caesarean birth is safer for almost all babies in breech presentation.

Signs and symptoms

Your baby lies sideways

A baby that's lying crosswise (horizontally) in the uterus is in the position called transverse lie.

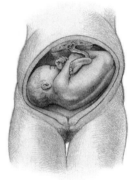

Treatment

Just as in breech presentation, an external version may be successful. All babies who remain in this position are delivered by Caesarean birth, and even laboring with a baby in this presentation may be harmful.

Transverse lie

Signs and symptoms

Umbilical cord prolapse

If the umbilical cord slips out through the opening of the cervix, blood flow to the baby may be slowed or stopped. Cord prolapse is most likely to occur with a small or premature baby, with a baby in a breech position or when the amniotic sac breaks before the baby is down far enough in the pelvis.

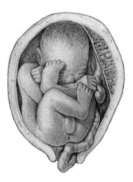

Treatment

If the cord slips out after you're fully dilated and ready to push, a vaginal delivery may still be possible. Otherwise, a Caesarean birth is usually the best option.

***Umbilical cord
prolapse***

Signs and symptoms

Umbilical cord compression

If the umbilical cord becomes squeezed between any part of the baby and the mother's pelvis, or if there's a decreased amount of amniotic fluid, the umbilical cord can become pinched (compressed). Blood flow to the baby is slowed or stopped during a contraction. This problem usually develops when the baby is well down the birth canal, close to the time of birth. If cord compression is prolonged or severe, the baby may show signs of decreased oxygen supply.

Treatment
To minimize the problem, you may be asked to labor in various positions, to take weight off the cord. You may be given oxygen to increase the amount the baby gets. It may be necessary for your health care provider to get the baby out with forceps or a vacuum extractor or, if the baby is too high, a Caesarean birth.

Fetal intolerance of labor

A fetus is considered to be intolerant of labor if he or she persistently demonstrates signs that suggest decreased oxygen supply. These signs are usually detected by studying the fetal heart rate on an electronic monitor. Decreased oxygen delivery to the baby usually occurs when blood flow from the placenta to the baby is reduced, meaning that he or she isn't receiving enough oxygen from the mother. This may mean that the baby will need to be delivered quickly.

Potential causes for this problem include compression of the umbilical cord, decreased blood flow to the uterus from the mother and a placenta that's not functioning correctly.

Signs and symptoms
During labor, your baby's heartbeat may be monitored regularly. If your baby's heart beats persistently very quickly or very slowly, it can mean that he or she isn't receiving ample oxygen. By using a fetal monitor, your health care provider can pick up heartbeat irregularities that may indicate concern. Two methods of fetal monitoring are:

External fetal monitoring
In external monitoring, two wide belts are placed around your abdomen. One is put high on your uterus to measure and record the length and frequency of your contractions. The other is secured across your lower abdomen to record the baby's heart rate. The two belts are connected to a monitor that displays and prints both readings at the same time so that their interactions can be observed.

Internal fetal monitoring
Internal monitoring can be done only after your water has broken or has been broken for you. Once your amniotic sac has ruptured, your health care provider

can actually reach inside your vagina and dilated cervix to touch the baby. To monitor the baby's heart rate, your doctor attaches a tiny wire to the baby's scalp. To measure the strength of contractions, the doctor inserts a narrow, pressure-sensitive, fluid-filled tube between the wall of your uterus and the baby. The tube responds to the pressure of each contraction. As in external monitoring, these devices are connected to a monitor that displays and records the readings, as well as amplifies the sound of your baby's heartbeat.

Other tests may be needed to indicate how well your baby is tolerating labor. These may include:

Fetal stimulation test

Ordinarily, when a baby's scalp is stimulated by the health care provider's touch, the baby will move around, and his or her heart rate will go up. A baby who doesn't have an increase in heart rate may not be getting enough oxygen.

Fetal blood sampling

A more precise test of the well-being of your baby can be done by checking the pH (acid-based balance) in a sample of the baby's blood. If the pH is low, it confirms the baby isn't getting adequate oxygen. In the test, a tube is inserted through the vagina and dilated cervix and pressed against the baby's head. Using a tiny blade on a long handle, the health care provider gently nicks the baby's scalp to obtain a drop of blood, which is sent to a lab and analyzed.

Treatment

A baby whose pH is very low must be delivered quickly and treated, if necessary. However, most babies whose fetal-monitoring findings cause concern are normal, and many abnormal heart rates return to normal with minor intervention.

There are ways to help a baby get more oxygen. Your health care provider may give you medication during labor to slow your contractions, which increases blood flow to the fetus. If your blood pressure is low, you may be given a medication to increase it. You may also be given oxygen, if necessary.

Very rarely, a severe lack of oxygen to a baby can result in brain damage. In extreme situations, oxygen deprivation can be fatal. Your health care provider is trained to identify the signs of these problems and to minimize the risk of any complications developing.

The majority of cases of nervous system (neurologic) damage occur before labor begins. Current high rates of Caesarean birth haven't decreased the risk of these problems. In most cases, labor should be allowed to continue, even when there are signs the baby is responding to temporary stress.

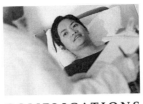

postpartum conditions

After your child is born, you're in the postpartum period. It's a transition time for you, both physically and emotionally. This section explains problems that can develop during the postpartum weeks.

Deep vein thrombophlebitis

A blood clot inside an internal vein, called deep vein thrombophlebitis (DVT), is one of the most serious potential complications following birth. If it's left untreated, a blood clot in the leg can travel to your heart and lungs. There, it can obstruct blood flow, causing chest pain, shortness of breath and, in rare cases, even death.

The hormonal changes of pregnancy increase every new mom's risk of developing DVT. That said, the condition is rare, occurring in only about one-half of 1 percent of all deliveries. However, your risk of developing a blood clot inside a vein in your leg is about three to five times greater after a Caesarean birth than after a vaginal birth. Clotting often occurs in the legs but can also occur in the pelvic veins. This, too, is more common after Caesarean births.

Signs and symptoms
Signs and symptoms of DVT include tenderness, pain or swelling in your leg, particularly around your calf. You may also have a fever. You're at increased risk of developing DVT if you have a body mass index (BMI) of 30 or greater, are over age 35 or can't walk around after surgery as much as recommended. In addition, recent studies indicate that many if not most people with DVT have a genetic predisposition for it.

DVT typically appears within the first few days after delivery and is detected in the hospital. It can, however, occur up to several weeks after you've been discharged. If you notice any signs and symptoms of DVT, call your health care provider immediately.

Treatment

If you have DVT, you'll probably have to be hospitalized with your legs elevated and given the medication heparin to thin your blood and prevent the development of any more clots.

Endometritis

Endometritis is an inflammation and infection of the mucous membrane that lines the uterus (endometrium). The bacteria that cause the infection usually grow at the site of the placenta. The infection then spreads through the uterus and, at times, even to the ovarian and pelvic blood vessels.

Endometritis occurs in 1 percent to 8 percent of all births. It's one of the most common infections that follow childbirth. The infection can develop after a vaginal or Caesarean birth, but it's far more common after a Caesarean. A long labor and early rupture of the membranes surrounding the baby in the uterus can contribute to endometritis.

Signs and symptoms

Endometritis usually occurs 48 to 72 hours after delivery. Signs and symptoms can vary depending on the severity of the infection. They may include:

- General discomfort
- Fever
- Chills
- Headache
- Backache
- Abnormal or foul-smelling vaginal discharge
- Enlarged and tender uterus
- Uterine pain

To diagnose the condition, your health care provider may press on your lower abdomen to check for tenderness. If an infection is suspected, a pelvic exam, blood tests and urine tests may be done. In some cases, your health care provider may take cultures from your cervix to check for sexually transmitted diseases or other organisms that could be contributing to an infection.

Treatment

Women with endometritis are commonly hospitalized and given antibiotics. Antibiotics typically are given intravenously for two to seven days in the hospital. Fluids are given either orally or intravenously. If you have a fever, you may be given acetaminophen (Tylenol, others) to help relieve it. You may be isolated from other new mothers, even though there's little likelihood that the infection will spread. If you're breast-feeding your baby, you usually can continue to do so during treatment. In mild cases, treatment may be done on an outpatient basis.

Antibiotics clear up most cases of endometritis. But if the infection goes untreated, it can lead to more serious problems, including infertility. Contact your health care provider if you develop signs or symptoms of endometritis.

Mastitis

Mastitis is an infection that can occur when bacteria enter the breast while breast-feeding. Nipples may become cracked or sore from breast-feeding. This can happen if your baby is not well-positioned when feeding or latches on to the nipple instead of putting his or her lips and gums around the area surrounding the nipple (areola). Mastitis can affect one or both breasts.

Signs and symptoms

When a breast becomes infected, it may feel sore, hard and hot. It may swell, become reddened and cause you to develop a fever. Typically, no tests are needed to confirm a diagnosis of mastitis in women who are breast-feeding. In women who aren't breast-feeding, a mammogram or breast biopsy may be performed to help determine the cause of an infection. If you develop any signs or symptoms of mastitis in one of your breasts, be sure to contact your health care provider.

Treatment

Antibiotics can be prescribed for mastitis. Your health care provider also may recommend acetaminophen (Tylenol, others) to help bring down any fever and relieve discomfort. Because mastitis can be painful, you may be tempted to stop breast-feeding. It's best to keep breast-feeding or breast pumping. Doing so will help empty your breast and relieve pressure. The infection won't spread to the milk your baby consumes. And the antibiotics you take won't harm your baby, although you may notice a change in the color of your baby's bowel movements.

To make yourself more comfortable, you may want to breast-feed for shorter periods of time. Applying warm compresses to the infected breast several times a day also can help. Dry your breasts between feedings and compresses so that they can heal properly.

Although breast infections can be painful, they typically aren't serious and can be successfully treated with antibiotics. Good breast care can reduce the risk of developing infections, but the problem probably can't be completely prevented. Watch for the signs and symptoms, and notify your health care provider promptly if they develop.

Post-Caesarean wound infection

Most Caesarean incisions heal with no problem at all. In some cases, an incision can become infected. Wound infection rates following Caesarean births vary. Elective, repeat Caesarean births generally have a wound infection rate of about 2 percent. Caesareans that follow labor, particularly if your water broke (membranes ruptured), have a wound infection rate of 5 percent to 10 percent. Your chances of developing wound infection after a Caesarean birth are higher if you abuse alcohol, have type 2 diabetes (formerly called adult-onset or noninsulin-dependent diabetes) or are obese, which is defined as having a body mass index of 30 or higher. Fat tissue tends to heal poorly.

Signs and symptoms
If the skin on the sides of your incision is newly painful, red and swollen, it may be infected, especially if the wound is draining in any way. Wound infection can also cause fever. If you suspect your incision has become infected, contact your health care provider.

Treatment
If your health care provider confirms that you have an infection, he or she will likely need to drain the incision to release the trapped bacteria. This is generally done as an office procedure.

Postpartum bleeding

Experiencing serious bleeding (hemorrhaging) after giving birth is not common. It occurs in about 5 percent of all births. It generally takes place during childbirth or within 24 hours of giving birth. This is what's known as early postpartum hemorrhage. In late postpartum hemorrhage, bleeding can occur up to six weeks after childbirth.

A number of problems can cause serious bleeding after birth. In the majority of cases, blood loss is the result of one of the following three causes:
- **Uterine atony.** After you've given birth, your uterus must contract to control bleeding from the placental site. In fact, the reason your nurse periodically massages your abdomen after delivery is to encourage your uterus to contract. With uterine atony, the uterine muscle doesn't contract. Why this happens isn't well understood. It's slightly more likely to occur when the uterus has been stretched by a large baby or twins or if labor has been long.
- **Retained placenta.** If the placenta isn't expelled on its own within 30 minutes after a baby is born, you can experience excessive bleeding.

Even when the placenta is expelled on its own, your doctor carefully examines it to make sure it's intact. If any tissue is missing, there's a risk of bleeding.

- **Tearing (lacerations).** If your vagina or cervix tears during birth, excessive bleeding can result. Tearing might be caused by a large baby, a forceps- or vacuum-assisted birth, a baby that came through the birth canal too rapidly or an episiotomy that tears.

Other, less common, causes of postpartum bleeding include:

- **Abnormal placental attachment.** Very rarely, the placenta attaches to the uterus more deeply in the wall than it should. When this happens, it doesn't readily detach after birth. These abnormal placental attachments can cause severe bleeding. They happen more frequently in women who have uterine scars from previous incisions, such as from a Caesarean birth.
- **Hematomas.** Hematomas result when bleeding occurs within tissue and can't escape through the skin. In the lower genital tract, swelling in the tissue can be very painful. It can be so severe that urination becomes difficult or temporarily impossible.
- **Uterine inversion.** In less than one in 2,000 births, the uterus turns inside out after the baby is born and placenta removed. This can happen without any risk factors, but it's somewhat more likely when there's abnormal attachment of the placenta.
- **Uterine rupture.** In about one in 1,500 births, the uterus tears during pregnancy or labor. If this happens, the mother loses blood, and the baby's oxygen supply is decreased. The tear can provoke serious bleeding.

Your risk of bleeding may be increased if you have had bleeding problems with past births. Your risk is also increased if you have a complication such as placenta previa, a condition in which the placenta is located low in the uterus and may partly or completely cover the opening of the cervix. This lower segment of the uterus doesn't contract as actively as the upper uterus, and bleeding may result.

Signs and symptoms

The body responds to hemorrhaging by diverting most of its blood supply to the brain and heart. This is a survival mechanism designed to protect these most important organs. But the body takes care of them at the expense of other organs. Because the oxygen supply going to body cells is greatly depleted, shock can set in.

With heavy postpartum bleeding, the following problems can occur:

- Pallor
- Chills
- Dizziness or fainting

- Clammy hands
- Nausea and vomiting
- Racing heart

These are the signs and symptoms the staff will look for if you have had bleeding. Blood loss is an emergency situation that requires immediate action.

Treatment

In most cases, you'll still be in the hospital when signs and symptoms of blood loss occur, and the medical team can take several steps to respond to the problem, including lowering the head of your bed and massaging your uterus. They'll probably also give you intravenous (IV) fluids and oxytocin — a hormone that stimulates uterine contractions.

Additional treatments can include everything from different medications to stimulate contractions to surgical intervention and blood transfusions. It all depends on the severity of the problem. Overall, the likelihood of a woman needing a blood transfusion after childbirth is less than 2 percent. Even Caesarean births need a transfusion only 3 percent of the time. Still, most treatment decisions will depend on the cause of the bleeding. Specific causes and treatments include the following:

- **Uterine atony.** If the uterine muscle is too fatigued to contract on its own, medication can be given to help the process. In addition, your health care provider may stimulate contraction of the uterus by pressing on your abdomen with one hand and on your uterus from within your vagina with the other. Medications to stimulate contractions also are very useful. If these measures aren't enough to control bleeding, surgery may be necessary.
- **Hematomas.** Small hematomas usually are allowed to heal naturally, but large ones might have to be drained. Vessels that continue to bleed can be tied off. If the loss of blood is too great, a blood transfusion may be needed. Occasionally, hematomas occur in the abdominal cavity and need to be drained surgically through an abdominal incision (laparotomy). Hematomas, especially those that must be opened, can become infected. Therefore, it's essential to keep the area clean. Antibiotics often are given to treat any infection that occurs.
- **Retained placenta.** If your placenta stays in your uterus after birth or is not fully expelled, your health care provider might have to reach in manually to remove the placenta or any remaining tissue from the uterine wall. If this doesn't work, the uterus can be scraped, a process called curettage, and suctioned to clean it out.
- **Tearing (lacerations).** Your health care provider will need to find and repair the tear.
- **Uterine inversion.** If the uterus turns inside out after delivery, your

health care provider will try to push it back through the cervix and into its proper place.

- **Uterine rupture.** If the uterus tears during pregnancy or labor, immediate surgical intervention is required to remove the baby and repair the tear. If your health care provider can't repair the tear, sometimes removal of all or part of the uterus (hysterectomy) is the only way to control the bleeding.

If the cause of excessive bleeding results in damage to the uterus, it may affect your ability to become pregnant again or to carry another baby. Blood transfusions can be lifesaving, and in the United States and Canada, they carry only a tiny risk of infectious disease.

In extremely rare cases, hemorrhaging can cause maternal death. In fact, in the United States, hemorrhaging is one of the leading causes of pregnancy-related death. These complications are the rare events that make delivering your baby in a well-equipped medical center important.

Postpartum depression

The birth of a baby can bring on many powerful emotions, including excitement, joy and even fear. But there's another emotion that many new moms may not expect: depression.

Within days of delivery, many new mothers experience a mild depression that's sometimes called the baby blues. The baby blues may last for a few hours or up to two weeks after delivery.

About 10 percent of new mothers experience a more severe form of the baby blues called postpartum depression. It can occur anywhere from weeks to months after giving birth. Left untreated, it can last for up to a year or longer.

In rare cases, women can develop postpartum psychosis within days to months after having a baby. Although some symptoms of this psychosis are similar to postpartum depression, they are more extreme. Postpartum psychosis may lead to thoughts and behaviors that can be life-threatening.

There is no one clear cause of postpartum depression. Instead, it's likely that a combination of body, mind and social interactions play a role. During pregnancy, labor and delivery, a woman's body experiences enormous changes. The levels of the hormones estrogen and progesterone drop dramatically immediately after childbirth. In addition, changes occur in the body's blood volume, blood pressure, immune system and metabolism. These changes can impact how a woman feels physically and emotionally.

Other factors that can contribute to postpartum depression and increase the risk in new mothers include:

- A personal or family history of depression
- An unsatisfying birth experience

- Postpartum pain or complications from delivery
- A baby with a high level of needs
- Exhaustion from caring for a new baby or multiple children
- Anxiety or unrealistic expectations about motherhood
- Stress from changes in home or work life
- Feeling a loss of identity
- Lack of social support
- Relationship difficulties

Signs and symptoms

Signs and symptoms of baby blues or mild depression include episodes of anxiety, sadness, irritability, crying, headaches, exhaustion and feeling unworthy. Often, these signs and symptoms pass in a few days or weeks. In some cases, baby blues turn into postpartum depression.

With postpartum depression, the signs and symptoms of depression are more intense and can last longer than those of the blues.

They include:

- Constant fatigue
- Lack of joy in life
- A sense of emotional numbness or feeling trapped
- Withdrawal from family and friends
- Lack of concern for yourself or your baby
- Severe insomnia
- Excessive concern for your baby
- Loss of sexual interest or responsiveness
- A strong sense of failure or inadequacy
- Severe mood swings
- High expectations and an overly demanding attitude
- Difficulty making sense of things

Many of the signs and symptoms of postpartum psychosis are the same as those of postpartum depression, but are even more extreme. With postpartum psychosis, women become severely depressed and anxious. They may experience intense anxiety, confusion and disorientation, feelings of paranoia or hysteria, and a fear of harming themselves or their babies.

If you're feeling depressed after your baby's birth, you may be reluctant or embarrassed to admit it. Or you may think that you can't be helped or that your problems won't be taken seriously. But it's important to inform your health care provider if you or a loved one — partners can feel this way, too — is experiencing signs or symptoms of postpartum depression. Reporting signs and symptoms of postpartum psychosis and seeking treatment is especially important if you suspect that you or someone you know is at risk of harming a life.

Self-care for postpartum depression

If you're diagnosed with postpartum depression, start your recovery by seeking professional care. In addition, you can aid in your recovery. Try these tips:
- Get as much rest as possible. Make a habit of resting while your baby sleeps.
- Eat properly. Emphasize grains, fruits and vegetables.
- Engage in moderate exercise.
- Stay connected with family and friends.
- Ask for occasional help with child care and household responsibilities from friends and family.
- Take some time for yourself. Get dressed, leave the house and visit a friend or run an errand.
- Talk with other mothers. Ask your health care provider about groups for new moms in your community.
- Spend time alone with your partner.

Treatment

To evaluate you for the possibility of postpartum depression, your health care provider most likely will want to review your signs and symptoms in person. Because a great number of women feel tired and overwhelmed after having a baby, your health care provider may use a depression-screening scale to distinguish a short-term case of the blues from a more severe form of depression.

Postpartum depression is a recognized and treatable medical problem. Treatment varies according to individual needs. It may include:
- Support groups
- Individual counseling or psychotherapy
- Antidepressant medications
- Hormone therapy

If you're breast-feeding, discuss this with your health care provider before taking antidepressant medications. Some of these drugs can be safely used during breast-feeding, but others can affect breast milk.

If you experience depression following childbirth, you have an increased risk of depression after a subsequent pregnancy. In fact, postpartum depression is more common in second-time mothers. With early intervention and proper treatment, however, there is less of a chance for serious problems and a greater chance of a rapid recovery.

Urinary tract infection

After giving birth, you may not be able to empty your bladder completely. The remaining urine provides an ideal breeding ground for bacteria, which can cause an infection of your bladder, kidney or urethra — the tube that transports urine from the bladder during urination. Urinary tract infections (UTIs) can occur after either vaginal or Caesarean births. They rank second to endometritis as the most common complication after Caesareans. You're at increased risk of developing a UTI if you have diabetes or if you keep a catheter in longer than normal after surgery.

Signs and symptoms

If you have a UTI, you may have a frequent, almost panicky urge to urinate, pain while urinating, a mild fever and tenderness over the area of the bladder. If you get home and experience any of these signs and symptoms, call your health care provider. You'll need to provide a urine sample so that it can be tested for bacteria.

Treatment

Treating a urinary tract infection generally involves taking antibiotics, drinking plenty of fluids, emptying your bladder regularly and taking acetaminophen (Tylenol, others) for the fever.

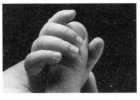

GLOSSARY

A

active labor. The phase of labor where steady progress in the dilation of the cervix can be expected, often accompanied by stronger contractions. This phase extends from 4 centimeters to full dilation at 10 centimeters.

afterbirth. The placenta and membranes discharged from the uterus after childbirth.

afterbirth pains (afterpains). Uterine contractions that help control bleeding.

alpha-fetoprotein (AFP) test. A specific protein produced by the fetus but not present to any degree in nonpregnant people. Testing the levels of this protein has implications for the baby's well-being.

amniocentesis. A test in which a small amount of amniotic fluid is removed from the mother. Used to detect various genetic characteristics, evidence of infection or lung maturity of the unborn baby.

amniotic sac (bag of water). A sac formed of two thin membranes that contains watery fluid (amniotic fluid) and the fetus. The membranes either rupture spontaneously during labor or may be ruptured to hasten labor.

anemia. A condition in which the blood has too few red blood cells. It can cause fatigue and lowered resistance to infection.

anencephaly. A neural tube defect that results in the abnormal development of the baby's brain and skull.

antibodies. Protein substances that the body makes to help protect itself against foreign cells and infections.

Apgar score. A rating or score given to a newborn at one and five minutes after birth to assess color, heart rate, muscle tone, respiration and reflexes. Zero to two points are given for each. Scores close to 10 are desirable.

apnea. Cessation of breathing.

areola. The circular, pigmented area around the nipple of the breast.

asphyxia. Organ malfunctions due to a lack of oxygen, a buildup of carbon dioxide and a low pH.

assisted birth. Delivery that is assisted by medical intervention, such as an episiotomy, forceps-assisted birth or vacuum-assisted birth.

assisted reproductive technologies. Medical intervention that aids conception, such as in vitro fertilization.

B

baby blues. A period of low mood (dysphoria), occurring in as many as 80 percent of new mothers.

biochemical testing. Use of chemical analysis of blood or amniotic fluid to detect a fetal condition. Examples include alpha-fetoprotein, estriol, inhibin and pregnancy-associated plasma protein testing.

biophysical profile. An assessment of fetal status based on heart rate testing and ultrasound findings.

birth plan. A written or verbal guide prepared by you and your health care provider that explains how you wish to deliver your baby.

blastocyst. The rapidly dividing fertilized egg once it enters the uterus, having cells committed to placental and fetal development.

bloody show. Blood-tinged mucous discharge from the vagina either before or during labor.

bradycardia. A sustained period during which the heart rate is slower than normal.

Braxton-Hicks contractions. Irregular uterine contractions that occur during pregnancy but do not result in changes in the cervix. Sometimes referred to as false labor.

breech position. A position in which the baby is positioned with feet or bottom toward the cervix at the time of birth.

C

Caesarean birth. An operative birth in which an incision is made through the abdominal wall and uterus to deliver the baby. Sometimes called Caesarean section or C-section.

cephalopelvic disproportion. A circumstance in which the baby's head won't fit through the mother's pelvis because the head is too large for the birth canal.

cervical incompetence. A condition in which the cervix begins to open without contractions before the pregnancy has come to term; a cause of miscarriage and preterm (before the 37th week) delivery in the second and third trimesters.

cervix. The neck-like lower part of the uterus, which dilates and effaces during labor to allow passage of the fetus.

chorionic villus sampling (CVS). A procedure that removes a small sample of chorionic villi from the placenta where it joins the uterus, to test for chromosomal or other abnormalities.

circumcision. A procedure on male infants that removes the foreskin from the penis.

colostrum. The yellowish fluid produced by the breasts until the milk "comes in"; usually noticed in the latter part of pregnancy.

congenital disorder. A condition that a person is born with.

contraction stress test. One of several tests designed to help evaluate the condition of the fetus and its placenta. It measures the fetal heart rate in response to contractions of the mother's uterus.

contractions (labor pains). The tightening of the uterine muscles.

D

deep vein thrombophlebitis (DVT). A blood clot inside a vein, which is a potential complication of childbirth.

dilation. Indicates the diameter of the cervical opening and is measured in centimeters; 10 centimeters is fully dilated.

Doppler. Commonly used to refer to a device with which your doctor can hear a fetal heartbeat by about the 12th week. Named for the Doppler effect, intrinsic to its function.

dystocia. Difficult labor for any reason.

early (latent) labor. The earliest phase of childbirth, during which uterine contractions begin to change the cervix, but changes are often gradual. This phase is almost always over when the cervix reaches 4 centimeters dilation.

ectopic pregnancy. A pregnancy that occurs outside the uterus; the most common variety is tubal pregnancy.

effacement. The progressive thinning of the cervix as its connective tissue is drawn up around the baby's head. It may be measured in cervical length in centimeters or as a percentage of thinning. 100 percent indicates total effacement.

embryo. The fertilized ovum from shortly after the time of fertilization until eight weeks of gestation.

endometritis. An inflammation and infection of the mucous membrane lining the uterus.

endometrium. The lining of the uterus, in which the fertilized egg embeds itself for nutrition.

epidural. An anesthetic method used to decrease or eliminate discomfort during labor. This is sometimes called an epidural block.

episiotomy. Surgical incision in the perineum to enlarge the vaginal opening.

external version. A doctor's attempt late in a pregnancy to turn a poorly positioned baby into a better birthing position.

F

fallopian tubes. Structures that pick up the egg as it is released from the ovary while propelling sperm toward its end where fertilization can take place. The fertilized egg is then nourished and delivered to the uterus through these tubes.

fetal alcohol syndrome (FAS). A condition caused by alcohol consumption during pregnancy. It can cause birth defects such as facial deformities, heart problems, low birth weight and mental retardation.

fetal fibronectin. A substance held between the fetal membranes and uterine wall. The substance can be tested to assess the risk of preterm (before the 37th week) delivery.

fetus. An unborn baby after the first eight weeks of gestation.

follicle-stimulating hormone. A hormone

that fosters the development of eggs in the ovaries.

fontanelles. The "soft spots" on a baby's head where the skull has not fused together. At birth, a baby has these soft spots on the top and back of the head. The back one closes about six weeks after birth, and the top one takes up to 18 months to close.

forceps. An obstetrical instrument that fits around the baby's head to guide the baby through the birth canal during birth.

fundal height. The distance from the top of the uterus to the pubic bone; used to help assess the growth of the fetus in the uterus.

G

genetic disorder. A condition that an individual can pass on through parentage and may have acquired from a parent.

gestational diabetes. A form of diabetes that develops during pregnancy, resulting in improper regulation of glucose levels in the blood.

glucose challenge test. A test that screens for gestational diabetes by measuring your blood glucose level after drinking a glucose solution.

group B streptococcus (GBS). A bacterium that is part of the normal floras of the genital tract in many women. This bacterium can cause severe infections in newborns if passed to the baby during birth.

H

human chorionic gonadotropin (HCG). A hormone produced by the placenta. Its measurement is the key to all pregnancy tests.

human placental lactogen (HPL). A placental hormone that alters your metabolism to make nutrients available for your baby and stimulates your breasts to prepare to produce milk.

hydramnios, or polyhydramnios. An excess of amniotic fluid.

hypoglycemia. A condition in which the concentration of sugar (glucose) in the bloodstream is lower than normal.

I

induction of labor. A means of artificially starting labor, usually by administering oxytocin, a prostaglandin medication, or by breaking the bag of water.

intrauterine growth restriction (IUGR). Significant slowing of fetal growth, usually defined as less than the tenth percentile for a given gestational age.

In vitro fertilization (IVF). The process by which eggs and sperm are combined in an artificial environment outside the body, then transferred back into a woman's uterus to grow.

J

jaundice. Yellow tinge to the skin and whites of the eyes caused by too much bilirubin in the bloodstream.

K

Kegel exercises. Exercises done to strengthen the muscles of the pelvic floor; can prevent urine leakage.

L

labia. Two sets of skin folds that surround the opening to the vagina and urethra. The outer set is covered with pubic hair, but the inner set is not.

Lamaze. A technique of physical and emotional preparation of the mother for childbirth to reduce pain and the use of medications during birth.

lanugo. Fine, downy hair growing on the skin of a fetus by about week 26.

lightening. The repositioning of the baby lower in the pelvis. This usually occurs several weeks before the onset of labor.

lochia. The discharge of blood, mucus and tissue from the uterus during the six weeks after childbirth (postpartum).

luteinizing hormone. A pituitary hormone that causes an ovarian follicle to swell, rupture and release an egg.

M

macrosomia. Larger-than-normal birth weight (usually more that 9 ¾ pounds, or 4,500 grams).

mastitis. An infection of the breast that occurs when bacteria enter the breast.

meconium. The product of a baby's first

bowel movements, characteristically green in color.

meconium aspiration. Situation in which a newborn inhales amniotic fluid mixed with meconium. This may cause partial or complete blockage of the airways and inflammation.

miscarriage. Premature, spontaneous termination of a pregnancy.

molding. The temporarily flat, crooked, elongated or pointy shape of the bones of the baby's skull while passing through the birth canal.

mucous plug. A collection of mucus that blocks the cervical canal during pregnancy to prevent entrance of germs into the uterus. The plug is loosened and passed when the cervix starts to thin out and open. This usually pink-tinged or bloody mucous discharge is called the bloody show.

N

neonatologist. A physician with advanced training in the diagnosis and treatment of problems of the newborn.

neural tube. The structure in the embryo that develops into the brain, spinal cord, spinal nerves and backbone.

nonstress test. A test that helps a doctor examine the condition of a fetus by measuring the heart rate in response to his or her own movements.

nuchal translucency. A normal structure seen on ultrasound between 11 and 14 weeks that may be enlarged in the presence of a variety of congenital disorders.

O

occiput posterior position. A position in which a baby faces the mother's abdomen rather than the preferred delivery position of facing the back.

ovulation. The release of an egg from the ovary. Fertilization can occur only within a day or two of ovulation.

P

Pap test. A test to detect cancer and precancer of the cervix.

pelvic floor muscles. A group of muscles at the base of the pelvis. They support the bladder, urethra, rectum, and (in women) vagina and uterus.

perinatologist. An obstetrician who specializes in diagnosis and treatment of problems of pregnancy.

perineum. The area between vaginal and anal openings in women.

pica. An uncommon craving during pregnancy to eat nonfood items such as laundry starch, dirt, baking powder or frost from the freezer. It strongly suggests iron deficiency.

placenta. The circular, flat organ that is responsible for oxygen, nutrient exchange and elimination of wastes between mother and fetus. It is also known as the afterbirth.

placenta accreta. An abnormal placental attachment in which the placenta adheres too firmly to the wall of the uterus.

placenta previa. An abnormal location of the placenta in which it partially or completely covers the cervix.

placental abruption. Separation of the placenta from the inner wall of the uterus before delivery.

postpartum depression. A type of clinical depression that can afflict a mother between two weeks and six months after a baby is born.

preeclampsia. A disease occurring during pregnancy marked by hypertension and protein in the urine. Formerly called toxemia.

premature labor, or preterm labor. Contractions that start opening the cervix before week 37 of pregnancy.

progesterone. A hormone that inhibits the uterus from contracting and promotes the growth of blood vessels in the uterine wall.

prostaglandin. A chemical produced by the lining of the uterus and fetal membranes at or near the onset of labor.

pudendal block. A local anesthetic injected into the vaginal wall to prevent pain during delivery or during repair of any vaginal tears or an episiotomy.

Q

quickening. The mother's first perception of fetal movements. These are usually felt between 18 and 20 weeks of pregnancy for first-time mothers, but often earlier in those with a prior pregnancy.

R

regional anesthesia. An anesthetic that numbs a segment of the body.

relaxin. A hormone produced by the placenta that softens connective tissues, which allows your pelvis to open wider during childbirth.

respiratory distress syndrome (RDS). Difficulty in breathing, caused by lack of surfactant in premature babies.

retained placenta. Failure of the placenta to be delivered within 30 minutes after birth; can cause excessive bleeding.

Rh immunoglobulin (RhIg). A drug used in Rh-negative women to prevent their immune system from recognizing Rh-positive blood, thus protecting future pregnancies.

Rhesus factor. A red blood cell protein very similar to the proteins that determine blood types A, B and O. It is generally considered to be present or absent in individuals; thus you are Rh positive or negative.

S

sciatica. A temporary condition caused by extra pressure on one or both sciatic nerves. This may cause pain, tingling or numbness running down your buttocks, thighs and lower legs.

spina bifida. A defect in the spine that results in failure of the vertebrae to fuse. This can occur in any vertebra but is most commonly found in the lower spine.

spinal block. An anesthetic technique in which medication is injected into the fluid surrounding the spinal nerves, resulting in nearly immediate anesthesia in a segment of the body.

station. A measurement of the descent of a fetus in the birth canal relative to a bony landmark that can be felt on pelvic exam.

stillbirth. The delivery of a baby who has died in the uterus.

surfactant. A substance covering the inner lining of the air sacs in the lungs that allows the lungs to expand normally during breathing.

T

tailor sitting. Sitting with the bottoms of your feet together. This position may strengthen your pelvic floor muscles and may aid recovery from childbirth.

teratogens. Agents that cause defects in a developing fetus, such as alcohol, certain medications, pollutants and recreational drugs.

transient tachypnea (wet lung). A mild, temporary respiratory condition of newborns characterized by rapid breathing.

transition. The portion of active labor in which contractions are most intense, typically between 7 centimeters and complete dilation.

transverse lie. A position in which a baby lies crossways in the uterus before birth. It is incompatible with a vaginal delivery.

twin-twin transfusion. The passage of blood from one identical twin into the other through connections of blood vessels within the placenta.

U

umbilical cord. The tubular structure that carries the fetal blood to the placenta, where oxygen and nutrients can be delivered and waste products removed.

umbilical cord compression. A complication in which the umbilical cord becomes compressed or pinched, which may cause blood flow to and from the baby to the placenta to slow or even stop.

umbilical cord prolapse. A complication in which the umbilical cord slips out through the opening of the cervix, often followed by compression of the cord by the baby's presenting part.

uterine atony. The lack of muscle tone in the uterus after birth, preventing contractions needed to control bleeding from the placental site.

uterus (womb). The female organ in which the unborn baby develops.

V

vacuum extractor. A tool with a rubber or plastic cup that can be held gently to the baby's head, providing suction that can aid in the baby's delivery.

varicose veins. Protruding, dilated veins, commonly in the legs or vulva.

VBAC. Vaginal birth after Caesarean delivery.

vernix caseosa, or vernix. A slippery, white, fatty substance covering the skin of a fetus.

Z

zygote. The result of the union of an ovum and sperm; a fertilized egg before it begins to divide and grow.

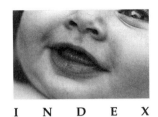

I N D E X

Bold-face page numbers indicate the most complete information on a topic

F

genes, 45
genetic amniocentesis, 300–301
genetic carrier screening tests, **269–276**
  family history based, 271–272, 274
  interpreting results of, 274–276
  population-based, 271
genetic counselors, 273, 309
genetic disorders
  autosomal recessive, 271
  chromosome rearrangements, 274
  defined, 270
  mitochondrial, 274
  preconception screening for, 269–276
  prenatal testing for, 299–311
  X-linked, 272, 274
genital warts, 529
German measles (rubella), **565**
  blood test for, 68
  exposure to, 33, 60, 565
  fetal growth restriction and, 551
  vaccination for, 5, 26
gestational age. *see also* premature babies
  determination of, with ultrasound, 296, 299
  prenatal testing and, 291, 292, 294
  weeks 1 to 4, 43–48
  weeks 5 to 8, 57–60
  weeks 9 to 12, 71–73
  weeks 13 to 16, 79–80
  weeks 17 to 20, 93–95
  weeks 21 to 24, 103–105
  weeks 25 to 28, 113–114
  weeks 29 to 32, 123–124
  weeks 33 to 36, 133–134
  weeks 37 to 40, 145–147
gestational diabetes, **547–549**
  age of mother and, 39
  macrosomia and, 191
  maternal obesity and, 8
  testing for, 118
ginkgo, 5
glucose challenge test, 118
glucose tolerance test, 118
glyburide, 549
gonorrhea, **529**
  eye infection from, 212–213
  tests for, 66
grief, 316–317, 543
grocery shopping and food safety, 15
ground meat, 16
group B streptococcus (GBS), 141, **563–564**
guided imagery, 151, **336**
gum disease, 448–449
gums, bleeding, 424
gymnastics, 18

H

hair
  coloring, while pregnant, 434
  maternal, fullness of, 128
  of newborns, 211, 248
  perming, while pregnant, 476–477
  postpartum loss of, 257
  prenatal development of, 80, 93, 94
hamburgers, 16
hands
  development of, 59, 113
  itching, **85, 459**
  newborn reflexes and, 233
  numbness of, 128, **429–430**
  reddened palms of, 85, 482
  swelling of, **490–491**
  washing of, 15, 34
hand-to-mouth reflex, 233
hand washing, 15, 34
hazardous substances at work, 33
HCG tests, **449–450**
head
  bruising of, 209
  crowning of, 161, 178
  engagement of, 161
  flat spot on, 243
  molding of, 168, **208–209**
  position of, in labor, 189, 573–574
  size of, 168, 187
  soft spots in, 209
  too large for pelvis, 575
headaches, 62, 74, **450–451**
  after epidural block, 331
  after spinal block, 332
health care (for baby)
  choosing a provider, 86, **359–362**
health care (for pregnancy)
  choosing a provider, 277–288
  first visit during pregnancy, 65–69
  follow-up appointments, 68–69
  good communication with, 68
  physical examinations, 66–67, 87, 141–142, 152
  planning birth, 158, **287–288**
  postpartum care, 251–266
  postpartum checkup, 259–260
  preconception visit, 5
  preparing questions for visits, 55
  types of providers, 279–285
health problems (maternal)
  asthma, 507–508
  cancers, 508–510
  diabetes, 513–515
  epilepsy, 515–517
  food poisoning, 14–17

R

racket sports, 18
radiation
diagnostic X-rays, 60
exposure at work, 33, 34
therapeutic, 509
ranitidine, 465
rashes
diaper rash, 246–247
during pregnancy, 480–481
raw milk, 15
"recreational" drugs, 22–23, 60, 67
rectal bleeding, 481–482
reflexology, 342
relaxation techniques
in labor, 151, 174–175, **333–337**
for stress reduction, 32
relaxin, 148, 168
respirators, 221
respiratory distress syndrome (RDS), 221
retained placenta, 184, 583
retinopathy of prematurity (ROP), 104, **224**
rheumatoid arthritis, 528
Rh immunoglobulin (RhIg), 118, 119, 560
Rhinocort (budesonide), 419
Rh (rhesus) factor
incompatibility of, 119, 302, **559–560**
maternal, 67–68
sensitization, from prenatal tests, 302, 307
rhythm method, 395–397
rib tenderness, 482–483
rooming-in, 208, 285
rooting reflex, 233
round ligament pain, **483–484**
rubella, *see* German measles

S

salivary estrogen test, 534
salivation, excessive (ptyalism), 62, **479**
salmonella poisoning, 15
salmon patches, 210
salt, 9
Sarafem (fluoxetine), 466
sausage, 16
scents and cologne, 29
sciatica, 127, **484–485**
screening tests, 213–215, 269–276. *see
also* prenatal testing
scuba diving, 19
seafood, 16–17
seat belts, 322
seborrheic dermatitis, 248
Seconal (secobarbital), 328
secondhand smoke, 22
self-hypnosis, 341–342
semen, 44
sepsis, 216

sertraline, 466
sex chromosomes, 45
sex of baby, 45, 298
sex organs, formation of, 71, 72
sexual abuse, 8
sexually transmitted diseases
circumcision and, 356
maternal, 528–530
tests for, 66
sexual relations
conception and, 44
conflicts over, 53–54
first trimester, 76
postpartum, 266
during pregnancy, 24–25
second trimester, 108–109
and starting labor, 162
shaking babies, 229
shark, 17
shellfish, 16–17
shingles, 430
shoes, 31, **445**
shortness of breath, 91, 125, **427–428**
shoulder dystocia, 548
shrimp, 16
"Siamese" (conjoined) twins, 92
siblings
adjustment of, to new baby, 411
hospital visits of, 411
planning for care of, 166
pregnancy loss and, 317
preparing of, for new baby, 410–411
sickle cell disease, 214, 275, 530–531
sight. *see* vision
sitting, at work, 30–31
sitting, in labor, 177
skiing, 18
skin
acne, 417–418
blotches, during pregnancy, 85
blue lines under, 425
cradle cap, 248
darkening, during pregnancy, 83, 85, 485
fetal, development of, 80, 94
growths or tags, 487
infantile acne, 210
itching, during pregnancy, 127, **459**
moles, 85
of newborns, 209–210, 249
of premature babies, 219
rashes, during pregnancy, 480–481
red blotches, on palms and soles, 482
red spots, postpartum, 257
stretch marks, 127–128, **489–490**
vascular spiders, 125, 485–486
skin tags, 487
sleep
in family bed vs. crib, 240